LEICESTER POLYTECHNI
CITY CAMPUS
Telephone 551551

Please return this book on or before the last date stamped below.

Fines will be charged on books returned after this date.

R570

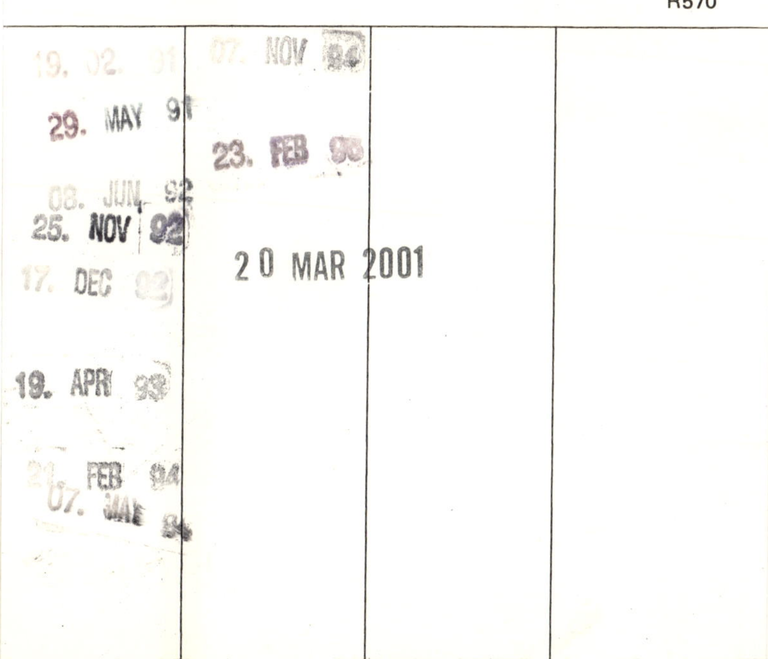

SOCIAL TOPICS SERIES

Society and Fertility

SOCIAL TOPICS SERIES

Society and Fertility

Malcolm Potts
M.B., B.Chir., Ph.D., D.Obst. RCOG
Executive Director
International Fertility Research Program
N. Carolina, U.S.A.

Peter Selman
B.A., D.P.S.A., Ph.D.
Lecturer in Social Studies,
University of Newcastle-upon-Tyne
England

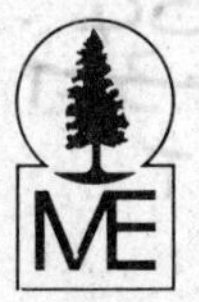

MACDONALD AND EVANS

Macdonald and Evans Ltd,
Estover, Plymouth PL6 7PZ

First published 1979

© Macdonald & Evans Ltd, 1979

ISBN 0 7121 1960 4

This book is copyright
and may not be reproduced in whole
or in part (except for purposes of review)
without the express permission
of the publishers in writing

Printed in Great Britain by
Butler & Tanner Ltd, Frome and London

LEICESTER POLYTECHNIC
LIBRARY
Acc. No.
Date 7-3-80 26-8-81
Loc./Form
Class. 301.321 304.66
POT

Preface

At some time in the mid 1970s the number of people alive on our planet passed the 4,000 million mark. By the end of this century the total will probably be approaching 6,000 million, as increasing numbers of women reach their reproductive years. Although the annual rate of growth in world population has been falling in recent years from the peak of 2 per cent per annum reached in the earlier part of the decade, each year a further 60 to 70 million is being added to our total numbers (a figure in excess of the total population of West Germany or Mexico in 1976). Growth rates of this order are a phenomenon of the post-war world and represent what must be a temporary deviation from the very slow rates of growth increase which have characterised most of man's history.

The roots of this so-called "population explosion" lie in the dramatic fall in mortality, especially amongst children, throughout the world over the past thirty years. In the words of a recent issue of the magazine *New Internationalist*, it is "not that we have started breeding like rabbits, but rather that we have stopped dying like flies". Nevertheless, if growth rates are to fall and population is to stabilise, without a return to very high levels of mortality, it is the pattern of human reproduction that must change, so that fertility is the key to the future of growth of world population and, many would add, to the future well-being of mankind.

It is not our aim in this book to offer yet another doom-laden prediction of a world with standing-room only, but rather to examine closely the patterns of human reproduction in an historical and cross-cultural perspective. We shall be looking at the problems of measuring fertility, at the biological and social factors which influence reproductive behaviour, and at the wide range of means by which people limit their fertility, covering not only contraception, abortion and sterilisation, but also less obvious, though equally important, practices such as sexual abstinence and breast feeding. In the latter part of the book, we also consider some of the personal and social consequences of fertility patterns and take a critical look at family planning programmes in both developed and developing countries.

We have deliberately chosen a broad definition of our subject matter, which takes us into a consideration of marriage patterns, sexual behaviour, infertility and adoption, as well as family size preferences, unwanted pregnancy and the use of contraception. In looking at the implications of fertility patterns, we have sought to link the needs and problems of individuals with the economic and social consequences of population growth. We have also tried to face the abortion controversy realistically, arguing that there is a genuine need for abortion, and indeed sterilisation, along with contraception if countries are to reduce their population growth and if individuals are to be offered the maximum choice in controlling the number and timing of births. The text gives many examples from history and the contemporary world, both industrialised and developing, of the problems of fertility control, and makes extensive use of published research and our own experiences.

One aim of the book is, therefore, to offer an introduction to the study of human reproduction, based on our knowledge as a doctor and sociologist (who have spent much of their working lives in the area of fertility and family planning). We hope that it will prove of value to those readers who have little previous knowledge of the subject and wish to gain some understanding of one of today's major issues, but also that there will be much to interest and inform those already working in family planning, and students of the social sciences, medicine and related disciplines, who wish to further their knowledge of population dynamics. The material we present has been gathered over many years from a variety of sources, including experience in international family planning, which has taken one of us to most corners of the globe as an advisor on birth control, and in teaching courses in Population Studies to honours Sociology students, which, together with empirical research into British fertility, has occupied the other for the past seven or eight years. We both owe huge debts to our colleagues in these various spheres and to those we have tried to advise or teach, and from whom we have ourselves learned so much.

Finally, it is our hope that anyone who reads this book—no matter what their previous knowledge of the subject—will find here some new insights and perhaps be stimulated to think afresh about some of the issues we discuss and to pursue further their study of the subject through the reading suggested at the end of each chapter. We cannot claim to offer any simple solution to the problems described, but it is our belief that they can be tackled, and eventually solved, if there is a genuine attempt to provide people with the means to control their fertility and a way of life which makes it meaningful for them to wish to do so. There are many barriers, some linked to the still limited technology of fertility control, but most arising from ignorance and prejudice on the part of those who should be offering help, and from the widespread poverty and inequality which is to be found in countries of the world. In recent years there has been a tendency for family planning to be seen either as a cure-all for the problems of the world, or as a dangerous irrelevance, diverting us from the true task of eliminating poverty through economic development. It is our view that the truth lies with neither extreme: persisting poverty does indeed present a major barrier to the reduction of fertility in many Third World countries, but likewise high fertility, and consequent rapid population growth, is a major factor in the persistence of poverty and malnutrition. We also believe that a majority of persons in *all* countries have a strong desire to be able to control their fertility, whether this be in order to limit their ultimate family size or to space children or avoid extra-marital births. Access to the means of fertility control is thus a fundamental right, denied to all too many individuals throughout the world. If we are to offer such people the opportunities many of us take for granted, and if we are to overcome the barriers to tackling the problems of poverty and overpopulation, one need is to develop a deeper understanding of the dynamics of human reproduction, based on an awareness of historical experience and cultural variation. It is our hope that this book, in exploring the relationship between society and fertility, may help towards such understanding.

April 1978 M.P.
P.S.

A man born into a world already possessed, if he cannot get substance from his parents on whom he has just demands, and if society do not want his labour, has no claim of right to the smallest portion of food and, in fact, has no business to be where he is . . . at nature's mighty feast there is no vacancy for him. She tells him to be gone and will execute her commands.

Thomas Malthus, 1799

There are more hungry people in Asia than ever before in its history. The chain must be broken by drastic reduction in population growth. The opponents of family planning are motivated by a misguided sense of humanity and morality, misguided because they refuse to face startling changes in man's control over nature. . . . I believe it is better not to shed tears over those not born than to remain unmoved seeing millions come into the world where chronic hunger and death by malnutrition, disease and starvation must be their inevitable fate.

Lee Kuan Yew, Prime Minister of Singapore, 1977

There is no event in personal history more significant for the future than becoming a parent, and there is no pattern of behaviour more essential for societal survival than adequate fertility.

Norman Ryder, 1959

Contents

Chapter 1

Introduction

The birth of a child is an event of great social and individual significance and one that is recognised as such in all human societies. It marks the entrance into the world of a new actor, whose total life chances are often largely determined by the circumstances of that entry, and it has a profound effect on the social and personal situation of the parents and any previously born children in a family unit. Like the other great demographic events of death and marriage, birth is associated with social rituals and is increasingly subject to the requirement of official registration.

The birth of a first child is of especial importance as it signifies the transition of the parents into a new social status, with its related expectations, responsibilities and rights. It marks the sexual and social maturity of the mother and the visible consummation of the marriage. Until a child is born the marriage may be deemed in some sense incomplete and in almost all societies the "barren" wife is the subject of pity, if not condemnation, so that failure to bear a child may be seen as sufficient reason to dissolve the marriage or justify the taking of a second wife.

Indeed, in a few societies the impregnation of the wife may be deemed too important to be left to the husband—hence the ritual of *ius primae noctis*, or the search for divine parenthood. The fact of pregnancy may be crucial to the decision to marry, so that birth may occur in a socially acceptable context. A birth outside marriage may be at best a source of shame, stigma and dependency for the woman, and at worst a cause of her exile or death.

The implications of birth are not limited to the parents, but also create new roles and relationships in the wider family of aunts and uncles, grandparents and other relations. In many countries registration of the birth will set in motion the processes of assimilation into the social order and the mobilisation of a range of social agencies, from health to social security.

The significance of a birth may be enhanced by the sex of the child. The birth of a male child, especially the first son, is regarded as particularly important. The birth of second and subsequent children transforms the initial family unit into an ever more complex one in terms of sibling and child–parent relationships. The number and timing of births is crucial to the life chances of both parents and children. In different societies large families may be a source of prestige and prosperity; alternatively, a cause of poverty and social disadvantage.

When mortality in childhood is low, fertility largely determines the size of a family. Where many children die young, there will be less significance in the relationship between the number of births and family size, and acceptance of the child as part of society may be delayed. The parents' perceptions of, and involvement with, their children will differ according to the probability of survival. In societies where most children survive the first years of life, the new-born baby is treated almost immediately as a full member of society.

In any circumstances, the importance of birth for both individual and society relates to the potential for growth to adulthood. While the demonstration of an ability to conceive in itself may be important to a mother, the continuing existence of the child establishes her status, so that any study of fertility must be concerned not only with the events leading up to the birth, but with beliefs and values about the consequences of the birth. In other words the study of human fertility must not neglect the fact that it is ultimately concerned with children in a society.

Populations are the product of birth, death and migration rates, so that the level of births is a key factor in determining the future size and structure of a society. Any change in the pattern of births implies long-term changes in the age-structure of a country, making differing demands on education services and housing provision, influencing the number of young workers entering the labour market or creating problems of dependency in old age. In the twentieth century it is the fertility rate, rather than mortality, which has come to affect the future shape of most populations.

Many countries of the developing world maintain high levels of births whereas those of deaths have fallen, leading to the rapid population growth witnessed in the world over the past few decades. At the same time, the last few years have seen a continuous decline in the fertility of many developed countries, so that some European nations, such as West Germany and Great Britain, are now experiencing a decline in population; while others, such as Japan, have a level of fertility which is approaching or below that of replacement, although because of the age-structure of the country this has not yet led to a falling population.

Man is a social animal who is actively concerned in the creation of the society in which he lives. The fascination of studying human fertility is that it is increasingly influenced by individual choices. On aggregate, these have important consequences for society as a whole and are so important that society often attempts to influence them one way or another. It is in the context of human society that decisions are made about fertility.

Human reproduction, therefore, is determined to a large extent by social factors, beliefs and attitudes towards sex and procreation, the structure of the family and economic and political considerations. In exploring these factors, we need also to look at the "social construction" of human reproductive behaviour—the way in which members of a society define themselves as parents and view their sexual activity. But we must not emphasise the importance of fertility for society, or the way in which society can influence fertility, to the exclusion of other viewpoints. As Mary Calderone has pointed out, people rarely behave reproductively, they rather behave sexually with reproduction as a by-product of their sexual behaviour. Such behaviour is regulated by social rules in all human societies, rules which govern the transition to adulthood, courtship, mate selection, extra-marital sexual behaviour and other events. Such rules have considerable influence on the pattern of reproduction and are rooted in the need for any society to regulate the bearing and rearing of children; nevertheless they are about sexual, not reproductive, behaviour. They may be most controlling of the reproductive element, simply because this tends to be more visible than the underlying sexuality.

As highly effective means of fertility control separate sex from reproduction, the rules governing sexual behaviour tend to wane, and social norms about reproduction may become more explicit, despite the fact that reproduction remains deeply rooted in human sexuality. Therefore, in exploring the factors determining the frequency with which people have children, we shall look at both individual and social aspects of sexual activity and the production of children.

One aim of this book is to stress the universality of sexual behaviour and its reproductive consequences. We shall argue that in all societies individuals have to face similar problems and develop comparable means of coping, determined by their definition of the situation. In other words, we seek to view fertility through the eyes of those whom it directly concerns and their perceptions of the costs and benefits of actions modifying sexual activity. To the outsider, for a poor person to have a large number of births is irrational, but a careful consideration of the realities of infant mortality, the economic value of children and the social status of parenthood may make that individual's choices a rational achievement. At the same time, we intend to emphasise the accessibility and acceptability of the available means of birth-control from the viewpoint of the potential user. Large families are often the result of inadequate means of fertility regulation. Parents who want several children may yet wish to space them. The sexually active unmarried girl will need birth-control to avoid the shame of an illegitimate child. Throughout the world, the millions of women who seek illegal abortions are testimony to a desperate need to avoid unwanted children.

It is self-evident that motivation to control fertility varies from country to country, and from individual to individual within a society, but we would argue that for all couples there are times when there is a need for birth-control and that, in most cases, this represents a large proportion of the total period in which a woman is exposed to the risk of pregnancy. The key is to understand how the individual defines his or her needs and to interpret behaviour in the light of personal perceptions, rather than in terms of outside definitions of how people should behave. When achieved fertility is viewed according to outside criteria, deviation from the average is easily misinterpreted as stupidity, irrationality or cultural oddity. In contrast, when fertility regulation is seen from the user's point of view, it is the paradoxes and imperfections of those attempting to offer family planning services that are often most apparent and in need of sociological exploration and analysis.

In summary, therefore, the aim of our book is to describe and discuss the experience of human fertility in different societies at different times, paying special attention to the way in which all societies have developed patterns of behaviour to keep fertility below its biological potential. We start with a consideration of the factors that influence human fertility at both individual and societal levels; we go on to describe in detail some examples of achieved fertility patterns in various human societies, and changes over periods of time; and we then consider the consequences for individuals and the society of this fertility experience. We survey the means of regulating fertility and end by looking at current efforts in both developed and developing countries. We assert throughout our belief that in most respects the individual actors are in advance of any of the attempts that society makes to assist them. Even today, most societies tend to be more concerned with denying the means of controlling reproduction to their members than with practical, realistic assistance. The saddest paradox of all is that this is often truest of the very countries most beset by problems of overpopulation and, on the surface, most committed to family planning programmes.

MEASUREMENT OF HUMAN FERTILITY

We will present our story in terms of the experience of individuals and groups of individuals, but in order to discuss differences in the fertility behaviour of various societies, or changes in such behaviour over periods of time, we must be able to characterise the level of such fertility in accurate and meaningful terms. Hence the need for statistical analysis of fertility which is part of the scientific measurement of population we know as demography (*see also* Chapter 3).

DEFINITION OF FERTILITY

A clear distinction needs to be made between "fertility" and "fecundity". Fertility refers to the actual bearing of children, the reproductive performance, and is measured in terms of live births. Fecundity is the capacity to bear children or the reproductive potential. Fertility is, in the words of a French demographer Alfred Sauvy, "a statistical concept with social relevance", whereas fecundity is a biological concept.

Unfortunately, confusion can arise because of the biological and medical use of the term "fertility" to refer to the capacity to reproduce (occurring especially in the use of the term "infertility"), and because the French terms *fertilité* and *fecondité* have reversed meanings, referring to potential and performance respectively. For this reason some demographers have preferred the word "natality", with its French counterpart *natalité* as the term for child-bearing.

A second necessary distinction is between the experience of live births and the experience of pregnancy, its inevitable precursor. Demographers use the term "parity" to refer to the number of live births experienced by an individual mother. Births in a population may be analysed by previous parity, referring to the previous number of live births experienced by the mother. To obstetricians in a hospital, however, the term "parity" refers to the experience of pregnancy, so that a "nulliparous" woman is one who has never conceived and a "grand multipara" a woman who has experienced five or more pregnancies, irrespective of the number of resulting live births.

Further difficulties may arise over the handling of multiple births. A woman who has had two sets of live-born twins has had four live births and this is the relevant fact in measuring her fertility or "parity" in the demographic sense—but she has achieved this as a result of only two pregnancies. The term "maternity" is used by demographers to denote a pregnancy which has terminated in the birth of one or more live or stillborn children. Demographic measurements of fertility are concerned only with live-born children, although data on total births and stillbirths is usually also recorded; these, of course, are important records for the practising doctor.

For most of us, the meaningful summary of fertility experience is the family size of an individual woman, or the mean family size of a group of women, but, again, different disciplines use different definitions. For the demographer "family size" is defined as the number of live births to the family unit under consideration, not the number of children surviving at the time of observation. Thus, reference to a decline in family size refers to changes in the number of live-born children amongst women born or married at different periods, not to changes in the number of surviving children. For the sociologist studying the effect of family size on the life chances of members of a family, it is usually the number of siblings (brothers and sisters) which is taken as a measure and this may be further restricted to take account only of those children still living in the family unit. The demographer's "family size" is therefore essentially an attribute of the mother and one which is irreducible, while for the sociologist it is a description of the "existential" family at a particular time. In advanced industrial societies, where childhood mortality is low, the difference between the two measures is usually small, especially in early marriage before children have grown up and left home. But in the developing world, where many children die in their early years, the number of live births is, typically, well in excess of the number of surviving children in the family unit at any time. This fact is of crucial importance in exploring women's attitudes towards their own fertility. If a woman is asked about her "intended" family size, her answer will be in terms of the number of living children she wants and should not be compared with measures of achieved family size, which relate to the number of live births.

If, therefore, we are to understand fertility as a subjective reality, we need to think beyond it as a statistical concept and see it rather as a process, the succession of live births experienced by an individual woman or group of women over a period of time, a process which is constantly being modified by the woman's experience of those births and by the fate of the children already born. To take a dramatic example, infanticide must be grouped alongside other means of fertility control, because it relates to a couple's perception of the actual number of children they will have to rear and care for, although in the real meaning of the word it is a method of death-control. But, having said this, it remains true that human reproductive behaviour, at a societal level, is most accurately and clearly defined by accepting fertility as a measurement of live births. Fertility, thus defined, together with migration and mortality, determines the future size and shape of any population.

AVAILABILITY OF DATA ON POPULATION

The basic requirement for measuring fertility patterns effectively is reasonably accurate data on the number of live births occurring in a society over a specified period, together with data on the number of people living in the society over the same interval. Ideally such data should also provide information about the characteristics of parents (e.g. age, marital status, previous reproductive history) and of the total population (especially its age and sex structure). Such demographic data can be obtained from a variety of sources, the most important of which are the population census and vital registration systems. A World Fertility Survey is currently in progress, largely initiated by U.S. Aid to International Development.

The term "census" refers to a nationwide counting of population, usually carried out at regular intervals of five to ten years. Although the count is of individual persons, enumeration is more often by "households", the head of such units being expected to provide data on all those present at a specified time. Censuses are taken in all regions of the world and now cover over 90 per cent of the world's population.

The range of data required by censuses varies. In addition to providing basic personal characteristics such as age, sex, marital status, place of birth and occupation, recent U.S. censuses, for example, have extended the list to cover such things as race, native language, residence five years earlier, employment status, place of work, means of transportation to work, income, ownership of a radio, number of living children and whether an individual is sick, how they get to work and what fuel they use to heat water. In recent years there has been a move to cover some of the more detailed data by means of sub-samples, whereby one in ten census forms are much more detailed; or by alternative methods of regular sampling, such as the Household Survey in Britain.

Information so gathered is seen as essential by national governments for the planning of social and economic policy. In developed countries the history of census-taking is a long one, dating back to the eighteenth and early nineteenth century. In developing countries censuses are more recent. For most of Africa there is no data available prior to the twentieth century and, until the Second World War, population counts were often derived from estimates based on tax registers or other administrative counts, and had little statistical value. Even today there are large areas such as Ethiopia where no accurate figures on total population are available. But even with censuses of limited coverage, the *United Nations Demographic Year Book* is able to present population data for most countries, covering total size of national and city population, trends in national population size, age–sex composition and rural–urban distribution.

Even the basic count of total population in an area presents numerous difficulties, especially in areas where inhabitants are unfamiliar with census-taking. There are often serious risks of underenumeration, as in India. Careful post-census evaluation studies sometimes enable demographers to make corrections to estimates, but it is no easy task. There can also be cases of overenumeration, associated with political pressures, as in the 1963 census in Nigeria which revealed a biologically impossible rate of population increase over ten years (even allowing for a 10 per cent underenumeration in the 1952/3 census), because some groups were attempting to establish political dominance.

A national census is costly and time-consuming and only gives a picture of population at a single time. The need to update census data can be met by the continuous registration of demographic events—births, deaths, marriages and migration. The importance of adequate national vital registration cannot be overemphasised. It provides the raw data from which to compute the level of fertility or mortality in a particular period and, if there is sufficient data, to develop sophisticated measures of those events linked to census-based population data. Vital registration is usually based on a system of compulsory certification of births, marriages and deaths and is crucial to the running of most societies, in that it legitimates the rights of citizens to various claims on the state and in turn defines obligations to the state.

Vital registration as a continuous process is more difficult to establish than a census and the introduction of civil registration usually occurs after the initiation of census-taking. In many parts of the world there is still no effective system of vital registration.

In England and Wales the first census took place in 1801 and the civil registration of births and deaths commenced in 1838, but there was a long history prior to this of the recording of baptisms, burials and marriages in parish registers. Therefore, before 1838, estimates of vital rates depend on assumptions about the ratio between baptisms and burials in parish records and total births and deaths, as we know that not all births and deaths were followed by the relevant religious ceremony and that not all such ceremonies were accurately recorded. Various ratios have been suggested based on census estimates for the period of overlap between parish and civil registration, but their validity is questionable, not least in the assumption of a fixed ratio applying throughout the eighteenth and early nineteenth century. One specialist has suggested that the system of parish registration collapsed at the turn of the nineteenth century, so figures derived from the use of constant ratios may distort the pattern of fertility and mortality for earlier periods which, in turn, may encourage historians to look in the wrong places for factors associated with population growth in the eighteenth century.

Doubts about such estimates and about the parish register abstracts on which they are based have led English historical demographers to concentrate on describing local patterns, either using aggregate data, like Chambers's study of the Vale of Trent, or by the technique of family reconstitution, used first in France by Louis Henry and later adapted by Wrigley in his classic study of Colyton in Devon (*see* p. 168). In this technique, the life history of individuals is reconstructed by linking baptisms, marriages and burials, in order to show changes over lengths of time in age at marriage, family size and life expectancy for men and women born in different periods, using the "cohort" approach to the analysis of demographic data discussed in Chapter 3.

The quality of vital statistics is very poor in most developing nations. Vital statistics from civil registration for most of Asia and many parts of Latin America are not widely available, which seriously limits international comparisons. In much of tropical Africa there is no effective universal system of civil registration, and although there is limited coverage in most countries, there is no immediate likelihood of nation-wide recording. Developed countries also have their limitations and even the Republic of Eire, for example, does not require the registration of stillbirths, although this is an important public health measure. Where demographic studies cannot depend on current vital statistics, estimates of trends have to be based on cross-sectional reports on the size and structure of population and on retrospective reports on vital events during a specified period, or over the lifetime of the individuals studied.

CONCLUSION

Today we are faced with a challenge. Whatever the academic limitations of population data, there can be no doubt that the world has experienced unprecedented population growth since the end of the Second World War. The "population explosion" is a meaningful term and is acknowledged to be one of the most important events of the twentieth century. Population growth is most rapid in the least developed parts of the world (*see* Fig. 1): it is the result of technical changes, such as better water supplies, improved transport systems and the invention of D.D.T. and antibiotics, and modified by political and cultural factors: it is an event with profound implications for problems of unemployment, the division of the world's non-renewable resources and, ultimately, the capacity of the planet Earth to support the millions of people to whom it is host.

In the coming decade the world will add more to its numbers than the total global population in 1800. Whatever happens to fertility

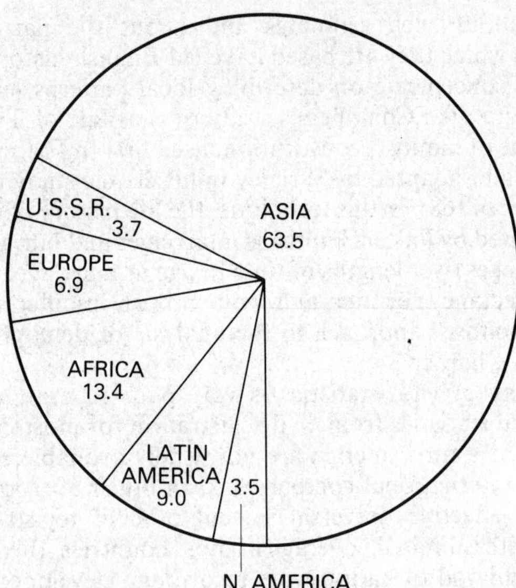

Fig. 1. *Percentage distribution of global births* (*not including Oceania* (0.4)).

rates, the ratio of young people in the populations of all developing countries is now so high that, even if they all have small families, the global population will double and then still continue growing for at least the first half of the next century (*see* Fig. 2).

The next chapter will analyse several aspects of human fertility and provides the background for understanding statistics which, on aggregate, are overwhelming. The aim of the succeeding chapters is to review the biological and social variables controlling fertility and to establish a comprehensive framework for exploring cultural norms and individual preferences about family size and spacing. Subsequently, we will discuss variations in achieved fertility in different societies over periods of time and the consequences of these for individuals and society.

SELECTED REFERENCES AND BIBLIOGRAPHY

Chambers, J. D. "The Vale of Trent, 1670–1800: A Regional Study of Economic Change." *Economic History Review* Supplement no. 3 1957

Freedman, R. "The Sociology of Human Fertility." *Current Sociology*. 10, 35 1961

Glass, D. V. and Eversley, D. E. C. *Population in History*. Edward Arnold, London 1965

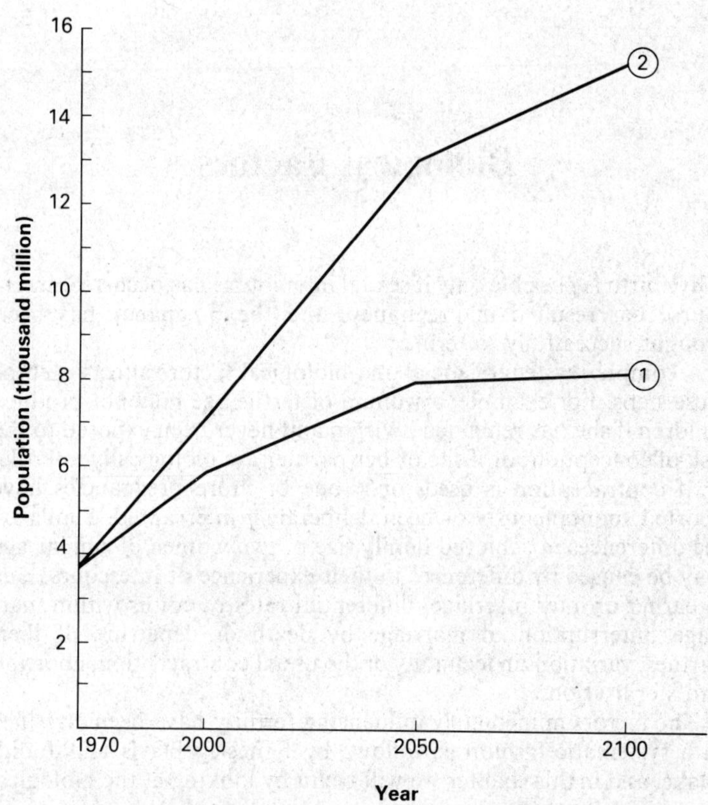

(*Source:* Frejka, T. *The Future of Population Growth.* Wiley, New York 1973)

Fig. 2. *Global population* (*A.D. 1970–2100*). Projection 1 assumes the developing world reaches biological replacement levels of population growth in A.D. 2000–05. Projection 2 assumes the developing world reaches biological replacement levels of population growth in A.D. 2040–45.

Hauser, P. H. and Duncan, O. D. *The Study of Population: An Inventory and Appraisal.* University of Chicago Press, Chicago 1959

Hawthorn, G. *The Sociology of Fertility.* Collier-Macmillan, London 1970

Petersen, W. *Population.* Collier-Macmillan, London 1975

Sauvy, A. A. *General Theory of Population.* Weidenfeld & Nicolson, London 1969

Wrigley, E. A. *Population and History.* Weidenfeld & Nicolson, London 1969

Wrong, D. *Population and Society.* Random House, New York 1967

Chapter 2

Biological Factors

A live birth is possible only if sexual intercourse has occurred, intercourse has resulted in pregnancy, and the pregnancy has been brought successfully to term.

A complex system of social and biological factors affects each of these steps. For example, a woman of fertile age may not produce children if she has remained a virgin and never been exposed to the risk of conception; or if she or her partner are biologically infertile, or if contraception is used, or if one or more pregnancies have aborted spontaneously or been deliberately interrupted. Similarly, the differences in achieved family size of two women of similar age may be caused by differences in their experience of intercourse due to earlier or later marriage, differential rates of coitus within marriage, interruption of marriage by death or departure of their partner, variations in fecundity or the use of contraception, abortion and sterilisation.

The factors immediately influencing fertility have been classified in a systematic fashion as follows by Kingsley Davis and Judith Blake, and in this chapter we will begin by looking at the biological variables.

Factors Influencing Human Fertility

Exposure to intercourse

(*a*) Formation and dissolution of unions in the reproductive period:
- (*i*) age of entry into sexual unions;
- (*ii*) permanent celibacy: proportion of women never entering sexual unions;
- (*iii*) amount of reproductive period spent after or between unions,
  - (a) when unions are broken by divorce, separation or desertion;
  - (b) when unions are broken by death of husband.

(*b*) Exposure to intercourse within unions:
- (*i*) voluntary abstinence;
- (*ii*) involuntary abstinence (from impotence, illness and unavoidable but temporary separations);
- (*iii*) coital frequency (excluding periods of abstinence).

Exposure to conception
(*a*) Fecundity or infecundity, as affected by biological (involuntary) causes;
(*b*) Use or non-use of contraception,
(*i*) by mechanical and chemical means;
(*ii*) by other means;
(*c*) Fecundity or infecundity, as affected by voluntary causes (sterilisation, subincision, medical treatment, etc.).
Gestation and successful parturition
(*a*) Foetal mortality from involuntary causes;
(*b*) Foetal mortality from voluntary causes.

Homo sapiens is an animal that is unusually active sexually but relatively slow and inefficient in its reproduction. Puberty occurs later than in many other animals of comparable size and even the blue whale is sexually mature many years earlier than man. Yet, as Freud demonstrated, human sexuality is present and important in infancy and childhood: at adolescence it becomes even more dominant and is capable of expression in successful reproduction.

MENARCHE AND MENOPAUSE

At puberty, the adult pattern of sex hormone secretion begins and the well known bodily changes of enlargement of the gonads (testes in males and ovaries in females), growth of the internal and external genitalia, the changes in body form, growth of sexual hair and the development of the mammary glands takes place. We are the only species in which the breasts develop in the female at puberty rather than during the first pregnancy and the only species in which the male caresses the breasts of the female during coitus. This is another indicator of the way in which sexual behaviour is socially significant to human beings, as well as being important from the point of view of reproduction.

Puberty in both sexes is a process extending over a number of years. In girls, the breasts begin to develop some time before the peak growth in body size, which itself precedes the onset of menstruation. The growth of the sexual hair is one of the last phases of the menarche. In boys, the growth in the size of the testes and of the penis precedes the growth of sexual hair and the fully established body and voice changes of the mature male. Viable sperm occur relatively early in puberty in the male.

Menstruation is the outward and visible sign of inward and hidden changes taking place in hormone output. The time of the first menstruation is called the menarche.

There is good evidence from a variety of countries that the age of the onset of the first period in girls has declined in the past hundred years, in the most developed countries (*see* Fig. 3). The simplest explanation to be put forward for this change is that the onset of puberty is related to body weight; the American physiologist Rose Frisch has suggested that girls menstruate when their body reaches a critical weight of approximately 48 kilograms—in the same way

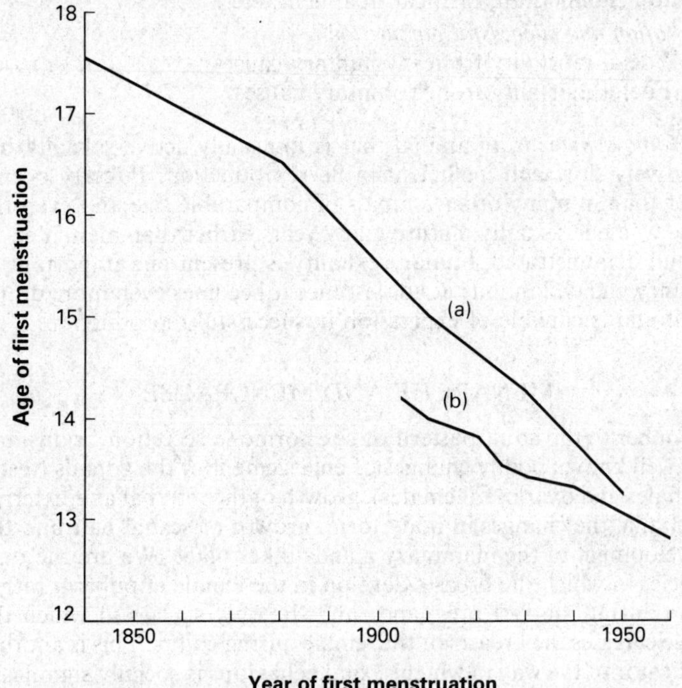

(*Source:* Tanner, J. M. in Meade, J. and Parkes, A. S. (eds) *Biological Aspects of Social Problems*. Oliver and Boyd, Edinburgh 1965)

Fig. 3. *Declining age of menarche*. (a) Norway; (b) U.S.A.

that an atomic bomb explodes when it reaches a critical mass. There may be additional variation between ethnic groups, but whatever the explanation, there is an outstanding conflict between biological change and social needs. In other animals, for example rats in overcrowded conditions, high densities of population and over-utilisation of the surrounding resources are associated with delay in the onset of sexual maturity. The bringing forward of sexual majority, particularly in girls, has occurred at a time when social demands on the human reproductive system have resulted in a tendency towards lower and lower fertility. In addition, in many Western societies there have been social trends which have exacerbated the problem. Whereas, one and two generations ago, Western society made an effort to prolong adolescence, upholding the virtues of education, withholding anything but the minimum pocket money from adolescents, accepting patterns of parental authority and partial chaperonage, today in Europe and North America there is a great pressure for young people to behave as adults at a much earlier age. In style of clothing, disposable income and in independence of decision-making the social pressures on them are those of the adult world. Yet girls in particular are poorly adapted both emotionally and physically to child-bearing, even though they may be biologically capable of becoming pregnant at or before the early teens.

It may be this tension which is at the root of the currently high incidence of anorexia nervosa in the Western world. In this condition, which in Britain in some form may affect up to 1 in 100 girls who have reached the age of puberty, a girl begins to eat less and less, loses weight and eventually ceases to menstruate. In a sense, it represents a physical mechanism by which a girl can escape the challenges of emerging adulthood. It is a serious condition and can be fatal. Again, it seems there is a critical weight at which menstruation ceases; in different societies where loss of weight is not self-inflicted but due to malnutrition, women may cease to menstruate and become infertile at times of hardship. Here, evolution seems to have created a situation where a woman must attain a certain body weight, and in particular, a certain level of fat stores, before pregnancy is possible.

Of the apparently critical body weight of 48 kilograms which seems to initiate menstruation, approximately 16 kilograms are body fat; this is no doubt intended to act as a store of energy to carry a woman through the stresses of pregnancy and, in particular, the one to two years of lactation following delivery. It represents nearly 150,000 calories and would be sufficient in itself to carry a woman through pregnancy and the first three months of lactation where food was in short supply. Perhaps it is a sad comment on the modern world and the stresses it produces that an evolutionary mechanism designed to carry the human race through times of extreme hardship should in some cases be overridden by an impulse towards self-destruction apparently triggered by an environment of affluence. The girl who gets anorexia nervosa often comes from the middle or professional classes, she is typically sixteen or seventeen years old and of above average intelligence. She may disguise the early stages of her self-restriction of food intake as health or food fads. She may hide her food or even force herself to regurgitate it when nobody is looking, until she becomes emaciated and ceases to menstruate. Interestingly, her own image of her body is often that of a well-covered person and she may become worried about being overweight long after she has become exceptionally thin and is perhaps even approaching a situation where her life is at risk.

Following normal puberty, the initial menstrual cycles may occur without ovulation taking place. Some waxing and waning of ovarian hormones at this stage will take place at a sufficient level to lead to menstrual bleeding at the end of the month, but will be insufficient to bring about ovulation. The variation in the length of the menstrual cycle (a cycle which itself provides a rough guide to the degree of probability of ovulation at particular times) is greatest at the extremes of fertile life.

For boys there is no single landmark in puberty as dramatic as the menarche, but the appearance of viable sperm in the ejaculate indicates fecundity. This occurs at about the same time as girls commence menstruation. It would not be reasonable to ask adolescent boys to collect semen by masturbation, as is done with older men, but if urine is centrifuged and if spontaneous ejaculation has taken place in the previous twenty-four hours, then microscopic specimens of sperm can be collected.

The female's reproductive life ends with varying degrees of suddenness, with the menopause, a largely human phenomenon. The time taken to conceive and the degree of foetal wastage rises with age in a great many species, but few or none have the total break of reproductive capacity that occurs in a woman. The evolutionary significance of the menopause is open to dispute, but one explanation could be that in traditional societies which lack the benefits of scientific medical care, giving birth is a particularly dangerous process for an older woman. We are a species where family care extends over more than one generation and, perhaps, it is in the interests of survival of the group that there should be a few experienced grandmothers about. It is also known that the rate of foetal abnormality rises rapidly in women who are in the forties and this is another reason why it may be an advantage to the species to curtail female reproduction at a certain age.

In the male, fertility wanes with age but comes to no finite end. The production of sperm is a continuous process and hundreds of millions of new sperm are manufactured each day. In women, however, the production of eggs is not continuous. All the eggs that will ever be available for fertilisation are produced and undergo the halving of the chromosomal number necessary for reproduction while the female is still in her mother's womb. These eggs are then merely packaged, as in a cold store, for monthly release from the ovaries throughout the female's fertile life. Incidentally, it is this biological difference between the two sexes which has made it easier to develop pharmacological methods of family planning for women but not, to date, for men. The Pill merely imitates the normal switching off of egg release which occurs during pregnancy.

SEXUAL INTERCOURSE

Man, unlike most other mammals, does not have a defined breeding season but is sexually active throughout the year, and intercourse occurs much more frequently than is necessary for conception. This last aspect of behaviour is not confined to man, but occurs in a number of species which have the ability to modify their environment greatly. For example, lions copulate much more frequently than is necessary for conception and their relatively inefficient reproduction, together with the high infant mortality that is known to occur in a pride of lions, probably reflects an evolutionary adaptation which acts to keep their numbers low in comparison to the game animals on which they prey. It would be easy for a large number of lions to overexploit their food supply. The lethargy of the adults who spend a great deal of time sleeping is probably another aspect of the same biological need. Man also has the power to destroy his environment and, like the lion, copulates more frequently than is necessary for reproduction, although he is not a lazy species in other ways.

The social factors which restrict sexual intercourse to certain mates will be discussed in Chapter 4 but, within a sexual partnership, the frequency of intercourse is not the important factor in achieved fertility that it is sometimes assumed to be. At the extremes of coital patterns, where a couple may have intercourse two or three times a day or only once a month, there will be an effect on time taken to conceive. In both cases, the time taken to conceive is likely to be extended, as both infrequent intercourse and exceptionally frequent intercourse (which is associated with a low sperm count in each ejaculation) will decrease the probability of fertilisation at ovulation. There is no evidence that sperm production is linked to the frequency of sperm ejaculation. But, within most sexual partnerships, once the novelty of the new relation is overcome, normal patterns of intercourse (from several times a week to once a week) only alter the time taken to conceive from three to six months (*see* Table 1). Social factors altering frequency of intercourse are discussed on pp. 73–6. There is a decreasing frequency of intercourse as age increases, although it is normal for coitus to continue far beyond the

TABLE 1: COITAL FREQUENCY AND TIME TAKEN TO CONCEIVE

Reported coital frequency (per month)	*Months taken to conceive*	
	age of marriage	
	14–17	*18–27*
less than 10	8.2	6.1
11–20	7.5	5.6
21–30	7.1	5.4
over 30	5.5	3.1

(*Source:* Yaukey, D. *Fertility Differences in a Modernising country*. Princeton University Press, Princeton 1961)

menopause. Kinsey found that teenage brides reported having intercourse on average 3.7 times a week which dropped slightly to 2.6 by thirty, 2.1 at forty and 1.5 at fifty (*see* Table 11). At sixty, however, coitus was still reported on average once in twelve days. Sex is a normal part of human life for the aged as well as the young. When an older person discontinues coitus it is, as Alex Comfort has pointed out, usually for the same three reasons that a person might discontinue riding a bicycle—they have not the energy, they fear looking ridiculous or they cannot get hold of a bicycle!

THE MENSTRUAL CYCLE AND PREGNANCY

Mammalian reproduction requires a co-ordinated series of changes in the mother's body to prepare for, and sustain, pregnancy. The attachment of the fertilised egg to the wall of the uterus involves complex changes.

In the human species, a sequence of pituitary and ovarian hormone changes build up to the release of an egg from the ovary; these changes begin to prepare the uterus for pregnancy. Another equally necessary series of changes occurs to ensure the passage of the egg from the fallopian tubes (where fertilisation takes place), and completes the changes in the lining of the uterus necessary for the attachment of the egg, which take place five days after fertilisation. In other mammals, and probably also in man, the uterus will only permit the egg to attach for a period of twelve hours or so. Within a few days of beginning to develop, the egg produces hormones that are virtually identical to the woman's own pituitary and ovarian hormones and which have a similar effect on the woman's body. The embryo is like a parasite; it takes over and begins to control much of the woman's hormone system to its own advantage.

Hormones are chemical messengers. There are a great many types; insulin, for example, is a hormone unrelated to reproduction but essential for normal body action. The hormones made by the ovaries and the testes are called steroids, because they have a common chemical structure based on four hexagons of carbon and hydrogen atoms. Like insulin and other hormones, they are secreted into the blood-stream and act upon a number of "target" organs. In the female, steroid hormones affect the uterus, the fallopian tubes, the breasts, the brain, the skin, the heart and the circulatory system.

Both sexes make basically the same hormones, although in different proportions. Women have a small amount of circulating "male" hormones, such as testosterone and compounds related to it. It is thought, for example, that these are responsible for a woman's libido. A normal man will also have small amounts of circulating "female" hormones, such as oestrogen.

A second series of hormones control the release of ovarian steroids in women and testicular steroids in men. These come from the pituitary gland at the base of the brain. They, in turn, are controlled by a third series of hormones called "releasing factors", which come from the brain itself and travel a few millimetres through special blood vessels connecting the brain with the pituitary gland.

Steroid hormones can be made artificially. They are the basis of the Pill and a related series of hormones called "cortisone" which are made in the adrenal gland. The pituitary hormones, or gonadotrophins, are not so readily available. In theory, they could be the basis of a contraceptive Pill, but such a method has not yet been developed. One pituitary hormone, oxytocin, is used clinically to induce labour in women. The releasing factors have only been isolated relatively recently. They are quite simple chemicals and one of them (thyroid releasing hormone) has already been tried as a method of increasing milk production in lactating women. In theory, these releasing factors also could form the basis of a contraceptive Pill, and such a method might be devised in the next decade or so.

QUALITY OF REPRODUCTION

For the layman, and unfortunately for many members of the medical profession, pregnancy is thought to begin when a nice sperm meets a perfect egg in the protected, friendly environment of the fallopian tubes and uterus, and to end nine months later with a bouncing baby. The reality is different. Up to 15 or 20 per cent of the sperm production of a normal healthy man is abnormal and one way of regarding the female reproductive tract is as a series of hurdles designed to eliminate unhealthy sperm. The cervix hangs down into the top of the vagina—the opposite design to one that any intelligent plumber would make—and the tubes leave the uterine cavity by the smallest of openings; so of the hundreds of millions of sperm deposited in the vagina, only a few hundred make it as far as the egg. It is reasonable to believe that the abnormal sperm are screened out in the process.

Probably many eggs are also abnormal when first ovulated, although a study of this is more difficult than in the case of sperm. What is certain is that many of the products of conception are lost at varying stages of pregnancy. Of all the eggs fertilised, up to half prove abnormal and are lost before the first week or ten days of pregnancy. Biologically this wastage can be classified as abortion although it takes place before the woman misses her period or suspects that she is pregnant. It is a reasonable speculation that many women conceive during every cycle of unprotected intercourse, although pregnancy diagnosed by menstrual delay takes an average of several cycles of coitus.

Once menstrual delay has occurred (and in the modern world pregnancy may have been proved with a pregnancy test) a further 10–15 per cent of embryos will be lost through spontaneous abortion. Spontaneous abortion is a key factor in the natural processes of human reproduction. Induced abortion, as will be shown later, is one of the oldest, most universal and powerful means of volitional family planning.

When very early embryos are studied by the microscopic inspection of the uteri removed at hysterectomy (in a woman who was unknowingly pregnant at the time of the operation, or who was using it as a form of abortion), or when the products of conception are collected at spontaneous abortion, and chromosome patterns studied, then it is found that much or most foetal wastage involves the loss of abnormal embryos. In other words, spontaneous abortion is a natural, necessary, healing process without which pregnancy would be a nightmare of concern. At present, approximately one in fifty new-born babies has a congenital abnormality; but, fortunately, in nearly all cases these are mild biological anomalies, such as extra digits or a cleft palate. However, if abortions did not take place, then up to half of all new-born babies would be congenitally abnormal and most of the defects would be severe.

For example, in Down's syndrome (the mental and physical defect commonly known as mongolism) each cell, instead of having a particular pair of chromosomes, has one extra chromosome—a so-called trisomy. The pair involved is one of the smallest in the human cells. Trisomies also occur involving larger, more important pairs of chromosomes, but all such abnormalities appear to be aborted. In other words, mongolism is a defect that in biological terms is so slight that it fails to stimulate the natural processes of abortion.

When spontaneous abortion occurs later in pregnancy it can be a messy process involving many hours of uterine contractions. These can be very painful, and, if all the contents of the uterus are not expelled, infection may ascend from the neck of the womb. Sometimes hospital admission and artificial scraping of the uterus is necessary. Unless the woman is willing to give an honest history, it can be difficult for a doctor to distinguish between an accidental spontaneous abortion or miscarriage and a deliberately provoked abortion.

BREAST FEEDING

Pregnancies in animals that breed throughout the year (such as mice, red kangaroos and man) are spaced out mainly by lactation. The hormonal control of milk production begins with the partnership established between the mother and foetus during pregnancy, and continues after delivery in response to suckling. The breasts are prepared for milk production during pregnancy; the flow of milk, however, begins with the fall of hormone levels that occurs once the placental source of hormone production is removed at delivery.

At the time of delivery, the nipples become extremely sensitive, and suckling by the baby stimulates a nervous reflex that passes to the brain and in turn releases oxytocin and prolactin—two pituitary hormones. Oxytocin makes the uterus contract and this is one reason why a new-born child should be put straight to its mother's breast. The mother herself may feel uterine contractions when the suckling baby stimulates oxytocin release. Prolactin is a hormone which has only recently been fully understood. Among its actions is the inhibition of ovulation. Prolactin is nature's contraceptive.

In evolutionary terms, the use of lactation as the main element in the spacing of pregnancies has the two-way benefit of protecting the child that has already been born from the competition of a sibling conceived too quickly, and of returning the woman to regular ovulation if the pregnancy should end in a stillbirth or the baby should die in infancy. The natural adjustments of breast feeding may extend to an added protection of the mother in cases of malnutrition. A poorly nourished woman has poor quality milk; consequently the baby must suckle harder and longer to get sufficient milk and this may well add to the reflex stimulation which plays on the brain of the mother, enhancing the suppression of ovulation and spacing pregnancies more.

In pre-agricultural societies and in contemporary traditional rural societies, breast feeding lasts for nearer to two years than one and these intervals, which seem prolonged to Western observers, must be considered biologically normal. For most of the breast feeding period, ovulation (or from the woman's point of view the onset of menstruation subsequent to ovulation) is suspended (*see* Fig. 4). When ovulation resumes it may take several cycles to conceive the pregnancy which will itself last for nine months. Therefore births

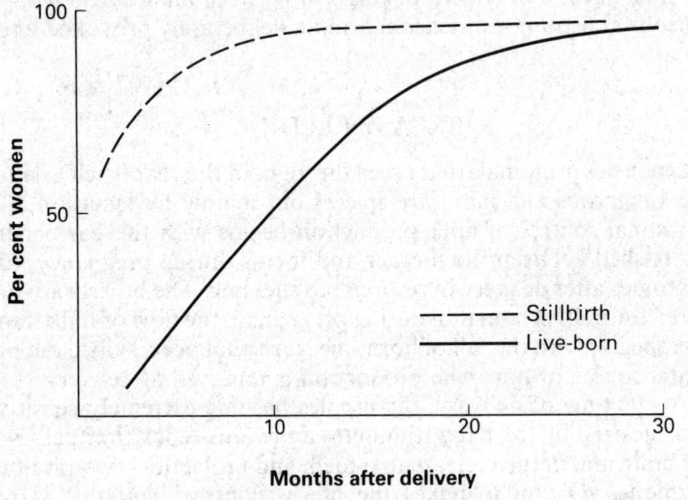

(*Source:* Wyon, J. B. and Gordon, J. E. *The Khanna Study*. Harvard Press, Cambridge, Mass. 1971)

Fig. 4. *Resumption of menstruation after delivery* (*traditional society with breast feeding*).

can easily be eighteen months to two and a half years apart. Seen from this perspective, much of contraceptive practice in industrialised nations, for the purpose of spacing pregnancies, is doing no more than substituting modern contraceptives for the biological control once exerted by lactation.

A well known paediatrician tells the story of a woman in a developing country sitting on a pavement with an infant less than one year old at one breast, and a child of five or six standing nearby, occasionally sucking at the other breast. This in itself is not uncommon, except for the fact that in this case the older child was also holding a cigarette behind its back and having a quick draw between sucks! A less amusing but physiologically more informative example concerns a woman in a very overcrowded, insanitary community who obtained milk from her breast and put it on a mosquito bite on the child's leg. "It prevents a sore developing," she commented, although she could not have known that milk contains antibodies that transfer to her child the mother's immunity to several infections. This, together with the finely balanced and changing pattern of fats and other nutrients that milk possesses, is why artificial feeding, at least in the early months of life, is biologically second-best to breast feeding.

In developing countries where artificial milk (always an import from temperate countries) is relatively much more expensive than in the West, and where even the most conscientious mother has difficulty sterilising the bottle and purifying the water for the feed, bottle-fed babies are much more prone to gastro-intestinal infections and have a demonstrably higher death rate. It is one of the many paradoxes of health care and family planning that governments of developing countries permit widespread advertising of artificial feeds, but restrain comparable advertisements of contraceptives.

Lactation puts a heavy burden on the mother's nutrition, but she is partially prepared for this by her stores of body fat. During lactation a woman will draw on these resources. This is the reason why, with the modern curtailment of lactation, women often complain of putting on weight with every child they have. Perhaps if this was more widely appreciated, those women who avoid lactation because it might "spoil their figures" (itself a myth) might be more inclined to breast feed.

Breast feeding is said to deepen the emotional bond between mother and baby, and although this may sound like well-intentioned idealism, recent data from animals and man should give pause for reflection. In some animals, for example goats, if the mother is prevented from seeing or smelling her new-born kid for the critical first few minutes after delivery, she will reject it altogether. If the human species requires a similar imprinting process it certainly takes place over a longer interval; nevertheless a number of studies suggest that where mother and child are artificially separated (as in most hospitals around the world) in the first few hours after delivery, breast feeding is less adequate, and emotional problems are possibly more common later. Battered babies are more likely to have been delivered by Caesarian operation, or to have been nursed in the artificial environment of the incubator.

The curtailment of breast feeding which has occurred in the Western world, and is occurring in the developing world, has been dubbed the biggest uncontrolled experiment in human physiology—perhaps modern obstetric practices are the biggest uncontrolled intervention in human psychology. These practices are odd because the separation of mother and baby at delivery is done for no other reasons than habit, administrative tidiness and to provide a temporary division of labour for the nursing staff.

THE PREGNANCY INTERVAL

The time from the birth of one child until the birth of the next is called the pregnancy interval (*see* Fig. 5). It consists of three parts:

(*a*) the time taken to conceive;
(*b*) the duration of pregnancy;
(*c*) an interval without ovulation after delivery or abortion.

The pregnancy interval can vary from less than a year to the extremes of a fertile lifetime. There is a great deal of evidence from many different societies (*see* p. 223) to show that babies can be too close together (and to a lesser extent too far apart) for the optimum welfare of the children and the mother. It takes some time for the reproductive system to recover from the stress of pregnancy and delivery, but

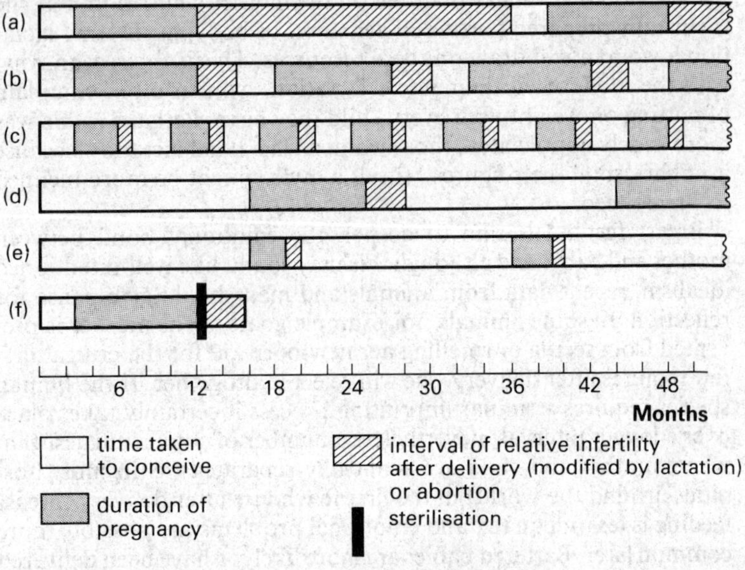

Fig. 5. *Patterns of human reproduction*. (a) Term delivery followed by breast feeding; (b) term delivery followed by artificial feeding, wet-nursing or stillbirth; (c) spontaneous or induced abortion; (d) use of contraceptives followed by term delivery; (e) use of contraceptives and spontaneous or induced abortion; (f) sterilisation of one or other partner.

it is concerning nutrition and the allocation of what can only be called "mother love" that babies born too close together suffer the greatest disadvantage.

Figure 5 illustrates a number of possible cycles of human infertility during a fixed number of years of a woman's life. The facts that require emphasis are that, in the absence of contraceptives, it can take two or three abortions to consume the same interval of a woman's life as conceiving, bearing and breast feeding a baby do. However, when abortion or delivery follow the use of contraception, the time periods involved with each are more nearly equivalent in length because, of the three factors that make up the pregnancy interval, the time taken to conceive is now the longest, and outweighs the other two in relative terms.

INFERTILITY

Both men and women can be infertile. There are biological reasons for infertility, as, for example, in cases of chromosomally abnormal individuals where the body cannot form viable sperm or eggs. Some diseases such as mumps in a sexually mature man or tuberculosis in a woman may cause sterility. Venereal disease is another cause of sterility. In women, gonorrhea can block the tubes, even though the disease itself may not have been very serious. Other forms of female infertility are consequent upon previous deliveries or abortion. Infection after childbirth, or after an unlucky abortion, can block the fallopian tubes.

The incidence of sterility increases with age, particularly in women. For women who attempt to conceive before the age of twenty, infertility is a rare problem. A woman who attempts to conceive her first child in the late thirties will be subject to a significant risk of sterility. A woman who is never able to conceive a child is said to have "primary" infertility, and a woman who has one or more pregnancies and then is unable to conceive again, is said to have "secondary" infertility.

A number of environmental and dietary causes can alter human fertility. Alcohol, as Shakespeare knew, has the effect of "increasing the desire but diminishing the performance". The chronic alcoholic often has degenerative changes in his testes. Marijuana depresses the sperm count. Sometimes factors which adversely effect sperm production also reduce reproductive performance in the female, by damaging embryos that have been conceived; in addition both alcohol and marijuana are under suspicion as teratological (embryo damaging) agents.

In laboratory animals fertility can be altered by a number of environmental factors. Deficiencies of Vitamin E can cause male infertility in rats but no such effect has been discovered in man. Gross malnutrition in human society as a result of protein deficiency can affect male fertility, although in the modern world obesity is a more common cause of reduced fertility. Severe anaemia and malnutrition can lead to anovulation in the woman. Amenorrhea was common, for example, in Nazi concentration camps and during the post-Second World War famine in Holland.

Mountain living, with its resultant lowering of oxygen levels in the blood, can affect reproduction in mammals. In the Andes, some domestic animals will become infertile if taken to very high altitudes. It is said that certain groups of Peruvians come to a lower level each year to sleep with their wives; perhaps this is a cultural adaptation to a physiological need. However, man and his domestic animals can adapt to height over periods of months and years. But the overwhelming majority of the world's population do not live in the high Andes. For the bulk of people involved in rapid population growth at the present moment, diet, coital frequency and altitude are not major factors determining fertility. The similarities between human patterns of sexual behaviour and biological performance are greater than the differences. The woman in a traditional society who has six, seven or eight children is not very far removed from our own great-grandparents in the way in which her reproductive system is used. The change which has taken place is one in death rates, not birth rates, and the challenge which remains is to bring modern birth-control into the life of traditional societies as successfully as certain aspects of modern death-control have diffused into those societies.

TECHNOLOGY AND BIOLOGY

The scientific manipulation of the biological variables controlling human fertility has proved difficult and it is useful to contrast the means available for bringing down death rates with those invented for slowing birth rates.

Since the end of the Second World War, death rates in the developing world have fallen dramatically. For more than a decade, in a country such as India, the average expectation of life increased by about one year every year; in a statistical sense, people almost stopped dying. As is always the case when death rates fall, the major changes were in infant mortality.

The dramatic and welcome changes that have been achieved came about without a major medical input of the sort that we are familiar with in the West. Hundreds of millions of children who have survived infancy in the developing world will never have been near a Western trained doctor in their life. They will have been vaccinated in some mass programme (which their parents may not have understood, or possibly even objected to). Perhaps they have had one or two illnesses which previously might have been fatal ones, but their lives were saved by an untutored use of antibiotics from the local "quack" doctor, who is rarely averse to taking effective therapies into his practice. In addition, there has been improvement in the water supply. Piped water involves not only clean water for drinking, avoiding gastro-enteritis and parasitic diseases, but water for washing. If you have to carry water a long way from a well, it ensues that your body cleanliness will be poor.

In the field of obstetrics many problems remain and 70 per cent of mothers delivering their babies in the developing world are attended only by untrained traditional midwives. However, in urban areas, very large hospitals often provide care which is unsophisticated but saves many lives. Sometimes the hospitals are so busy that women are only in them for the hours of labour and for a few hours afterwards, as in the great obstetric hospitals of Caracas, Tehran or Kinshasa. Often the women lie two in a bed, head to toe with their babies between them, before being discharged to make room for the next woman. In Saigon, women used to sit in the street during the first stage of labour and were only admitted into the hospital after an examination to prove that the cervix had begun to dilate. Even when it is not possible to deliver the babies of urban women in hospitals, at least some of those women who have a prolonged labour and serious complications get professional care, which ensures that their lives, and/or the lives of their babies, are saved.

Contrary to what might be thought, even wars have become less costly in human lives. The catastrophe and horror of the Vietnamese war, which went on for more than three decades, was associated with rapid population growth in North and South Vietnam.

The fatal effects of war, the third of the traditional Malthusian checks on rapid population growth, were always rather in epidemics and the social disruptions that followed the fighting, than in the deaths caused by the use of swords or atom bombs. One macabre way to review the present growth in the world's population is to compare it with the horrendous mortality which accompanied the use of atomic weapons in Hiroshima and Nagasaki. Each of these killed more than 100,000 people; but if the world's population was to be kept in check by atomic warfare, it would require an atomic bomb to be dropped more than once a day, week in week out, year in year out. Indeed, the world would run out of urban areas on which to use these fearful weapons, and the polluting effects of radiation would probably destroy humanity before their direct fatal effects could achieve a balance in population.

There have been nearly three decades of relative peace at a global level. The world has acted, for the first time, as a unit and when famine has threatened or arrived (as in sub-Saharan Africa, or the Indian sub-continent) food has been shifted from the great grain reserves of the West, particularly North America, to the affected areas. There has been greed, incompetence and lack of planning; nevertheless millions of people who would have previously starved to death are now competing for employment and the annual share of the world's harvests. In contrast to the success of public health measures in altering death rates, contraceptive measures are clumsy and costly; they require repetitive use and often carry with them minor inconveniences and occasionally real hazards. These problems are well known and will be highlighted later. At this point the only emphasis to be made is that, all sociological considerations apart, the technology of fertility control remains at a disappointing level.

CONCLUSION

Men and women have been evolved to have coitus much more frequently than is required for the purposes of conception, irrespective of the season and the likelihood or possibility of ovulation. Whereas in several of these characteristics we are unlike many other mammalian species, we share with other living creatures a reproductive capacity programmed to allow for the wastage which occurs at every stage of reproduction, from the preparation and release of sperm and eggs to the death of individuals between birth and the time when they themselves become parents. Sufficient overproduction has been possible at each stage to ensure that, on average, and allowing for long term vicissitudes as well as pregnancy wastage and infant and child mortality, each parent is succeeded by another in the next generation. This has been the pattern of affairs throughout most of history and the whole of prehistory. Until recently, in order to achieve biological replacement, women began intercourse at or around puberty and bore on average ten children in a fertile lifetime, two years or more apart if lactation took place, and closer if the infant died.

In the past 100 years and with accelerating pace since the Second World War, profound changes have taken place in the survival of infants and young children, and some lesser, but still important, changes in the life expectancy of adults. These have changed the balance and structure of human populations, creating a number of economic and social problems at a crucial moment in history, when technology has developed the means to enhance or degrade the human environment to unprecedented degrees.

The biological details of human reproduction, which over millions of years have been part of a profoundly different environment from that in which we find ourselves today, now require modification.

In natural populations of animals, reproduction is regulated by changes in some, or all, of three important variables. When over-crowding occurs it is usual for the age of sexual maturity to be delayed, the interval between pregnancies to increase and the mortality rate at birth and in the immediately succeeding interval to rise.

In the modern world, man has reversed these three natural regulators. The age of sexual maturity, the menarche, has declined from 17–18 in nineteenth century communities to 11–12 in many contemporary ones. The interval between pregnancies is being reduced by the shift away from the normal patterns of breast feeding. Finally, the neo-natal mortality rate (babies that are stillborn or die within the first week of life) is falling throughout the world.

SELECTED REFERENCES AND BIBLIOGRAPHY

Austin, C. R. and Short, R. U. *Reproduction in Mammals* Vols. 1–5. Cambridge University Press, Cambridge 1972

Davis, K. and Blake, J. "Social Structure and Fertility: An Analytic Framework." *Economic Development and Cultural Change*. 4 (3), 211 1956

Frisch, R. E. "A Method of Prediction of Age of Menarche from Height and Weight at Ages 9 through 13 Years." *Pediatrics*. 53, 384 1974

Harrison, R. G. and De Boer, C. H. *Sex and Infertility*. Academic Press, London 1977

Kinsey, A., Pomeroy, W., Martin, C. and Gebhard, P. *Sexual Behaviour in the Human Female*. W. B. Saunders and Co., Philadelphia 1953

Parkes, A. S. *Patterns of Sexuality and Reproduction*. Oxford University Press, London 1976

Parkes, A. S., Thomson, A. M., Potts, M. and Herbertson, M. A. (eds.) "Fertility Regulation during Human Lactation." *Journal of Biosocial Science* Suppl. no. 4 1977

Chapter 3

The Measurement of Human Fertility

The second half of the twentieth century is proving to be a period of unusual and significant change in human populations. Biologically, a number of variables have altered. These changes tend to increase human fertility at the very time when most societies are struggling to exercise a more rigorous control on achieved family size. The next step in the argument involves understanding the magnitude and nature of population change more fully, and appreciating the problems involved in population predictions.

Fertility analysis is concerned with the number of births occurring in a specified population unit in a specified time period. The crucial questions involve the choice of unit and period. The unit can vary from an individual female, a married couple, or a specified group, to a total population or subgroup of that population. The period may range from the lifetime of an individual, or a specific period of marriage, to a calendar year or group of years.

For the most part, interest centres not on an individual's isolated experience but on aggregate measures whereby the typical experience of a large number of people can be described. Two main approaches are possible:

(*a*) fertility may be measured as a "vital rate", based on the birth and population data of a calendar year, or a consecutive number of years. Such measures, expressed in terms of the frequency of births to the population or a relevant subgroup in it, are usually referred to as "period rates". Period rates include part of the reproductive performance of many different women of varying ages during the specified period;

(*b*) fertility may be described as the actual number of births per woman during the child-bearing period, expressed in terms of achieved family size, or as the average number of children borne by a woman at a particular stage of her reproductive career. If we are studying a group of women who have reached the end of their fertile years, we talk of "completed" family size, expressed as an average of distribution of live births. Such measures represent the total reproductive performance of one group of women, defined by their dates of birth or marriage and conventionally referred to as a "cohort". It must be stressed that *cohort rates* always refer to actual or historical cohorts and not to hypothetical cohorts, synthesised from age-specific rates in a given period (which represent short segments of many actual cohorts and are the equivalent of period rates).

PERIOD RATES

The "crude birth rate" is the number of live births per 1,000 people per year. This is calculated by dividing the number of births in a year by the mid-year population and multiplying by a constant factor (usually 1,000). Crude birth rates are the most commonly used aggregate measure of fertility. Table 2 gives examples of differences in level and trends of crude birth rates in various countries over a period of forty-five years. Industrialised nations have medium to low birth rates that are static or falling, as in Japan. Developing countries

TABLE 2: CRUDE BIRTH RATES, SELECTED COUNTRIES, 1930–74

Period	*Mexico*	*Singapore*	*Japan*	*Canada*	*England and Wales*
1930–34	44.5	38.5	31.8	22.2	15.3
1935–39	43.5	46.0	29.2	20.4	14.9
1940–44	44.2	44.9	30.1	23.2	15.5
1945–49	44.4	46.4	30.2	27.0	18.0
1950–54	44.1	45.5	23.7	27.7	15.5
1955–59	44.9	42.8	18.2	27.8	15.9
1960–64	44.4	35.6	17.2	25.2	17.9
1965–69	45.5	26.9	17.7	23.7	17.2
1970–74	43.0	22.3	19.1	16.2	14.7

(*Source: U.N. Demographic Year Book*. 1969 and 1974)

have high birth rates which either remain high, as in Mexico, or are falling to more modest, but still not low, levels, as in Singapore.

Crude birth rates are available for most nations of the world and so provide an easy way of reviewing fertility levels. In conjunction with "crude death rates" (the number of deaths per 1,000 people per year), they allow a simple calculation of the rate of natural increase in a population, if we exclude consideration of net migration.

Table 3 gives some indication of the wide variation in crude rates throughout the world and the consequent levels of natural increase. The implications of different rates of natural increase can be seen by relating the percentage growth per year to the time it takes for the population to double. Mexico's crude rate of natural increase

TABLE 3: CRUDE BIRTH, DEATH AND CRUDE RATES OF NATURAL INCREASE PER 1,000 POPULATION, SELECTED COUNTRIES, 1974

Country	*Births*	*Deaths*	*Natural increase*
Nigeria	50	23	27
Mexico	40	10	30
India	36	16	20
Taiwan	23	5	18
Singapore	18	5	13
United States	15	9	6
West Germany	10	12	−2

(*Source: Population and Family Planning Programs: A Factbook*. Population Council, New York 1976)

of 30 per 1,000, an annual growth of 3 per cent, entails a doubling of the population in twenty-three years.

There is a dramatic difference in the implications for a society in which the population doubles in a generation and for a society in which it doubles in a century (*see* Fig. 6), as is the trend in most industrialised nations. These differences are obvious and important and will be explored further in Chapter 10.

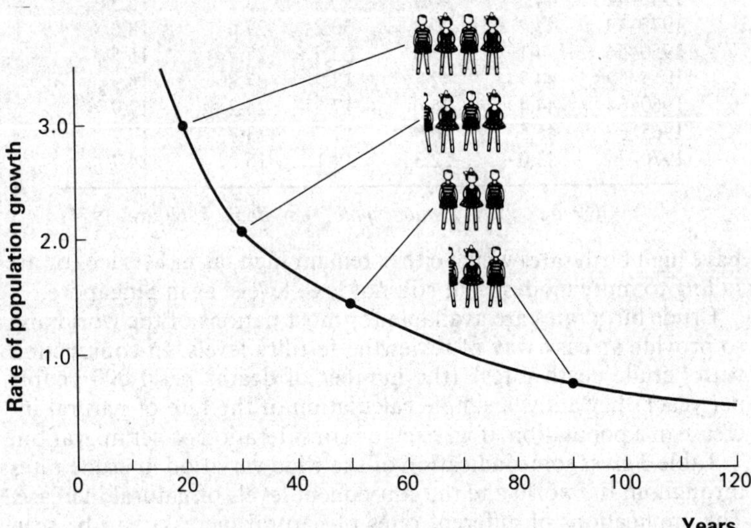

Fig. 6. *Average family size (Western mortality rates) and population doubling time.*

The crude birth rate can be useful in charting changes within a country over a period of time (*see* Table 3) or as a step in calculating the rates of natural increase (*see* Table 4); it can, however, be misleading if comparisons are made between countries with differing age-structures. Because of this, various refinements have been made which relate births more closely to the population at risk. The simplest step is to relate the number of births in a specific year to the population of women of reproductive age (conventionally taken as women aged fifteen to forty-four or fifteen to forty-nine). This is the "general fertility rate". As a further refinement, we can look separately at legitimate and illegitimate births in relation to the number of married or unmarried women of reproductive age. Thus the general "illegitimate fertility rate" is the number of illegitimate births per 1,000 single, widowed and divorced women aged fifteen to forty-nine. Illegitimacy is also sometimes measured by relating illegitimate births to total live births by the "illegitimacy ratio", which indicates the proportion of all births which are registered as illegitimate.

More accurate comparisons are possible with "age-specific fertility rates", or the number of births during a year to women of a given age per 1,000 women of that age. These too can be restricted to illegitimate or legitimate births and to married or unmarried women. For example, in England and Wales in 1972, there were 62,511 illegitimate births, 35 per cent of which were to women under the age of twenty. However, the illegitimacy rate at this age is low, because the population at risk is large and many women are not sexually active. In contrast, the illegitimacy ratio is the highest for any age-group, as there are relatively few legitimate births.

In order to obtain a single measure of period fertility which allows for age structure we may add up the age-specific fertility rates for women, allowing for the period of exposure to child-bearing at each age; this gives the "total fertility rate". This provides a measure of the average number of live births per woman which would result if the prevailing age-specific fertility rates were maintained over a reproductive span of thirty years. It can be thought of as the number of children a hypothetical average woman would have if, during her lifetime, her child-bearing behaviour were the same as that of a cross-section of women at the time of observation. As an approximation of average actual completed family size associated with current fertility rates, it is a useful measure, because it gives an indication which is easy to picture (although it also has limitations which we discuss below).

The difference between "crude birth rate" (C.B.R.) and "total fertility rate" (T.F.R.) can best be illustrated by looking at two

TABLE 4: AGE-SPECIFIC FERTILITY RATES, TOTAL FERTILITY RATE, AND CRUDE BIRTH AND DEATH RATES, ENGLAND AND WALES AND JAPAN, 1965

Age of mother at time of birth	*England and Wales*	*Japan*
15–19	23.9	1.8
20–24	176.3	112.3
25–29	178.1	203.1
30–34	101.5	86.4
35–39	48.4	19.3
40–44	12.5	3.0
45–49	0.9	0.2
Total	541.6	426.1
(Allowing for 5-year age-groups)	× 5	× 5
Total fertility rate		
1) per 1,000 women	2,708	2,131
2) per woman	2.71	2.13
Crude birth rate	18.1	18.6
Crude death rate	11.9	6.5
Crude rate of natural increase	6.1	12.1

(*Source: U.N. Demographic Year Book*. 1969)

countries where crude rates are similar but age-specific and total fertility rates are very different, as in England and Wales, and Japan (*see* Table 4).

In 1965, the crude birth rate was slightly higher in Japan, but the total fertility rate was substantially lower and age-specific rates were lower at all ages except 25–29—a five-year interval accounting for nearly half of the births to Japanese women. The reason for this is that women of child-bearing age, and especially women aged 15–34, represent a larger proportion of the total population in Japan, and so contribute a larger number of births relative to total population size, despite having a lower fertility per woman.

Differences in age-structure also affect the crude death rates. There are fewer old people in Japan, with the result that the crude death rate for the country in 1974 was 6.5, in contrast with 11.9 for England and Wales, although life expectancy was only marginally higher.

The other point of interest in the fertility patterns of the two countries is the concentration of Japanese fertility in the late twenties. Ravenholt of the U.S.A.I.D. Office of Population has devised a useful means of graphic representation of age-specific fertility rates which brings out such points by means of "fertility silhouettes". Figures 7 and 8 show the data from Table 4 presented

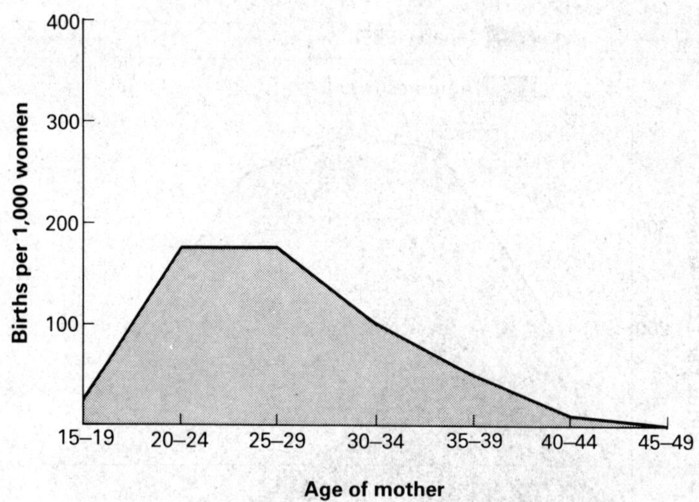

(*Source: U.N. Demographic Year Book*. 1969)

Fig. 7. *Age-specific fertility rates for England and Wales* (*1965*). Total fertility rate: per 1,000 women = 2,708; per woman = 2.7. Crude birth rate = 18.1.

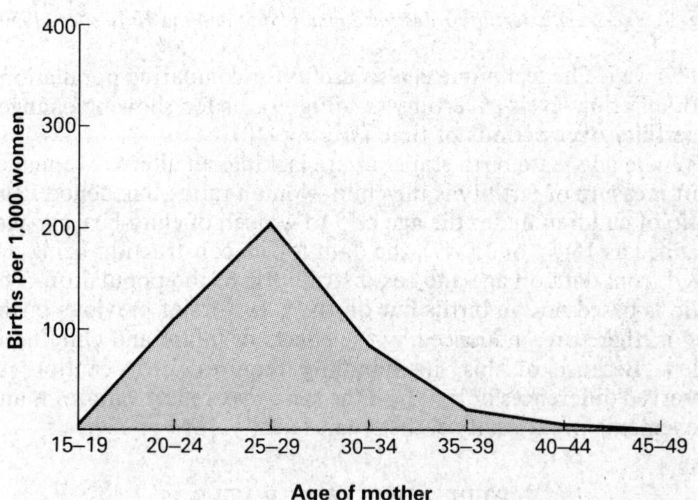

(*Source: U.N. Demographic Year Book*. 1969)

Fig. 8. *Age-specific fertility rates for Japan* (*1965*). Total fertility rate: per 1,000 women = 2,131; per woman = 2.1. Crude birth rate = 18.6.

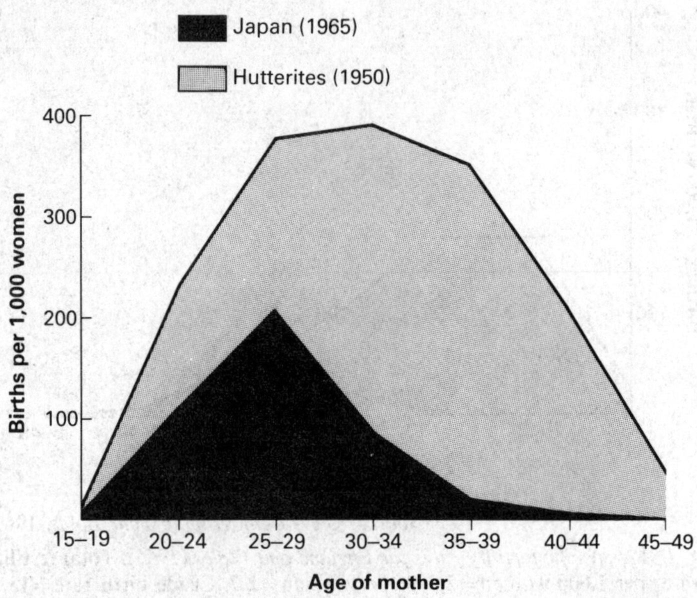

(*Source:* Eaton, J. and Mayer, A. *Human Biology*. 25, 206 1953; *U.N. Demographic Year Book*. 1969)

Fig. 9. *Age-specific fertility rates for Japan (1965) and the Hutterites (1950).*

in this way. The technique is also useful for comparing populations with differing levels of fertility (*see* Fig. 9), or for showing changes in fertility over periods of time (*see* Fig. 10).

Where adequate birth statistics are lacking, an alternative makeshift measure of fertility is the child–woman ratio; this denotes the ratio of children under the age of 5 to women of child-bearing ages (defined as 15–44 or 15–49), the data for its construction being derived from data on age and sex distribution of the population. The ratio is based not on births but on the survivors of previous births and is, therefore, influenced by the effects of infant and child mortality. Because of this, its handling requires great caution, as observed differences or trends in the ratio may reflect variations and movements in mortality rather than fertility. [*See* p. 177.]

REPRODUCTION RATES

The total fertility rate represents the number of live births which would occur to a hypothetical cohort of women subject to the age-specific fertility of the year(s) studied. The "gross reproduction rate"

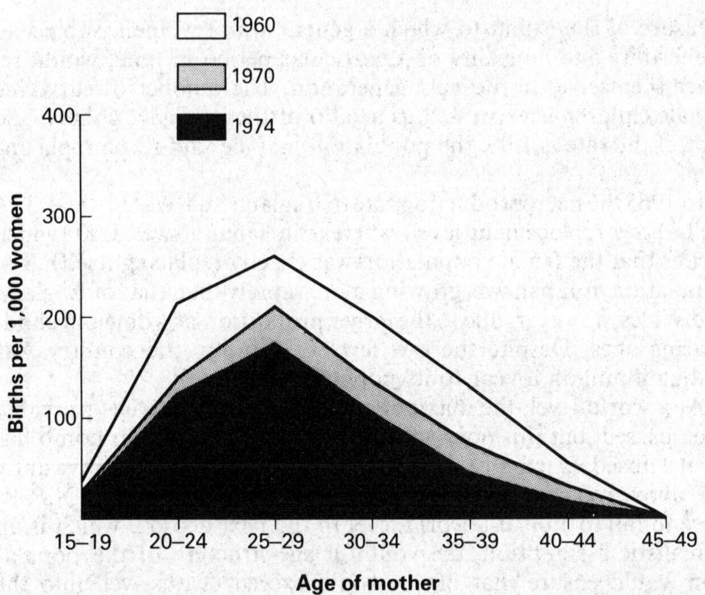

(*Source:* Anderson, J., Cheng, M. and Fook-Kee, W. "Component analysis of Recent Fertility Decline in Singapore." *Studies in Family Planning.* 8 (11) 1977)

Fig. 10. *Age-specific fertility rates for Singapore.*

(G.R.R.) is a measure of the number of female children born to such a cohort: it is calculated in the same way as the total fertility rate but considers only female births and so yields a value about half as large. In the absence of data on female births, the T.F.R. may be multiplied by 0.49 to allow for the higher proportion of male babies.

The "net reproduction rate" (N.R.R.) involves a further adjustment, to take into account the likelihood of a woman dying before she can complete her reproductive years. Female age-specific fertility rates are multiplied by the proportion of women surviving from birth to the mid-point of the relevant age range, and these are then summed and multiplied by five, as in the computation of the T.F.R. Alternatively, the G.R.R. may be multiplied by the proportion of women surviving to median child-bearing age, conventionally taken as twenty-seven in developed countries.

The net reproduction rate indicates the number of daughters born to each woman who survive at least to the age of their mother at the time of their own birth. It can, therefore, be thought of as a measure of the extent to which a generation of women, subject to the fertility and mortality of a particular period in time, would replace themselves in the next generation. The number of surviving female children is expressed as a ratio of the original "cohort", so that, if the rate is 1.00, the population may be said to be replacing itself.

In 1965 the net reproduction rate in England and Wales was 1.329, well above replacement level, whereas in Japan it was 1.00 (which means that the female population was exactly replacing itself). The population of Japan was growing more rapidly than that of England and Wales, however, due to the larger proportion of women in child-bearing ages. Despite the low level of fertility, the country was adding a million a year to its population.

At a world level, the maximum annual growth rate has probably been passed, but this does not mean that the population bomb has been defused. Currently, net reproduction rates are well above unity (i.e. above replacement level) in most countries. Even if the N.R.R. were to fall to 1.00 at a world level in the next decade, which is an unrealistic assumption, the youthful age-structure of the population would ensure that births would exceed deaths well into the twenty-first century (*see* Fig. 2).

Conversely, the achievements of a developing country in reducing its fertility may be grossly underestimated if crude rates alone are taken into account. It is often pointed out that the sharp fall in the crude birth rate in countries such as Singapore still leaves this rate above the level of most Western nations, and there is a rate of natural increase which will entail a doubling of population every sixty years. Nevertheless, the net reproduction rate for that country in 1974 had fallen to 1.119, lower than that for England and Wales in the period from 1957 to 1971. This represents a clear "modernisation" of fertility behaviour and a potential for replacement-level fertility, and an eventual stabilisation of population.

A serious limitation of measures such as the total fertility rate and the reproduction rates is that, although they seem to approximate to actual family size and to predict future reproductive performance, they remain "period" rates and so are affected by the timing and spacing of births. Consequently, they may not accurately reflect long-term fertility patterns of actual groups of women over their child-bearing period. In so far as they describe the fertility of a single year only, they predict nothing about the future levels of fertility.

The dangers inherent in the use of such measures can be seen by looking at British experience between the two World Wars, when net reproduction rates remained below unity from 1920 to 1945, leading to many prophecies of an impending decline in population. In fact, throughout the period births exceeded deaths, and after the Second World War fertility increased, with more women marrying and a higher proportion of those doing so having at least two children, so that by the 1960s concern had switched to that of excessive population growth.

It is only in the last few years that the net reproduction rate has again fallen below unity and only in 1976 that the crude birth rate fell below the death rate, resulting in a natural decrease in population. These problems underline the need to look at the actual reproductive performance of women during their child-bearing years, using the second approach referred to above, the "cohort" analysis of fertility. But before we look at the use of cohort analysis, it will be useful to consider briefly the effect of fertility on the age structure of populations, as we have already seen that this can have an important influence on the level of fertility in a country.

FERTILITY AND POPULATION AGE-STRUCTURE

The size of a population is determined by the combined effects of fertility, mortality and migration, and the rate of natural increase is determined by the gap between births and deaths for the population in a particular year. The number of births occurring in a population is influenced by the age-structure of the population, notably by the proportion of the female population who are in child-bearing ages. Thus in Japan in recent years, and in Britain and other European countries in the 1930s, population has increased in size (despite a level of fertility which is below replacement) as a result of the substantial number of potential mothers in those countries.

Likewise, the number of deaths in a population is influenced by the proportion of the population who are in age-groups which face a relatively high risk of mortality. For example, the crude death rate in England and Wales has been about 12 per 1,000 for the past fifteen years—twice the level found in developing countries such as Singapore, Mauritius and Jamaica. However, the age-specific death rates are lower at all ages in England, and the higher crude death rate results from the larger number of old people in the population. If the age-specific death rates of Singapore in 1968 are applied to the age-structure of England and Wales in the same year, the resultant "standardised" death rate for Singapore is about 18 per 1,000, i.e. 50 per cent higher.

Therefore the age composition of a population is a significant factor determining the level of births and deaths. However, it is equally important to recognise that the age composition is itself the result of past trends in fertility, mortality and migration. Of these three influences, fertility is the most important.

In order to demonstrate this, we need to look at populations with different demographic histories and consequently differing age-structures. The most graphic way of representing the age distribution of a population is by an "age pyramid" in which the proportion of men and women in each five-year age-group is represented by bars on each side of a vertical axis divided into such age-groups. Because the pyramids are based on proportions, all have the same "area", despite differences in the size of the country portrayed. This enables us to compare countries with varying total populations.

In a hypothetical population of 1,000 people equally divided into males and females, all of whom died on their 100th birthday and in which there were 10 births each year to replace the 10 resulting deaths, the "pyramid" would become a rectangle in which there would be 25 men and 25 women in each five-year age-group. In reality, people die at all ages, and in particular they die with increasing frequency at older ages, so that the top of a pyramid tends to be sharply pointed, with few surviving to die at the age of 100.

The actual shape of the pyramid depends on the patterns of fertility, mortality and migration over the lifetime of the population represented. Distinct and predictable patterns ensue from differing past levels of mortality and fertility as can be seen in Figs. 11–17 which represent countries with differing demographic histories.

Figure 11 (India, 1951) shows the classical pyramid shape of a growing population with high fertility and mortality. A similar shape was found in nineteenth century Britain and U.S.A. There is a high proportion of young people (35–40 per cent) but relatively few above the age of 65 and population growth is modest.

Such an age-structure is unusual today, even in developing countries, where the more usual pattern is of high fertility and falling mortality as in Fig. 12 (Costa Rica, 1963), where the recent experience of a sharp decline in infant and child mortality leads to a flared base and a "pinched" profile. Population growth is rapid and the proportion of the population under 15 is high (45–50 per cent) ensuring rapid growth for years to come as the women in these age-groups enter the reproductive ages. As in Fig. 11 the proportion of old people is small.

Figure 13 (Singapore, 1968) indicates the effect of a recent dramatic decline in fertility. The total number of births has been falling in the previous five years, with the result that the base of the pyramid narrows, but the proportion of old people remains low. Figure 14 (Japan, 1965) shows the impact of a continuation of this pattern over a longer period. The proportion of young people has

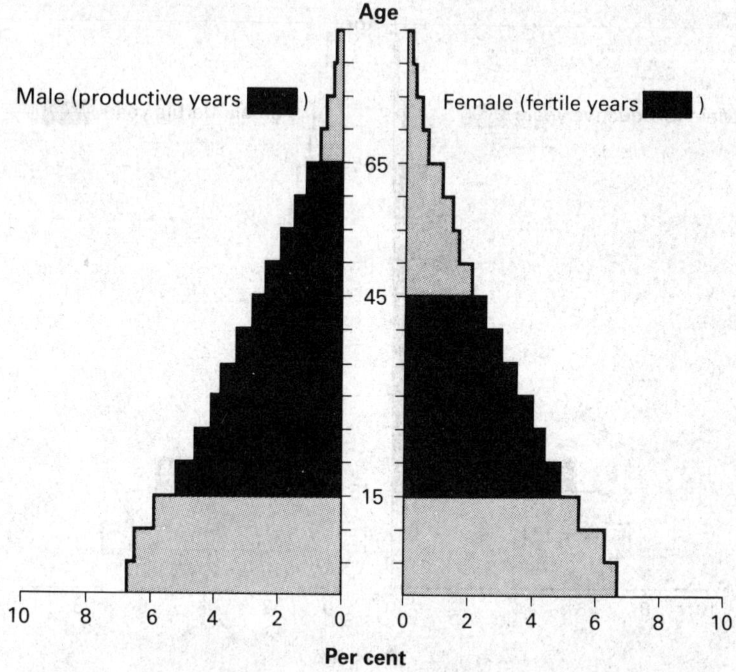

(*Source:* Census of India. 1951)

Fig. 11. *Population age pyramid for India* (*1951*).

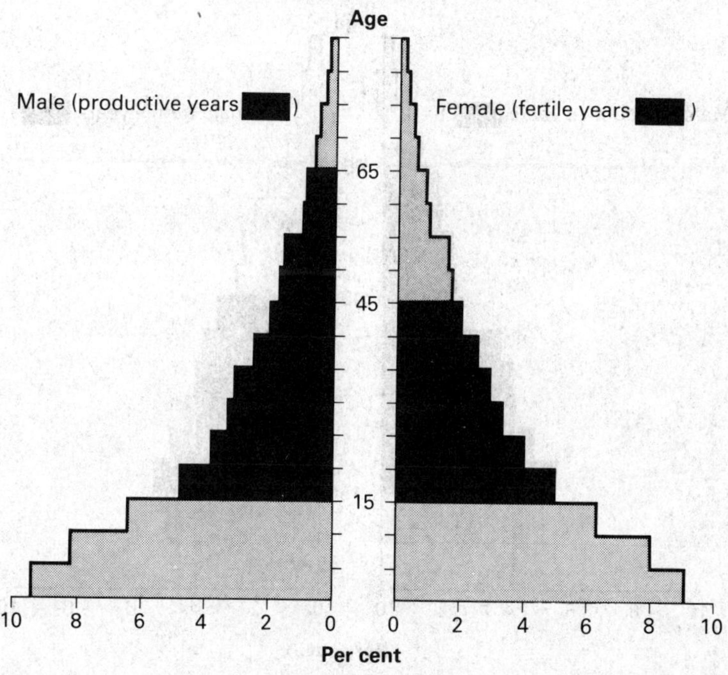

(*Source: U.N. Demographic Year Book*. 1965)

Fig. 12. *Population age pyramid for Costa Rica* (*1963*).

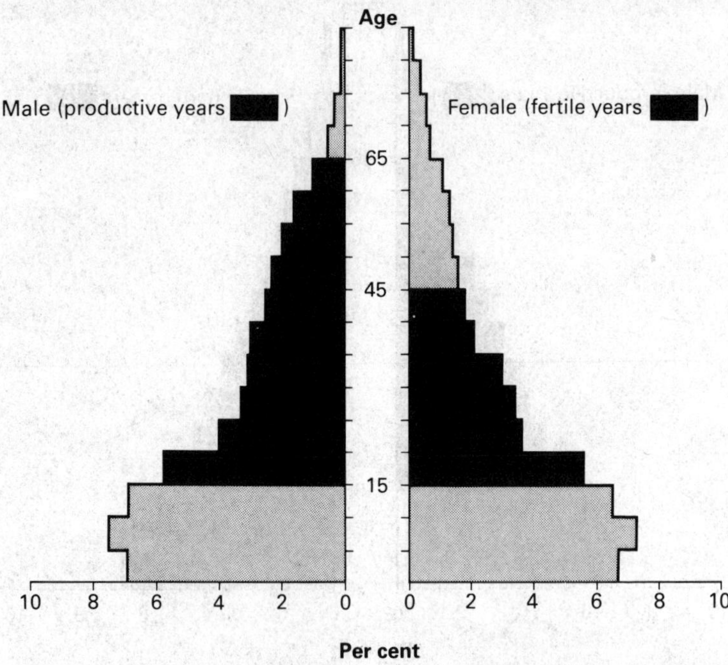

(*Source: U.N. Demographic Year Book*. 1969)

Fig. 13. *Population age pyramid for Singapore* (*1968*).

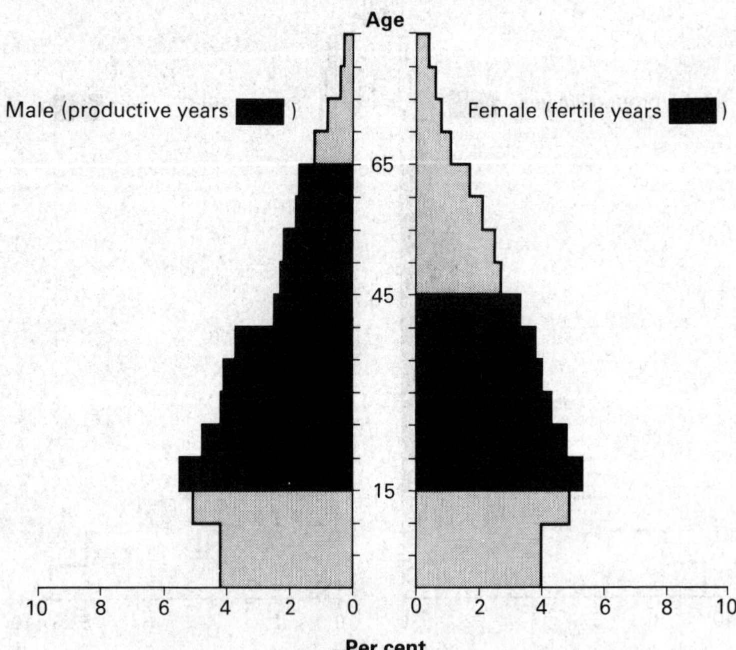

(*Source: U.N. Demographic Year Book*. 1965)

Fig. 14. *Population age pyramid for Japan* (*1965*).

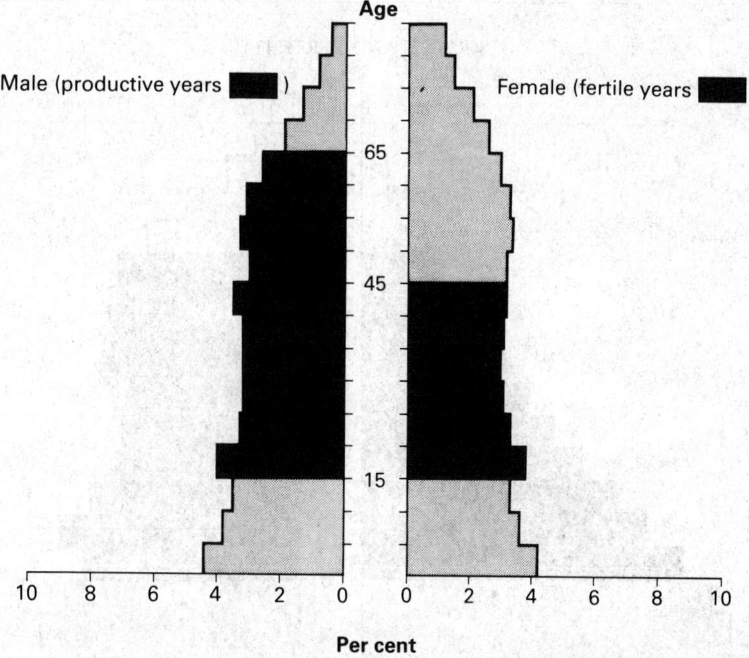

(*Source: U.N. Demographic Year Book*. 1965)

Fig. 15. *Population age pyramid for England and Wales (1965).*

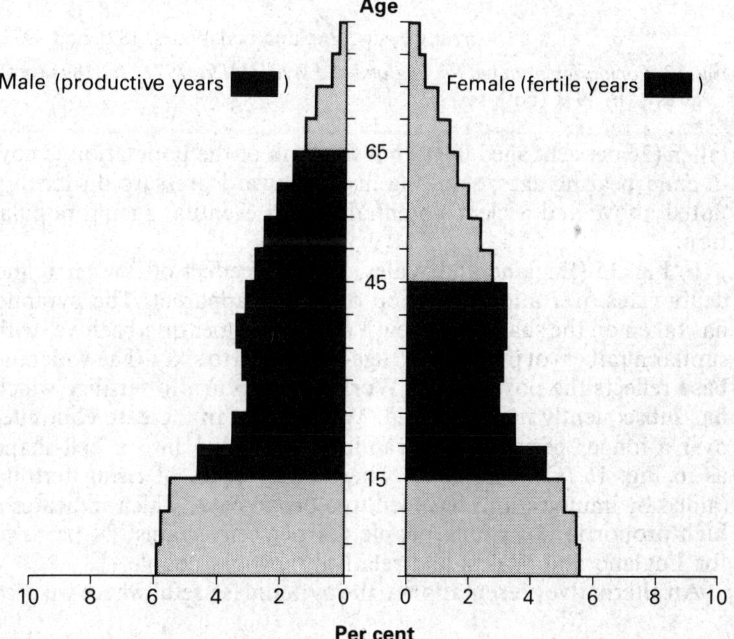

(*Source: U. N. Demographic Year Book*. 1965)

Fig. 16. *Population age pyramid for Canada (1965).*

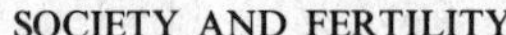

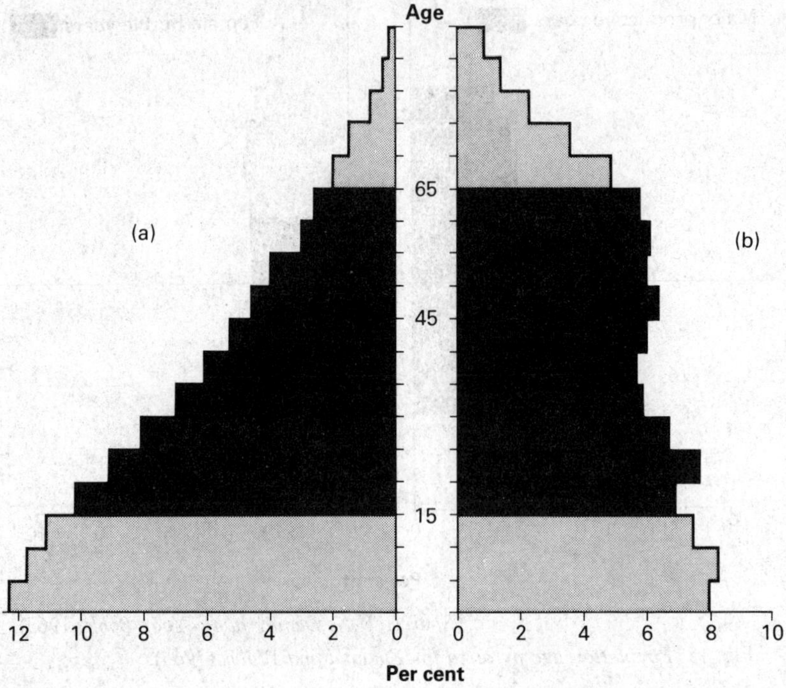

(*Source:* Census, England and Wales. 1891 and 1971)

Fig. 17. *Population pyramid for England and Wales (1891/1971).* (a) 1891 (both sexes); (b) 1971 (both sexes).

fallen (26 per cent aged 0–14) but the bulk of the population is now in child-bearing ages, resulting in the upward pressure on fertility noted above and a clear potential for an eventual ageing population.

In Fig. 15 (England and Wales, 1965) the effect of low birth and death rates over a longer period of time is apparent. The pyramid has taken on the shape of a New York skyscraper or a beehive, with similar numbers of people in all age-groups up to sixty. The widening base reflects the post-Second World War upturn in fertility which has subsequently been reversed. Where such an increase continues over a longer period, the pyramid can develop into a bell-shape as in Fig. 16 (Canada, 1965) where thirty years of rising fertility (aided by immigration) have led to a broad base, which indicates a high proportion of young people (34 per cent against 24 per cent for England and Wales) and relatively few old people.

An alternative presentation to the pyramid is useful where we wish to contrast countries or to show change over periods of time. In Fig. 17 the left-hand side of the pyramid represents the population of England and Wales in 1891, and the right-hand side the population in 1971. Sex distribution is ignored.

Common sense suggests that the ageing population represented in Fig. 15 must be the result of increased longevity, but in fact it is a declining fertility which most influences the move from a simple pyramid (Figs. 11 and 12) to the "beehive" or "artillery" shell of Fig. 15, via the narrow-based pyramids of Figs. 13 and 14 in which we see the "bulge" moving up the age-structure. Figure 16 likewise reminds us of the potential effect of a reverse in fertility decline.

It becomes clear, therefore, that the age-structure is very dependent on trends in fertility. As Ansley Coale has written, "whether a national population is young or old is mainly determined by the number of children women bear. When women bear many children, the population is young, when they bear few, the population is old." Coale has demonstrated this point by showing that if Sweden had followed its historical pattern of fertility decline over the past 100 years, but mortality had remained at 1860 levels, its age distribution in 1950 would have differed very little from that resulting from the falling mortality actually experienced. This is because a fall in mortality affects many age-groups, while changes in fertility affect only those entering at the bottom of the pyramid.

The "bars" in a population pyramid can also be thought of as representing survivors from the birth cohorts of the previous 100 years. Thus the 0–4 age-group represents survivors from the live-born children in the five years prior to the date on which the age pyramid is based, expressed as a proportion of the total population. Five years hence the survivors from this group will be represented by the 5–9 bar, and so on. On reaching the age-group 15–19, the surviving female members of the original cohort will begin to contribute towards the births which will form the base of the pyramid, creating a new cohort which will follow the same process.

Of course, age distribution can also be represented numerically. This is usually done by reference to the proportion of young and old (conventionally taken as 0–14 and 65 plus) as we have done above in discussing the pyramids. A useful single measure related to this is the burden of dependency in which the total population in these two groups is expressed as a ratio of the remainder of the population (aged 15–64) who are seen as representing the potentially economically active. Table 5 shows the age distribution and "dependency ratio" for selected countries in the 1970s.

TABLE 5: AGE-STRUCTURE AND DEPENDENCY RATIO IN SELECTED COUNTRIES

Age-group	*Morocco*	*Bangladesh*	*Cuba*	*New Zealand*	*U.K.*	*Japan*
	%	%	%	%	%	%
(A) 0–15	46	46	38	30	24	24
(B) 15–64	49	51	56	61	62	68
(C) 65+	5	3	6	9	14	8
Dependency ratio $\left(\frac{A+C}{B}\right)$	104	96	79	64	60	48

(*Source: Population and Family Planning Programs: A Factbook*. Population Council, New York 1976)

COHORT ANALYSIS OF FERTILITY

The measures of fertility considered so far are "period" rates, which summarise the fertility experience of women of various ages and at different stages of their reproductive career. However, the actual experience of child-bearing in an individual woman can cover a period of many years, so that demographers have been interested in evolving measures of fertility which take this into account. This approach is usually termed the "cohort" analysis of fertility, in which a group, or cohort, of women in the society are followed through their actual reproductive career. Cohorts are usually defined in terms of women born or married in the same year(s), with only legitimate births being considered in the latter case. There is, however, potential in the use of "parity" cohorts, e.g. women who have had a first birth by a specified date, for studying subsequent child-bearing in groups who have already started their child-bearing.

The value of this approach lies in its ability to isolate the actual fertility of women over their lifetime from the factor of the timing and spacing of pregnancies which can affect period rates. In this way interpretations of high and low fertility which are associated with short-term social and economic pressures, such as the post-war baby boom or the delayed child-bearing of the depression years can be avoided. This approach is able to describe not only the eventual completed family size of the women involved, but also the process by which this was attained, i.e. the timing and spacing of births, and the distribution of eventual family size, or the amount of child-bearing completed by a particular age or marriage duration. Such analysis is only feasible where the ages at which a woman bears her children are recorded, or by means of a special investigation, such as the classic cohort studies of Glass and Grebenik for the British Royal Commission on Population. With cohort measures it is possible to link variations in fertility for particular cohorts to a time series for economic and other social phenomena. Cohort analysis has proved of great value in explaining certain facets of the rising birth rate in developed countries after the Second World War, in terms of the postponement of births by older generations and earlier child-bearing by younger cohorts.

One limitation of cohort analysis is that a full picture of the cohort's fertility can only emerge when women have reached the end of their child-bearing, so that it can only fully describe past trends. However, measures of cumulative fertility after specified marriage durations can be used to explore more recent changes in the timing of births, and also to estimate eventual fertility of a marriage cohort where, as in Britain today, over 90 per cent of legitimate births occur within the first ten years of marriage.

Cohort and period measures are often alternative presentations of the same data. When we compute a "period" total fertility rate, we sum the fertility rates in a particular year for the women in each age-group, whereas the "cohort" total fertility rate for the women born in 1920 would include the fertility rates of 16-year-olds in 1936, 17-year-olds in 1937 and so on up to and including 49-year-olds in 1969. Table 6 sets out age-specific fertility rates for cohorts of British women who started their child-bearing between 1946 and 1970. The bold figures represent the period age-specific fertility rates for the years 1946–50 and 1961–5, which include segments of the fertility experience of several different cohorts. The total period fertility rate for 1961–5 is 2.85, higher than that achieved by any of the cohorts, reflecting the coincidence of early high fertility in the 1956–65 cohorts and the delayed child-bearing of earlier cohorts.

Summary measures of cohort and period fertility can be related to each other by plotting the generation (cohort) total fertility rates against the period T.F.R., which coincides with the mean age of child-bearing for the cohort. If this is done, it is possible to show that period rates fluctuate over periods of time much more than cohort rates do, reflecting the influence of timing and spacing of births on the former. Where successive cohorts are having their children at progressively earlier ages, as in the post-war cohorts in Table 6, this leads to period rates being artificially high, because the earlier child-bearing of the later (younger) cohorts coincides with the higher fertility at older ages of the earlier cohorts. The opposite phenomenon occurs when successive cohorts have children at progressively later ages. Consequently large movements upwards or

TABLE 6: AGE-SPECIFIC FERTILITY RATES FOR GIVEN COHORTS OF WOMEN

(*Births per year per 1,000 women*) (*Great Britain*)

Age segment of life in years of age	*Period when cohort started child-bearing* 1926–30	1931–35	1936–40	1941–45	1946–50	1951–55	1956–60	1961–65	1966–70
15–19	(16)	(16)	(16)	16	**20***	22	31	**41†**	49
20–24	(93)	(93)	102	**132***	133	158	**178†**	161	(154)
25–29	(115)	122	**151***	139	162	**182†**	162	(152)	
30–34	92	**107***	89	96	**105†**	89	(79)		
35–39	**58***	46	47	**50†**	41	(34)			
40–44	13	13	**13†**	10	(8)				
Total generation fertility rate (average number of live births per woman)	1.94	1.98	2.09	2.22	2.35	2.44	(2.40)		
Gross reproduction rate of cohort	0.94	0.96	1.01	1.08	1.14	1.18	(1.17)		

(*Source: Report of the Population Panel*. H.M.S.O., London 1973)

NOTE: Figures in bold type: * indicates the post-war baby boom, 1946–50 and ‡ indicates the post-war peak period for births, 1961–5 (T.F.R. = 2.85).

downwards in births from period to period may be consistent with a relatively constant level of cohort total fertility. For this reason, we cannot yet be certain to what extent recent declines in period fertility in the West represent a move towards a very small completed family size rather than a temporary postponement of child-bearing during years of perceived economic hardship.

Cohort fertility can be measured as the mean completed family size for women who have passed the age of child-bearing, or as the average number of live births by a certain age or marriage duration. It can also be presented in tabular form, showing the distribution of live-born children for different cohorts. Table 7 presents an excellent summary of the transition from high to low fertility for British women marrying between 1860 and 1960. There is a continual decline in the number of women having five or more live births, and a gradual emergence of two children as the modal family size. A feature of local interest is the comparison of the range of family size in the 1920–4 and 1955–9 marriage cohorts. The increase in fertility in the post-war cohort, from the 1935–9 level, can be seen as primarily due to the reduced proportion of childless and one-child families, rather than to any return to families of five or more.

TABLE 7: DISTRIBUTION OF FAMILY SIZE IN GREAT BRITAIN (BIRTHS OCCURRING TO FIRST MARRIAGES)

Number of children live-born in marriage	*Women married in period*				
	c. 1860	*1900–9*	*1920–4*	*1935–9*	*1955–9**
0	9	10	16	15	9
1	5	14	24	26	18
2	6	18	24	29	34
3	8	16	14	15	20
4	9	12	8	7	(11)
5+	63	30	14	8	(8)
	100	100	100	100	100
Average number of children	6.16	3.53	2.38	2.07	2.38

(*Source: Royal Commission on Population, Report* H.M.S.O., London 1949; *Report of the Population Panel.* H.M.S.O., London 1973)

NOTE: partly estimated figures.

CONCLUSION

In understanding the relationship between society and fertility, it is essential to consider fertility as a process and not as a static set of data. No single measure tells the full story of population change. Period measures, such as the crude birth rate, can identify short-term trends in fertility but often give a misleading picture of the achieved fertility of a particular cohort of women over a generation. Cohort analysis is particularly relevant to such questions as the total number of children born, the timing and spacing of births and age of marriage. It encourages exploration of such factors as the use of birth-control and family size preferences.

The changes which have taken place in successive cohorts of women as fertility declines in a population are an intrinsic part of the social and economic development of a twentieth century industrialised nation. It is the same series of changes that developing nations are attempting to achieve.

We have laboured the comparison between period and cohort rates, because the public in general and political leaders in particular tend to overreact to changes in the crude birth rate, while not understanding cohort changes. Thus there is a flurry of interest in the low period rates of contemporary industrialised nations but a possible waning of interest in the population problems of developing nations, now that their crude birth rates are eventually beginning to fall. Unfortunately, such an interpretation is the reverse of the real priority.

SELECTED REFERENCES AND BIBLIOGRAPHY

Barclay, G. *Techniques of Population Analysis*. Wiley, New York 1958

Benjamin, B. *Demographic Analysis*. George Allen & Unwin, London 1968

Bogue, D. J. *Principles of Demography*. Wiley, New York 1969

Cox, P. R. *Demography*. Cambridge University Press, Cambridge 1970

Frejka, T. *The Future of Population Growth*. Wiley, New York 1973

Hawthorn, G. *The Sociology of Fertility*. Collier-MacMillan, London 1970

Pressat, R. *Demographic Analysis*. Edward Arnold, London 1972

Ryder, N. B. "The Measurement of Fertility Patterns" in Sheps, M. and Ridley, J. (eds) *Public Health and Population Change*. University of Pittsburgh Press, Pittsburgh 1965

Chapter 4

Sociological Factors

Having considered the biological limits to human reproduction, we can now turn to the social factors restricting a woman's exposure to sexual intercourse during her child-bearing years; factors which help to keep achieved fertility below its biological potential. These factors consist of the proportion of women in their reproductive years who enter sexual unions, the age at which they do so, and any subsequent intervals of sexual inactivity arising from the dissolution of such unions (or from separation and abstinence within continuing unions). We will be concerned therefore with the age and extent of marriage and other sexual unions, the frequency of divorce, widowhood and subsequent remarriage, and the existence of periods of prescribed abstention from sexual intercourse. We will also consider the social factors affecting the frequency of coitus when intercourse is permitted.

RITUALS OF ADOLESCENCE

To signify entry into adulthood, many societies mark the biological transition occurring at puberty with social rituals. In traditional societies, the social division often coincides with the biological potential to become a parent. In industrialised nations legal majority, the right to vote and other symbols of adulthood are usually postponed for some years after the adolescent is biologically capable of becoming a parent.

For many girls, especially in the developing world, the first menstruation is a frightening event which they have not been warned about. "I thought I had a serious disease, I dare not tell my father and I stood up for the rest of the day," remarked one Filipino Muslim girl. In richer families, where children have separate sleeping rooms from their parents, they may be kept in considerable ignorance concerning sexual behaviour. It is not uncommon for the marriage night to be described as "rape".

The social rites of puberty in traditional societies vary from a happy festival to ferocious sexual mutilation. In Bali, Indonesia, the girl before menstruation wears her hair hanging down her back, but after the menarche she keeps her hair in a bun. In parts of South India menstruation is celebrated as a time of joy and a girl is given presents of jewellery and begins to wear a sari like an adult woman.

In other areas of India, which are more conservative, a girl's first period is a more frightening episode. She is separated, without explanation, and kept from other adults, except for married women among her close relations, who alone are permitted to feed and wash her. At the end of four or five days she is given a ritual bath. Her body is submitted to a painful scrubbing and covered in saffron. Subsequently, she is treated as a woman eligible for marriage, kept from her previous playmates and confined to the house. Ultimately, she will be married to a partner of her parents' choice, commonly to her mother's brother. When the marriage does take place, the newlyweds are locked in a small room with only a ventilation grill and the girl may still not know what is expected of her. Many women do not even have the vocabulary to describe any piece of anatomy between the navel and the knees.

A conversation took place between two upper class Indian girls, the daughters of a medical practitioner, some months after the second one followed her elder sister into marriage. The younger one said "Why didn't you tell me about *it*?" To which her elder sister replied "Because you didn't ask me about *it*!" In Mexico, the daughter of a wealthy family was convinced she had lost her virginity when, as a fourteen-year-old, she was kissed on her forehead by a boy.

Words often acquire an almost magical property because they give power over the things they describe. The gap between a modern couple who sit up in bed reading *Forum* and the Indian woman who cannot describe, anticipate or, least of all, discuss the closest of human relationships is very great. Just as religion is partly the establishment of a language to describe forces that are not fully understood, so the availability of words and concepts to handle sexual facts and emotions removes fear and myth from human sexual experience.

Sometimes the inability to handle adolescent sexuality and transmit useful information between the generations provokes acts of horrifying emotional and physical pain. In certain areas, mutilation of the genitals remains an all too common practice. Male circumcision is universal in some ethnic and religious groups such as the Jews. Fortunately it is a relatively simple operation, although somewhat uncomfortable if delayed until puberty. In the Philippines circumcision is almost universal amongst Catholics as well as Muslims. Commonly, the boy seeks circumcision of his own volition, as he feels that the operation is a symbol of manhood: it is done by a traditional practitioner, without an anaesthetic, but with tolerable skill.

Female circumcision is a different and more formidable undertaking. It can vary from removal of the clitoris to a horrendous attack on the female, removing both the *labia majora* and *minora*—that is, all the tissue around the entrance to the vagina. In much of sub-Sahara Africa, minor forms of female circumcision are practised, but in the Sudan the so-called "Pharonic" circumcision is still widespread. This involves the removal of the entire external genitalia. The operation is performed at or around puberty. Although the government of the Sudan has made it illegal for many years, even the daughters of higher social class and professional families are likely to disappear to the villages for this extremely painful, dangerous and highly mutilating procedure. The girls are aware of some of the aspects of the horror that faces them. Subsequent to the operation, the woman is very unlikely to have any degree of sexual satisfaction or pleasure whatsoever. The rationale from the male side seems to be twofold: the operation is supposed to reduce the likelihood of wifely infidelity (a hypothesis which may well be true) and to increase the husband's physical satisfaction (a hypothesis which is highly unlikely to be true). From the gynaecological and obstetrical point of view, the operation has a number of consequences. It can be associated with serious haemorrhage, retention of urine, or infection at the time of the procedure, and with subsequent difficulty during labour. The toughened scar tissue of the original wounds is likely to tear during delivery. In a country where most births are not attended by a trained person this can leave long-term wounds. Sometimes birth is protracted when the vagina fails to transmit the baby's head, and in such cases fistuli or holes may develop in the bladder or rectum, as a result of the prolonged pressure of the baby's head on the soft tissues involved.

However, some degree of hesitancy in the flow of information at adolescence between parents and children, and the significance of peer groups in modifying and transmitting sexual information, are both such common factors in human societies that it is necessary to pose the question as to whether these trends could also have a positive effect on behaviour. Perhaps human sexuality benefits from some degree of secrecy and is made more exciting if there is an element of the unknown.

MARRIAGE AND SOCIETY

In all known societies a special relationship is recognised between a man and one or more women—or, more rarely, between a group of men and one woman—whereby the offspring of such unions are deemed legitimate. This "marriage" relationship is rooted in the idea of the family and is intimately associated with the pattern of family and kinship of the society.

Marriage is a reproductive union and in most societies reproduction is normatively restricted to married couples. It is expected, or regarded as desirable, not only that those who want children will marry, but also that those who marry will want and have children. As a corollary of this, it is also usually expected that those who do not marry will neither want nor have children. Hence the dual tendency to stigmatise illegitimacy and, at the same time, to tolerate pre-nuptually conceived legitimate births.

Marriage is thus seen as essential for the bearing and rearing of children in a manner acceptable to society. Child-bearing is regarded as an essential part of marriage, so that a wife's failure to bear children may be seen as a reason for the dissolution of a marriage, and the presence of children as a reason not to accept such a dissolution. Voluntary infertility is still not widely accepted socially, despite recent attempts in developed countries to assert the concept of the "childfree" as opposed to the "childless" couple. Adoption, which is discussed in more detail in Chapter 9, aids the norm by providing a means whereby the childless married couple may obtain children and the illegitimate child may be integrated into a "normal" family.

The age at marriage and proportion of women marrying are fundamental determinants of fertility. The mean age at marriage in a society may vary from puberty to the late twenties, but there is usually both a legally prescribed minimum age for marriage, and a socially acceptable range of ages (which may vary from group to group with society). Each society also develops its own set of rules as to who may marry and whether more than one partner is permitted at one time (polygamy) or in succession (the serial monogamy found in countries with high divorce and remarriage rates).

Marriage may normatively precede reproduction, with extra-marital conception virtually unknown (as in Pakistan or Iran) or may be associated with a high degree of extra-marital intercourse and pregnancy. This may lead to marriage (as in pre-industrial Britain) or to illegitimate births, which in turn may occur to a greater or lesser degree within recognised consensual unions, or be accepted as a normal precursor to marriage.

Marriage is also associated with a wide variety of family forms and structures. Norms about age and extent of marriage, or the permissibility of divorce and remarriage will vary according to whether there is a pattern of patrilineal (through the father, as in Europe) or matrilineal (through the mother, as in parts of Sumatra) descent, and whether residence is patrilocal (with the husband's family), matrilocal (with the wife's family) or neolocal (where the couple form a new residential group).

The main aim of the rest of this chapter is to look at patterns of marriage and other sexual unions as they influence a woman's exposure to sexual intercourse. The actual relationship of such patterns to fertility within society will vary according to the degree of deliberate control over child-bearing within marriage. Where there is little control, age at marriage may be a key determinant of fertility; but where contraception or abortion is widely practised, age at marriage will be less directly associated with achieved family size.

AGE AND EXTENT OF MARRIAGE

Age at marriage and the proportion of the female population ever marrying are important factors in determining the potential level of marital fertility in a society. The actual potential for child-bearing is affected by the extent of pre-marital and extra-marital intercourse; so from the viewpoint of reproduction the age when sexual activity commences and the proportion of women who remain permanently celibate, are the real variables. However, in most societies reproduction is closely linked to marriage; data on marriage, unlike that on pre-marital intercourse, is relatively reliable and easy to assemble (*see* Fig. 18).

In Asian countries, such as India, Pakistan and Nepal, or African countries, such as Niger, Mozambique and Algeria, the majority of women are married by the age of twenty. In contrast, such early marriage is very much the exception in other countries such as Ireland and Japan; while in Caribbean societies a large number of women never enter legal marriages.

In India, the majority of women marry before the age of twenty; many of these marriages take place before the wife has reached puberty, although sexual relations are deferred until after first menstruation. In 1961 the mean age at marriage was 15.8, but the age of effective marriage (the time of the nuptial rites marking the consummation of the union)—according to data from the National Sample Survey of 1959/60—was 16.41 for rural women and 17.42 for urban brides. The fertility of girls marrying at, or near to, puberty is limited in the early years of marriage by adolescent subfecundity. However, the social pressures to become pregnant are great, which means that child-bearing under the age of 20 is common, and the motivation to avoid pregnancy is slight. A recent computer simulation indicated that an increase in mean age at marriage

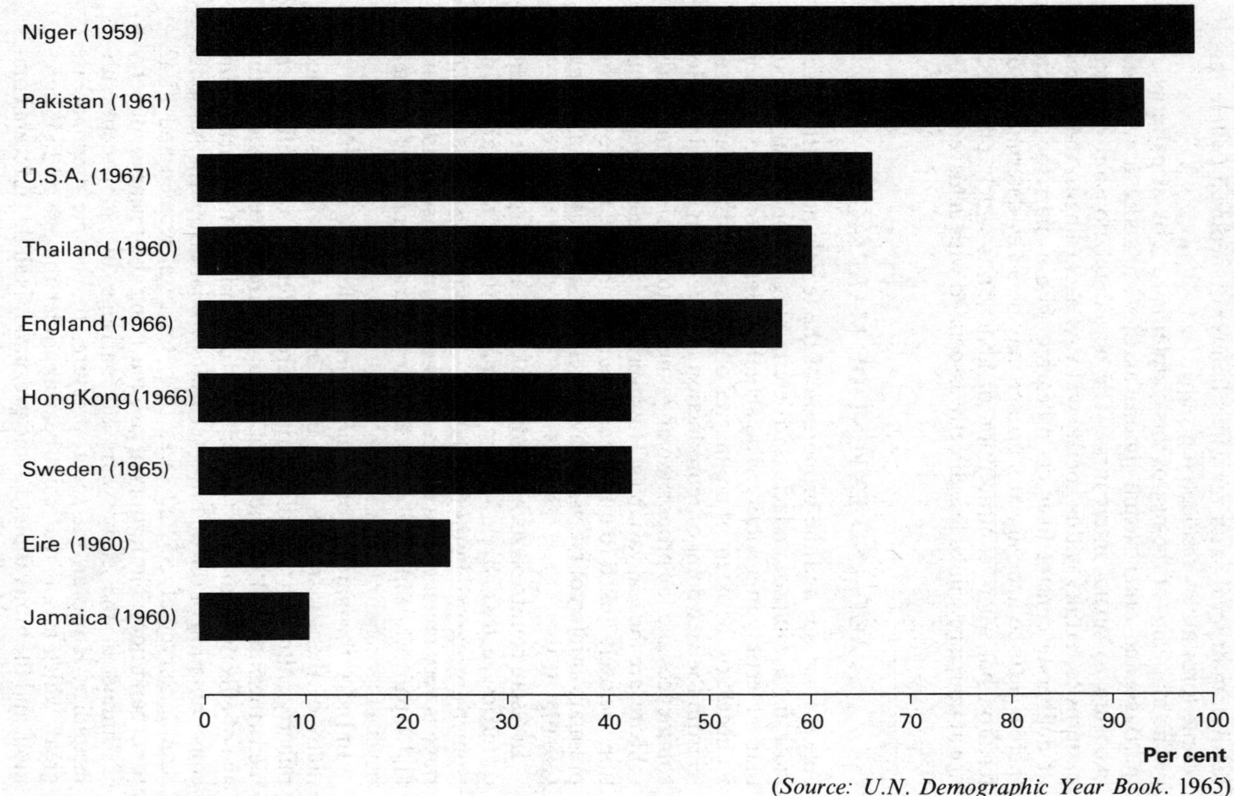

(Source: U.N. Demographic Year Book. 1965)

Fig. 18. *Proportion of women ever married at ages 20–24.*

to 20.5 could result in a 23 per cent reduction in the Indian birth rate, but such a delay in marriage would only be effective in reducing (as opposed to postponing) fertility if accompanied by a change in other sociocultural factors that support high fertility.

In tropical Africa most women marry before 20, although marriage is usually delayed until after puberty. There is, however, a wide variation in mean age at marriage—from 16 in Ghana to 19 in Mozambique, 20 in Nigeria and 22 in Burundi—although, interestingly, there is no simple correlation with the generally high levels of fertility.

In contrast to such patterns of early marriage, we find other societies where marriage is typically late. In Eire, the mean age of brides in 1969 was 25.3 and this itself was substantially lower than in previous decades. However, late marriage was still associated with high levels of marital fertility, so that the birth rate is above average compared to other countries in Europe.

In Caribbean countries such as Jamaica age at marriage and extent of marriage is a poor guide to the pattern of exposure to sexual intercourse, although it does explain the low level of marital fertility. Such countries have a low rate of legal marriage and late age at marriage, but sexual relationships begin when women are young. Child-bearing is common and acceptable (though classified as illegitimate) in other types of socially-recognised unions. Non-marital unions can be divided into two types: visiting unions, in which the woman is visited regularly at her own or her parents' home, with no shared household; and "common law" unions in which there is a common household, often within the wife's parental home, but no legal marriage. Visiting unions are particularly unstable and a woman may go through several in a lifetime. They may lead to a common-law union, which in turn may lead to legal marriage, but such a smooth transition seems rare. Reasons given for the persistence of common-law unions include the inability of the man to save sufficient money for proper marriage celebrations or the purchase of a house. Legal marriage is seen as the ideal, but the poor in Jamaica, Barbados and the other Caribbean islands "stretch" their value system to accept the reality of non-marital unions and widespread illegitimacy.

In general, the lower the mean age of marriage the greater the percentage of women who ever marry. Early entrance into marriage in Asian countries or in North and sub-Sahara Africa is associated with nearly universal marriage. Birth rates are typically high in such regions. This is due not only to the high potential exposure to conception during the years of maximum fertility, but also to the implication which early marriage has for a woman's role in society and in addition the common association of poor education for women in such a situation.

In contrast, late age at marriage may be associated with universal marriage, as in Japan, or with a significant proportion of women never marrying, as in Ireland and Jamaica. In the latter case, there may or may not be substantial exposure to non-marital intercourse, and late age at marriage does not in itself ensure low fertility. Likewise, countries such as Hungary and Belgium achieve low fertility despite a majority of women marrying before their mid-twenties.

From an evolutionary standpoint, early marriage and sexual partnership can be seen as necessary to the survival of the species whenever infant mortality is high. Not only do human beings reproduce slowly in comparison with most other animals, but their offspring need prolonged care. However, the main supports for early marriage are cultural, so that the pattern tends to survive, even when adult and infant mortality falls. Early marriage is especially common in societies with a joint household or clan organisation. Here marriage does not involve splitting an extended family and financial independence is not a prerequisite of marriage. Marriages tend to be arranged by the elders, often before a girl reaches puberty. A daughter is most in demand as a prospective bride when she is young, because she is more attractive sexually, has greater potential fertility and fits into a subordinate role in her husband's parental home, where there is a system of patrilocal residence.

In societies based on a nuclear family organisation, especially if this is linked to neolocal residence, the pressure is towards later marriage, as in Ireland, where marriages had to be postponed until land was obtainable for the couple. This resulted in an average at marriage as high as 29 for women in 1926. Early marriage is also less attractive to individuals when it competes with opportunities for education and female work-force participation, although this factor may be modified by access to contraception and the consequent possibility of delaying child-bearing after marriage.

In most contemporary developed countries, the majority of women marry in their late teens and early twenties. This results in a relatively low proportion of teenagers being married, but over half the women aged 20–24 having entered wedlock. Today, there are few countries where less than a third of the female population of this age remain single, whereas this was the common experience of most Western European countries at the turn of the century, as seen in Table 8 which is based on Hajnal's classic work on European marriage patterns. Late marriage in nineteenth century Europe ensured that birth rates there, prior to the decline in fertility in the West, were at a much lower level than is common in developing countries today. Or to put it the other way, as a result of a low age of marriage, developing countries are going to demand even more contraception, abortion and sterilisation than the Western world has done.

In Western Europe the age of marriage has fluctuated, being very high before the Industrial Revolution, then coming down as former agricultural workers migrated to the expanding nineteenth century cities, rising in the late nineteenth and early twentieth century, and falling after the Second World War. Today, the age of marriage in the West is rising again. In Ireland, before the potato famine of the 1840s, marriage was early; today Ireland displays the pattern of late marriage, but moderate to high achieved fertility, which was formerly found all over Western Europe.

TABLE 8: PROPORTION OF FEMALE POPULATION EVER MARRIED AT SELECTED AGES, EUROPE C. 1900

Country	*Age-group*		
	20–24	*25–29*	*45–49*
Hungary	74	85	96
Italy	40	70	89
Great Britain	27	58	85
Sweden	20	48	81
Ireland	14	41	83

(*Source:* Hajnal, J. "European Marriage Patterns in Perspective." Glass, D. and Eversley, D.E.C. *Population in History*. Edward Arnold, London 1965)

In Ireland an additional factor is the high incidence of celibacy associated with those men and women who enter religious orders. The move to earlier marriage affected most of Western Europe and was a major factor in the upturn of fertility after the Second World War. It is also important to note that the new pattern of earlier marriage was not reversed when birth rates began to fall in the early 1960s. From the mid-1970s, the mean age of marriage in Britain and the U.S.A. has risen marginally, but it is too early to say if this makes a new trend or is merely random variation. What does need to be emphasised is that Western marriage patterns are variations on a theme and that there has always been, and remains, a big gap in fertility (and in social terms) between adolescent marriage at puberty and marriage in the upper teens and twenties.

However, just as European countries have moved towards an earlier age at marriage, so many developing countries have moved towards later marriage. The proportion of married teenagers in Hong Kong and South Korea is now similar to that found in Sweden. Such rises in age at marriage have been important factors in the falling fertility in these countries, and in others such as Taiwan and Singapore. Table 9 shows the decline in the proportion of married women in younger age-groups in Taiwan between 1961 and 1972. In South Korea a rising age of marriage (itself partly an accidental side-effect of the two-year national service which is compulsory for all men) accounts for approximately one-third of the recent fertility decline in that country.

The only developing country to make a consistent public effort to alter the age of marriage has been China, where people are encouraged to delay marrying until 24 for women and 26 for men.

TABLE 9: PROPORTION OF WOMEN CURRENTLY MARRIED, SELECTED AGE-GROUPS, TAIWAN, 1961–72

	Percentage of Women by Age-group		
Year	*15–19*	*20–24*	*25–29*
1961	12.5	60.9	89.3
1965	9.2	58.3	88.8
1972	6.6	46.4	86.4
Per cent change 1961–1972	−47.2	−23.8	−3.2

(*Source: 1972 Taiwan Demographic Fact Book*. Taipei 1973)

Continuing early marriage remains an obstacle to fertility decline in many other Asian countries. Among the factors that will be difficult to overcome are the lack of alternative work roles for young girls, as in India, and the cultural obsession with virginity, as in Pakistan or the Lebanon. The latter is a controlling factor in the behaviour of many parents towards the upbringing of their daughters, and in decisions about marriage.

Just as late age at marriage exerts a downward pressure on marital fertility, so early marriage limits the potential for illegitimate childbearing. In most countries where marriage is early and universal, illegitimate fertility rates are low. The visitor from the Middle East who raises her eyebrows at Western problems of pre-marital pregnancy all too easily forgets that in her country most girls are married by the time they reach the age at which Western women are having illegitimate babies or pre-marital abortions. However, some of the lowest illegitimacy rates are also found in countries such as Ireland and Japan, where the proportion of unmarried women at risk of pregnancy is high. Only in the Caribbean community discussed previously are high levels of illegitimacy clearly associated with a low incidence of legal marriage. In many developed countries rising illegitimacy has been associated with a falling age at marriage, whereas in developing countries such as India the problem is emerging as marriage age rises.

There is no totally satisfactory social counterpart to the biological processes of puberty. Early marriage is associated with high fertility inappropriate to modern conditions and pre-empts a number of educational, work and emotional options which young women in particular may expect increasingly to enjoy. Late marriage is often associated with relatively high pre-marital conception rates, which are often perceived to be in conflict with society's desire to formalise sexual relationships within a marriage partnership. The conflict is exacerbated by the biological trend to earlier sexual maturity, which has occurred at the very time when an extension of educational processes is advantageous. In an increasingly sophisticated and technical world, the duration of education is now carried well into the child-bearing years. In addition, in an affluent society with long expectation of life and small family size, the reassortment of sexual partners is becoming almost as common as the maintenance of a lifelong marital partnership. There is a strong correlation between early marriage and the increased probability of divorce at a later date. This relationship reflects more than just a higher number of years in which marital breakdown is possible; the emotional expectations (and those concerning life-style) of people in the later teens and early twenties are still changing rapidly and it is not surprising that marriages made at this stage are less stable than those contracted in the middle and later twenties.

POLYGAMY

A polygamous society is one in which polygamy (whether polyandry, one woman with several husbands, or polygyny, one man with several wives) is socially permitted, not one in which it is the statistical norm. Polygamous marriages are usually in a minority, although they may involve up to half the married female population.

Polyandry is rare and there is no clear evidence on which to assess its effect on fertility. More attention has been paid to polygynous societies. Some studies, such as Nag's cross-cultural analysis, found no evidence for differential fertility between polygamous and monogamous marriages, while others, such as Dorjahn, claim that polygamy reduces fertility in African societies at least.

Various reasons are cited for the possible lower fertility of polygynous marriages:

(*a*) there is a lower frequency of coitus per wife and postpartum taboos on intercourse are more readily upheld;

(*b*) in most polygynous societies only older men can afford to take more than one wife and they may be less active sexually;

(*c*) polygynous marriages include a higher proportion of sterile women whose husbands have taken additional wives for this reason.

Polygamy is likely to afford the individual husband a greater number of offspring and this is one of its main functions; this, however, is achievable even if each wife has fewer children than the average woman in a monogamous union—and for every man with several wives there are likely to be, by simple logic, several men without wives. The possible depressing effect on total birth rates of polygynous unions therefore has to be set against the effect of the institution in encouraging earlier marriage and easier remarriage of widowed and divorced women.

High rates of polygyny are found in tropical Africa; in some areas up to 50 per cent of married women are involved. Even in the non-agricultural urban setting of Lagos in Nigeria a recent survey found that 31 per cent of wives were in polygynous unions. There was, however, evidence of a decline in the institution, with polygyny relatively rare in the more highly educated groups, and significantly less common amongst younger wives. Although polygyny was most common in Nigerian Muslims, about one-fifth of the Christian women were also in such unions.

DISSOLUTION OF SEXUAL UNIONS

The age of entry into a sexual union is one crucial determinant of a woman's potential exposure to conception over her reproductive years, but the actual exposure may be curtailed for a number of reasons. The woman herself may die before the end of her child-bearing period, or the union may end prematurely as a result of the death or departure of her partner. The actual impact of the dissolution of a union in any of these ways will depend on a number of factors:

(*a*) the frequency of widowhood or marriage breakdown;

(*b*) the age of the wife when this occurs;

(*c*) the incidence of subsequent remarriage or cohabitation;

(*d*) the length of interval before the formation of any new union.

WIDOWHOOD

In developing countries, where mortality is high, a substantial number of women die during their reproductive years, often as a result of child-bearing itself. Similarly, many women lose their husbands while still capable of having more children (*see* Fig. 19). The effect on fertility of such a relatively high probability of widowhood will depend largely on the institutional position of the widow as it affects her changes of remarriage. Social customs in relation to widowhood vary widely, from absolute prohibition on remarriage, and even immolation of widows (as in suttee in India), to compulsory remarriage (as in the Hebrew tradition of levirate, which obliged a man "to raise seed in his brother's widow"). Most societies fall between these extremes, but all will develop beliefs about the appropriateness of remarriage (influenced by the age of the woman, whether she has children, etc.) and the timing of such events. Even where remarriage is common among young widows, a period of three or four years may elapse between the death of the husband and the start of the new marriage, resulting in a significant loss of potential child-bearing.

Universal remarriage, associated with levirate, is most common in primitive societies characterised by strong clan or lineage organisation, where the widow is viewed mainly in terms of her potential production of children. Marriage to a kinsman ensures that if children are born they belong to the clan. In Africa, the death of the husband often does not sever ties between the two kinship groups involved and the inheritance of a widow by the kin of a deceased man is standard practice in many tribes.

In contrast, in stable agrarian societies, characterised by a joint household organisation, remarriage to a first degree relative may be forbidden as a threat to the importance of the father–son (as opposed to sibling) relationship and because it complicates any future possible dissolution of the family. At the same time, marriage outside the family may also be discouraged, as it would separate any subsequent children from the family. No-one is clearly responsible for the arrangement of such unions and when the widow is an older woman with several children she is seen as a less attractive marriage prospect, so that marriage at a suitable level would prove difficult anyway. Where remarriage is forbidden or rare, the widow is very dependent on her family for support and this reinforces the belief of many women in the need for sons to support them, not just in old age, but in the event of their husbands dying.

India is often cited as an example of a country where a ban on the remarriage of widows has significantly lowered fertility levels. Kingsley Davis estimated that in the period 1901–41 it curtailed the

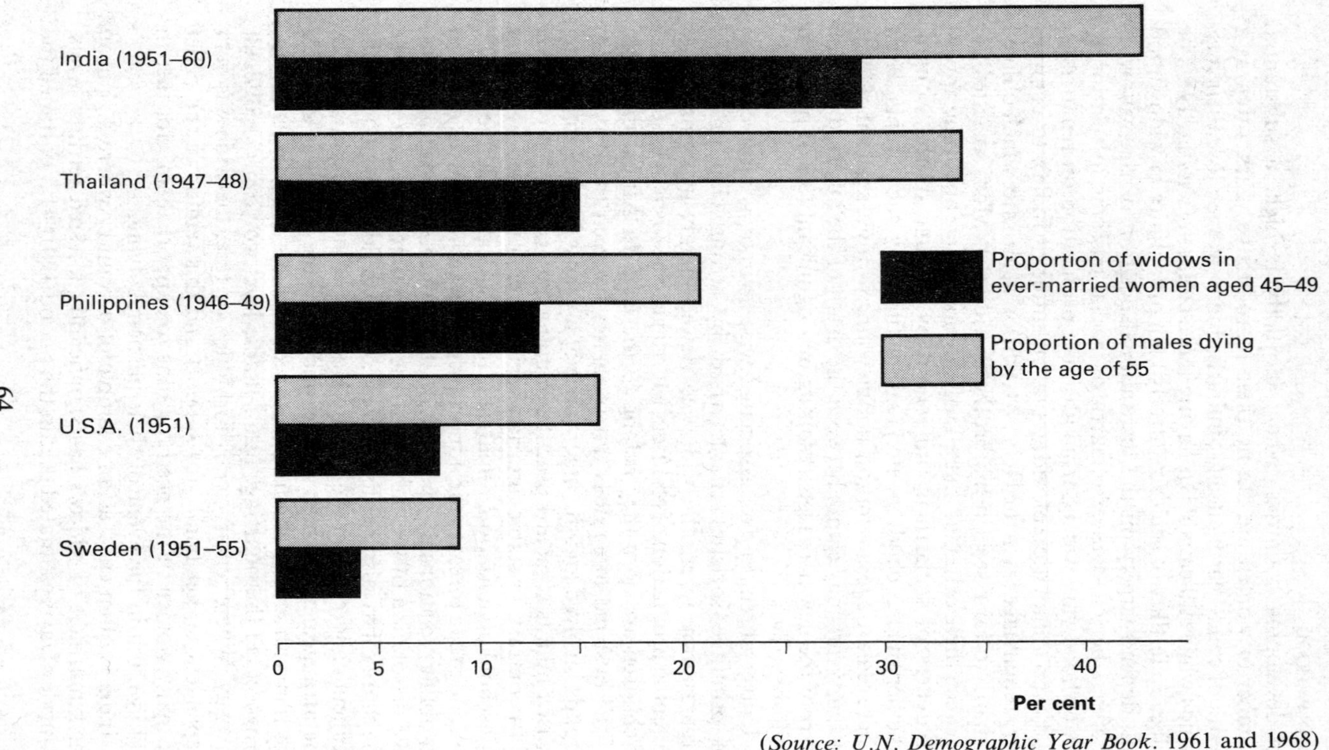

(*Source: U.N. Demographic Year Book*. 1961 and 1968)

Fig. 19. *Adult mortality and proportion of widows.*

Hindu birth rate by an average of 16.4 per cent. However, such a ban is totally effective only in certain high caste groups such as Brahmins. In other castes the chances of remarriage are good, especially if the widow is young and has only one or two children. In the Khanna area, which has been studied in particular social detail, it was found that the opposite custom, levirate, was common and that 60 per cent of those widowed before the age of thirty-five remarried. With the incidence of widowhood decreasing, as adult mortality declines, restrictions on widow remarriage are now probably of very little demographic significance.

In developed countries, the over-all impact of widowhood on fertility has been very slight during this century. Most women who lose their husbands during their reproductive period have probably completed their intended child-bearing. Younger women, who might have wanted more children by their husbands, are particularly likely to remarry and in some cases this can lead to them having more children than would have otherwise have been the case.

The exception to such a generalisation is in cases where there is exceptional mortality affecting younger husbands and unmarried males. A classic example is that of the Soviet Union in the years from 1916 onwards, when war, famine, and "collectivisation" decimated the adult male population, resulting not only in increased widowhood, with limited opportunity for remarriage, but also an adverse sex ratio which restricted the number of first marriages. In 1959 only 55 per cent of the female population aged 45–49 were married, in contrast with 96 per cent of the male population of similar age. The First World War had a similar, although less dramatic, effect in Western Europe.

DIVORCE AND SEPARATION

The impact of marital breakdown on fertility is more difficult to assess, as the occurrence and timing of such events is not accurately recorded. Most societies make some provision for divorce or separation, but records of these relate only to "legal" breakdown. The relevance of instability in non-marital unions, even those with some degree of social recognition, can be explored only through direct study of samples of such unions.

The effect of divorce is easiest to document, as it is a "legal" event, recorded with varying degrees of accuracy in many countries; nevertheless there can be difficulties of definition affecting compatibility, for example, in Egypt divorce figures include "revocable" divorces amongst Muslims, which are the equivalent of a "legal separation" in other societies.

The frequency of divorce varies considerably across societies and within societies over periods of time. Such variations often reflect differences in access to legal dissolution and, therefore, do not necessarily portray the true picture of marital breakdown and disruption of sexual activity. In some countries such as Ireland, Malta, the Philippines and several South American countries, there is no legal divorce, although re-allotment of partners occurs with particular frequency in Catholic developing countries such as Mexico and the Philippines. In other countries, there is provision, but divorces are rare due to legal barriers, cost or social disapproval. In a further number of countries, divorce is easy and common, with as many as one in three marriages ending in divorce, as in the contemporary U.S.A. One commonly used indicator is the number of divorces per 1,000 married couples a year. Such a "divorce rate" varies from nil in Ireland and less than one in Thailand and Portugal, to 9.4 for the U.S.A., 12.9 for the United Arab Republic and 15.1 for Puerto Rico in the years 1959–61. In England and Wales the rate, well below one before the Second World War, has risen from 2.1 in 1961 to just over 10 in 1976.

The legal dissolution of a marriage often takes place some years after the actual breakdown of the union, but even so a majority of women involved are still in their reproductive years. In the U.S.A. approximately half of all divorces involve women under the age of 30, whereas in the United Arab Republic in 1966, 49 per cent of women divorced were under 24. The potential impact of divorce on fertility is limited by the frequency of remarriage, especially by those in the younger age-groups. It has been estimated that in America well over 90 per cent of those divorced between the ages of 20 to 25 remarry, and recent increases in divorce in England and Wales are paralleled by a rise in remarriages involving divorced persons.

In the United Arab Republic in 1966, 16 per cent of all women marrying had been divorced; this proportion rose to 38 per cent for those marrying at ages 25–29 and to over 50 per cent in later marriages. The 50,000 divorces to women under 35 are matched by 40,000 remarriages involving divorcees. The over-all result in this Muslim country is that only 2 per cent of the population at ages 43–49 is divorced at any one time compared to 5 per cent in Sweden and 7 per cent in the U.S.A. Most divorces involve women without children, so that the main impact on fertility is through a postponement of child-bearing (*see* Table 10).

Even with extensive remarriage, some time will elapse between the two unions, although the interruption of sexual activity may be limited—a change of sexual partners often preceding or indeed precipitating a change of marital partners. Illegitimacy at later ages in developed societies often involves divorced and separated women.

There may also be a desire to have children by the new spouse, in women already having one or two children by their first marriage. But, over all, the loss of exposure to marital fertility after or between unions broken by divorce, does exert a downward pressure on fertility and data from the 1961 British Census showed that women in second marriages had slightly lower fertility than once-married wives, after standardisation for age and marriage duration (from date of first marriage).

A more important effect on fertility has been attributed to the instability of non-marital sexual unions in Caribbean countries, where a majority of children are born out of wedlock. Judith Blake has

TABLE 10: FAMILY SIZE OF DIVORCED WOMEN, EGYPT 1946

Number of children	*Percentage of divorced women*
none	77.8
one	15.0
two	4.2
three or four	2.8
five +	0.2

(*Source:* Hamed Ammar. *Growing up in an Egyptian Village: Silwa, province of Aswam* Octagon Books, New York 1966)

estimated that the fertility of women living in such unions in Jamaica was only two-thirds of what they would have achieved if they had been in unbroken marriages, the reduction being primarily due to conceptions averted during periods of celibacy between and after such unions. In a study of 124 Barbadian women, Nag found that the time spent between and after various types of union amounted to 20 per cent of the time spent within unions amongst women with several unions. He argues, however, that by reducing the extent of permanent celibacy which would otherwise have resulted from the high male emigration from Barbados (and the consequently unfavourable sex ratio), the existing conjugal patterns have advantages which offset the negative impact on total fertility of the reduced exposure to intercourse among women experiencing several unions.

EXPOSURE TO SEXUAL INTERCOURSE

Even when marriage occurs at an early age and continues uninterrupted throughout a woman's child-bearing years, there can be considerable variation in the amount of exposure to intercourse, related to periods of total abstention from sexual activity and the frequency of coitus at other times.

There is a general assumption that marriage will involve participation in sexual intercourse and failure to consummate a union may be seen as grounds for dissolution. It is assumed that those who are married should engage in regular intercourse and—to varying degrees—that those who are not married should not. At the same time, in most societies there are also beliefs about certain intervals during marriage when intercourse should be avoided, intervals which may be associated with the birth of a child, the age of the parents, religious ceremonies and other factors. Abstention from intercourse may also be forced on couples by the temporary absence or illness of a partner, or deliberately sought as a means of fertility control. Periodic abstinence (the rhythm method) as a contraceptive measure will be discussed in Chapter 6. Often the desire to avoid pregnancy will serve to reinforce adherence to societal taboos on sexual activity.

We shall start by looking at societally-prescribed periods of abstinence within marriage and then proceed to a consideration of the level of sexual activity during periods when sexual intercourse is permitted or possible.

ABSTINENCE

Some patterns of sexual abstinence are not associated with deliberate intentions to avoid conception, although these may still influence fertility and indeed affect society's need to limit population growth or affect the timing and spacing of births.

Post partum: the most important period of abstention from sexual activity is that following the birth of a live child. Some period of post partum abstinence is practised in nearly all societies, although in some poor societies and exceptional cases intercourse has occurred within hours of delivery. Typically, post partum abstinence is for a matter of weeks only and probably has very little impact on the reproductive potential of the woman, which is reduced (or non-existent if she is breast feeding). In other societies, however, the period may be extended for months or years, either in the form of an arbitrary time limit, or related to some developmental stage in the previous child, e.g. when he cuts his first tooth. In many cases, it is associated with the period of lactation (as in parts of Java) which may last two or three years. In this way, breast feeding is transformed from a moderate break in fertility to an absolute barrier. In such cases the practice is of profound importance in spacing live births and can restrict the potential fertility of a woman to an average of five or six deliveries in a lifetime. As such abstinence is practised only in the case of surviving children, any reduction in infant mortality may have the effect of reducing fertility, by increasing the number of women who avoid intercourse for significant periods after a birth. Such a pattern has been suggested as an explanation of recent fertility declines in Bangladesh. Conversely, such proscriptions can be perceived as an incentive to bottle-feed, as is occurring in the emerging middle classes in New Guinea. It is interesting to speculate whether a contraceptive method, such as a condom, might not be promoted as a more rational, modern alternative to such traditional proscriptions.

Numerous examples of post partum abstinence can be cited from the study of primitive societies. In the Mbuti pygmies the husband is prohibited from intercourse from the moment of birth until the child is weaned, a period typically extending to three years, so that most married women produce children only once every four years and few families are found with more than five or six living children. Many primitive societies show a great concern about motherhood and lactation and believe that intercourse during the weaning period is detrimental to the child's health. Amongst the Arapesh, Margaret Mead has described a taboo on intercourse lasting until the child takes its first steps and is felt to be able to cope with contact with parental sexuality. The effect on reproduction is recognised and welcomed. The practice seems particularly common in hunting and gathering societies where a woman must transport a child until it can walk well enough to keep up with the group. Such societies may also practice infanticide as a further means of spacing children. Such behaviour has been compared to that of other higher primates, such as the gorilla, which maintain a static population despite freedom from predators and who also have a need for the mother to be free to transport her offspring until they are able to travel independently.

In India a post partum taboo is observed in almost all groups, although the stipulated length varies considerably from just a few months to two years or more. Where there are longer periods of abstention, these are often reinforced by social pressures to avoid closely spaced births – a woman who has become pregnant too soon may become the object of village jokes. In Tamil a special term "savali" is used to refer to a child whose sibling is born soon after. A study in Bombay found that many women continued to avoid intercourse beyond the proscribed period, in order to avoid early pregnancy, and up to a third abstained from sex for over a year.

The practice may also be reinforced by a custom of husband and wife living apart for a year or more after a birth. A woman usually goes to her parental home for her first birth and remains there for many months, during which she will have no sexual contact with her husband, although the husband may be permitted access to another wife or to a concubine.

During pregnancy: clearly, abstinence during pregnancy cannot reduce a woman's chances of conception. Indeed, it may rather slightly increase that of other women, by encouraging her husband to seek sexual gratification elsewhere. Intercourse is often proscribed in later pregnancy, but seldom throughout—unless there is an individual decision related to medical advice, which in the West is as often ritualistic as based on scientific evidence. Increasingly, however, medical texts advocate a continuation of intercourse as essential to good marital relationships and often suggest the most appropriate positions for coitus. Among the extremes of cultural patterning is a general taboo on intercourse from the time a pregnancy is recognised, as in the case of some Indian communities, where the taboo against intercourse runs from the time a woman becomes pregnant until the child is at least two; on the other hand the Mbuti pygmies consider intercourse late in pregnancy to be beneficial in that it is thought to accelerate the onset of labour.

During menstruation: the widespread prohibition on coitus during menstruation can likewise have little negative effect on fertility and may be seen as having a positive effect on fertility, by concentrating intercourse on days when conception is most likely. A study of Mysore villages in India found that two-thirds of the women reported abstaining from intercourse for at least eight days after the onset of menstruation, and in some cases abstinence extended up to fifteen days, resulting in a resumption of intercourse at the time of maximum chance of conception. Sometimes intercourse is avoided until the woman has taken a bath that marks the end of menstruation, as in many Muslim societies.

Until the turn of this century students of Western medicine believed that ovulation occurred at menstruation, partly by analogue with the bitch, where vaginal bleeding accompanies ovulation. It is a strange fact of history that the theological legality of the rhythm method was argued on the basis of a physiological theory that made the middle of the cycle the "safe" period. Mbuti pygmies, like nineteenth century physiologists and theologians, also believe conception occurs at menstruation and those having intercourse at this time claim it is more pleasurable.

Occasional and ceremonial abstinence: in many non-industrial societies, restrictions on sexual intercourse are found relating to special ceremonies and holidays, tabooed days of the week or certain communal tasks associated with war and work. Often these apply only to single days and so may have the effect of concentrating sexual activity on other days rather than lowering the over-all level. However, field studies have shown the average number of tabooed days to be as high as twenty-five or more in a year. Such restrictions were common in medieval Europe when Fridays, Sundays and Wednesdays along with a large number of saints' days and the whole of Lent were proscribed days for intercourse.

More important are periods of prolonged abstention, especially where these are reinforced by physical separation of husband and wife. Amongst the Yap fishermen such restrictions last for six to eight weeks of the fishing season. The natives of the Mortlock islands proscribe any sexual intercourse in times of war on penalty of death, and amongst the Chaga of North East Tanzania, abstention from intercourse is traditionally imposed during certain ritual periods—when preparing for a sacrifice, before a hunt or expedition, and during initiation.

Abstinence associated with personal circumstances: certain other patterns of conventional abstinence affect expected patterns of sexual activity for people in special categories. The illness of one of the marital partners may result in enforced abstention, but in some societies there is a more general assumption that in such a case intercourse will not take place even if it is physically possible. This is related to beliefs that sexual activity causes debilitation, or that it increases the risk of the disease spreading. Such a belief has been noted in many Indian villages; therefore the relatively high incidence of intercurrent disease in such places may lead to a significant loss of exposure to pregnancy. In developed countries, the medical opinion concerning sexual activity amongst sufferers from heart disease is divided, and may well reflect a partial ritualisation of taboos about sex.

In many Asian communities, couples abstain from intercourse in the later years of marriage, even though the wife is still capable of producing children. This has been seen as a major factor in the falling-off in fertility at later ages in India, Pakistan and Bangladesh. On one level, this may simply represent the end point of reduced frequency of coitus, due to a decline in sexual energy and interest. Alternatively, it may be due to a conscious desire to limit family size, but seems also to be related to questions of role definition, as in cases where a woman is expected to cease bearing children when her daughter-in-law joins the household or when the couple become grandparents.

Many villagers in India believe that a woman whose children are old enough to become parents themselves is demeaned if she becomes pregnant again, especially if a daughter-in-law is present in the home. She is, therefore, expected to abandon sexual relations—or at least reduce their frequency—as the need for procreation is no longer present. The avoidance of late child-bearing by such abstinence seems to be motivated as much by feelings of shame as by any desire simply not to have another child.

In some Chinese communities, the supposed debilitative aspects of sex encourage the practice of *coitus reservatus* among older men, as it is the loss of semen which is assumed to sap a man's energy. But as with many sexual beliefs, other societies hold a contrary pattern of beliefs. In the Philippines the rejuvenating effect on an older man of sex with a young girl is summed up in the saying "the old buffalo eats the youngest and greenest grass!"

In most developed countries, late child-bearing is now rare, so that a woman in her forties faced with an unwanted pregnancy may well experience a similar sense of shame, especially if her children have reached or are approaching adulthood. The availability of alternative means of avoiding pregnancy and the high value placed on continuing sexual activity, means that abstinence is not widespread, but its incidence may well be underrated. A British study by Ann Cartwright in 1968 showed that 6 per cent of mothers with seven or more children were abstaining from intercourse in order to avoid further pregnancy—a figure that should be viewed in the light of the fact that over a third of such mothers had been sterilised. A later study by the same author found that more than one in five of mothers aged thirty-five and over had not experienced intercourse in the previous week. The role of abstinence in the history of Western fertility decline has probably been underestimated. It seems likely that many Victorian women limited their family size by deliberately abstaining from intercourse, especially in their later years. This pattern received cultural validation through the belief that women could not enjoy sex, and through the availability of other sexual outlets for middle class husbands thus deprived of their conjugal rights.

Moreover, we should not ignore the possible importance of alternative forms of sexual congress, such as anal intercourse or *coitus inter femora*. These alternatives may help to throw light on those primitive groups in which pre-marital heterosexual relations seem common, but pregnancy rare. Amongst the Luo of East Africa, young men practise *chode*, in which they place their legs outside the girl's almost closed limbs and achieve stimulation by means of a slight and partial insertion of the penis, without breaking the hymen. This allows adolescents of both sexes the opportunity for sexual experimentation with minimal pregnancy risks. Shorter describes practices which served a similar function in North America and Scandinavia in the eighteenth century, where "bundling" or "night-courting" brought young couples together in close intimacy, without actual intercourse taking place. A boy might spend the night with a girl, either sleeping on top of her bed—with the girl inside—or in bed with her, but with shorts and pants still worn. Studies of contemporary university students in several western nations have noted the widespread practice of mutual masturbation, especially prior to the advent of the Pill. A recent text on birth-control by David Delvin stresses the advantages of love-play, including oral sex, as a useful substitute for intercourse in the absence of effective contraception.

Enforced Separation: finally, there are examples of enforced abstinence arising from social necessities that separate husband and wife. The husband's absence due to business, war, the search for employment or the demands of his occupation will necessitate periods of abstinence from intercourse. In developed countries with low fertility, this may effect primarily the timing of pregnancy rather than the level of fertility. Indeed, groups such as deep-sea fishermen have been found to have above average fertility. This suggests that the pattern of separation may be associated either with a preference for a large family—either the wife's need for company or the husband's wish to ensure the wife's chastity—or with less effective contraception, which is perhaps linked to the segregated role relationships likely to develop in such groups.

In developing countries, such patterns may be more important in reducing fertility. It is common for rural men to migrate to the cities to find work, or even out of the country, as in the case of Indian house-servants and drivers in Singapore who may only return to their wives every three to five years. Sometimes migration takes place from one rural area to another, e.g. when highland Peruvians migrate to the coast for the sugar-cane harvest, or across borders, e.g. when Mexican labourers take seasonal agricultural jobs in the U.S.A.

Involuntary abstinence may also occur due to illness or impotence in one partner, or preferences for homosexual relationships. That impotence can be a factor in individual cases of infertility is certain, but there is no evidence for any significant impact at societal levels.

SOCIAL FACTORS INFLUENCING THE FREQUENCY OF INTERCOURSE

The biological relationship between coital frequency and the chances of conception have been reviewed (*see* Table 1). Are there cultural differences in the frequency of intercourse which alter achieved fertility?

There is a widespread belief that high rates of coitus are an important factor in the high fertility of many non-industrial societies, but the effect may be more in the culture of the observer than in the traditional society. It is a Western viewpoint to emphasise "primitive sexuality", to comment about sex as a "national sport" and to speculate on the "contraceptive effects" of introducing electricity. A book by Robbins entitled *Too Many Asians* includes the following passage:

> There are too many Asians for their own good. They have been breeding trouble for themselves and for the world as a whole.... When the sun goes down on an Indian village, the people are left to darkness. They have no books, no movies, no television. There is only one thing to do—go to bed. There they find their sole source of recreation and amusement, their brief escape from the hours of hard work of the day. At the roots of Asia's problem of population is copulation.

Such a view appeals to many Western observers who think of India only as the land of the Kama Sutra. But anyone who knows the villages or shanty-towns of the developing world might be rather inclined to guess that coitus would be less frequent there than in Western society. Children often sleep with their parents in overcrowded conditions, where the privacy most adults desire for sexual activity is hard to obtain. In addition, life in the paddy-fields is often extremely strenuous, particularly at certain seasons: "After a day planting rice you could explode a bomb beside me and I wouldn't wake up," commented one woman from a traditional village. In the Philippines one of the now disappearing courtship rituals at the *barrio* level was for the man to woo the girl while planting rice. Possibly the physical exhaustion at the end of the day also encouraged chastity between courting couples. The existence of tabooed days discussed in the previous section exerts a further downward pressure on coital rates. The myth of the sexually hyperactive peasant, like the cultural myth of the noble savage, is probably not something to be taken seriously.

Adequate objective evidence on variations in rates of intercourse between cultures is lacking. Ford and Beach, in their classic work on sexual behaviour, argue that in non-industrial societies adults normally engage in intercourse once daily in periods when coitus is permitted, but cite examples of much higher rates: "For Chagga men it is reported that intercourse ten times a night is not unusual."

Evidence for such levels is very slim and most data relate to hearsay or beliefs, rather than documented practice. They can also be matched by other accounts of apparently very low levels of intercourse. Likewise, beliefs vary from stress on the need for regular and frequent intercourse to an insistence that excessive coitus is harmful.

Turnbull's study of the Ik, the mountain people, presents a rare picture of a people whose level of sexual activity appears to be very low due to a lack of energy. Intercourse is not highly valued and

TABLE 11: MEAN COITAL FREQUENCY PER WEEK OF MARRIED WOMEN IN THE U.S.A. AND THREE RURAL BENGALI GROUPS IN INDIA

Age-Group	*American Whites*	*Hindu*	*Sheikh Muslim*	*Non-Sheikh Muslim*
15–19	3.7	1.5	1.7	2.3
20–24	3.0	1.9	2.4	2.6
25–29	2.6	1.8	2.4	2.7
30–34	2.3	1.1	1.8	2.1
35–39	2.0	0.7	1.4	1.5
40–44	1.7	0.2	1.0	0.8
Over 44	1.3	0.3	0.4	0.4

(*Source:* Nag, M. "Sex, Culture and Human Fertility: India and the United States." *Current Anthropology*. 13, 231 1972)

is seen mainly as a natural release comparable to defecation. It is occasionally consciously sought by young girls as a means of procuring food, by selling themselves to neighbouring hunters. Despite the fact that population growth amongst the Ik seems to be minimal, it is excessive for their environment, in the mountains of Northern Uganda.

The anthropologist Moni Nag, has compared data on coital frequency in Muslim and Hindu groups from three West Bengal villages with the findings of Kinsey for white married women in the U.S.A. Rates of intercourse are lower in the Indian sample at all ages (*see* Table 11), especially in the Hindu group. Nag offers several possible explanations, some of which we have already discussed:

(*a*) anxiety amongst men about loss of strength through loss of semen;

(*b*) traditional values about moderation, especially amongst Hindus;

(*c*) lack of privacy;

(*d*) abstinence on ritual occasions;

(*e*) beliefs that children should not be too closely spaced and that a wife should not become pregnant after her children marry;

(*f*) female inhibitions about sexuality.

In developed societies contraceptive practice has much more influence on fertility than coital rates, yet at times we seem to have a deep-rooted desire to believe that this is not so. Consequently we find stories about the American town where the high birth rate was supposed to arise from the disturbance of local sleep patterns by shunting trains. A classic illustration of this is the supposed effect of the great electricity blackout of 1965 on births in New York City.

...ut, which lasted ten hours from 5.27 p.m. on 9th ...o 4.00 a.m. on the 10th, led to a headline in the *New* ... on 10th August 1966 to the effect that a sharp increase ...ad been noted nine months later; one hospital reported ...nt births instead of the normal eleven, and others reported ...matic increases. A sociologist was quoted as saying, "The lights went out and the people were left to interact with one another instead." More cautious interpreters saw the explanation in terms of an interruption of contraceptive usage rather than increased sexual activity.

The story was widely believed and accepted, but later a detailed study of births occurring in New York City in the six-week period during which 10th November conceptions would have been most likely to reach term showed that the proportion of total births in the year occurring in this period was the same as for the previous four years, and that the number of births on the 267th day was not exceptionally high. Nevertheless such beliefs persist and in 1968 Chicago hospitals are said to have prepared for a baby boom following the great snows of 1967; similar myths arose over the strikes by miners and power workers in Britain in recent years. The wish to see such events as encouraging a return to copulation is clearly far from dead!

The timing of the fertilising intercourse in relation to ovulation may be a factor in determining the sex of the child. The data is difficult to gather and still disputed, but studies on natural intercourse, as recorded in the case of women taking their body temperature (which rises immediately after ovulation in response to the release of the hormone progesterone) suggest that more boys are conceived early in the cycle and more girls if intercourse and ovulation coincide (*see* Fig. 29). One explanation in biological terms might be that the male (XY) sperm survive longer in the female tract than the female (XX) sperm. In social terms, it is observed that after wars the sex ratio changes in favour of boys and a plausible explanation of this fact is that as soldiers are reunited with their wives there is likely to be a high frequency of intercourse for some months, increasing the possibility of coitus early in the cycle and a resulting male conception.

DESIRE TO CONFORM

No one knows the origin of female circumcision in the Sudan but logically there must have been a stage in history when, for the first time, parents subjected their daughters to what was always known to be an agonisingly painful and dangerous procedure. Presumably, they thought it was in the interest of their child to suffer the operation. And, even today, loving and reasonable parents continue to inflict this horror on their offspring, because they think that this is more preferable than for their daughter to join the minority of girls who have not had the operation. The pressure to conform in sexual behaviour with the rest of society is exceptionally strong. Perhaps it is even more demanding than the other pressures for social conformity which characterise the human species.

At a less dramatic level, coitus is usually an act limited to two partners, whose direct experience concerning other people (particularly of their own sex) in the same situation is often non-existent and commonly not transmitted verbally within their group. It is, in a way, a lonely human function. So we all seek reassurance that we are doing the same as relatives, friends and neighbours. If every one is circumcised, we wish to be circumcised. If most people believe coitus should only take place in a certain position we are embarrassed and reluctant to do it any other way ourselves. If everyone around you has six children you may want to conform by having six children; if everyone has two, you will feel guilty if you have three.

"Of course, in my mother's day people had big families," said a young medical graduate in Hungary.

"How many children did your mother have, then?"

"Three," replied the doctor with genuine emphasis.

The desire to conform in marriage and fertility may be particularly marked in siblings. Luker has observed that some of the women seeking abortions have sisters who have just had a baby, and (even when they knew a pregnancy could not be carried to term) they had yielded, consciously or unconsciously, to the desire to have a pregnancy themselves. The ideal age of marriage is another example of the desire to conform. A young Korean woman will cite the early or mid-twenties as a good age to get married, whereas a girl from Bangladesh would be astonished to think of delaying marriage for so long. The answer to the same question on the ideal age of marriage for a Western girl would change between 1950 and 1980.

In the contemporary Third World the desired family size is much larger than among industrialised nations (*see* Fig. 20), but the average number of children couples want is falling. In any village community there will be a small number of women who are desperate not to have any additional pregnancies and who will go through the pain and danger of criminal abortion to avoid them. There will also be a number of women, at least in the present generation, who are likely to go on having children at more or less the maximum reproductive rate that biology allows. Between these two extremes will

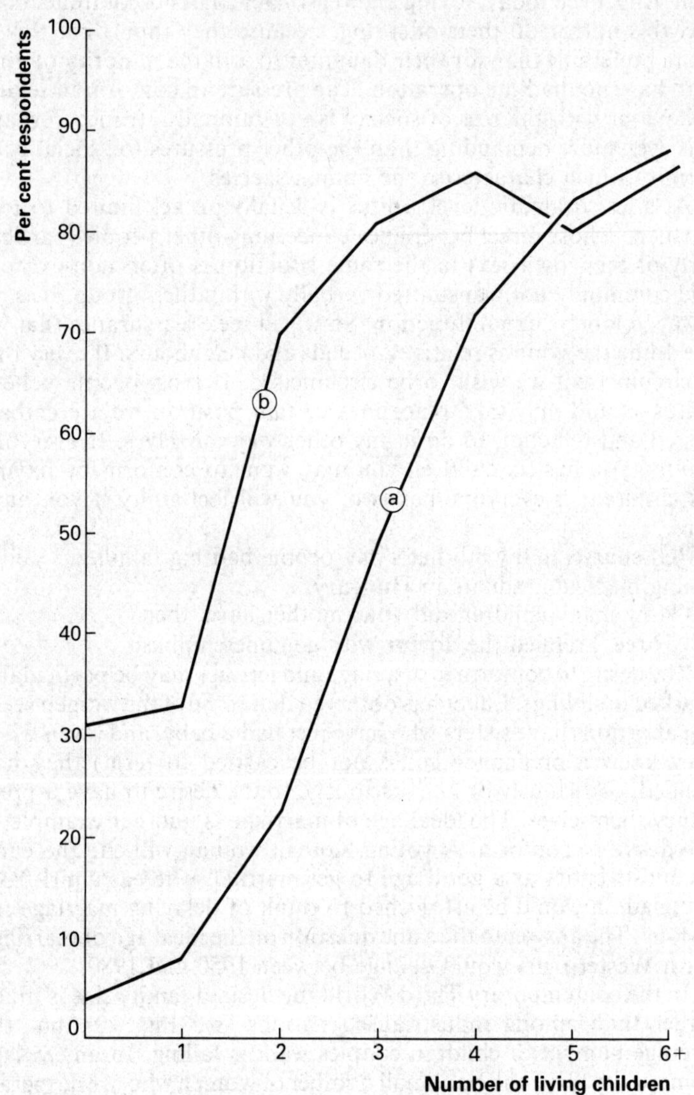

(*Source: Reports in Population/Family Planning*)

Fig. 20. *Couples wanting no more children*. (a) median of thirty-one surveys in the rural areas of sixteen developing countries (b) median of eight surveys in four developed countries.

be a large number of individuals whose achieved family size will be partly influenced by circumstances. Given access to abortion, sterilisation and the reversible methods of contraception, they are likely to attempt to conform to the minority in the village who will restrict their fertility whether the means are easily available or not. But if barriers are erected between those who might choose to use the services and the services themselves—barriers of distance, culture, economic cost—then the bulk of the people will probably conform to traditional patterns of high fertility within their communities.

As will be discussed later, there are examples of dramatic fertility declines within traditional societies in one to two decades, and there seems no reason why such changes should not take place throughout the developing world. All too often the recognition of sociological factors in patterns of sexual and fertility behaviour is used as a rationalisation for the failure of bad family planning programmes. In reality, it should be used as a tool in the provision of realistic and acceptable services, which can be and need to be created.

CONCLUSION

The preceeding review of the various factors which can influence the exposure of women to intercourse, and so to conception, indicates their considerable potential for reducing fertility levels. We have also seen that the variables have differing importance in different societies. In particular, potential fertility is higher in less developed countries due to early and universal marriage, reflecting a need to maintain high potential reproduction in the face of heavy and unpredictable mortality. After the formation of unions, such societies are more likely to have socially proscribed periods of abstinence, often for reasons not directly linked to any desire to restrict fertility, and in the case of post partum abstinence this can be of considerable demographic significance in extending the period between births. However, no society has achieved very low levels of fertility simply through the use of such restraints, although, given conditions of high mortality, modest rates of population growth may be attributable in certain circumstances to such controls over the spacing of children. In industrialised nations, delayed marriage has been an important factor in reducing fertility, but the achievement of replacement levels of reproduction has demanded extensive resort to other mechanisms, which reduce the chances of conception and birth in sexually active women. We must, therefore, now turn to look at ways in which the potential level of fertility associated with any particular pattern of exposure to intercourse can be further restricted. We will also consider the risk of pregnancy amongst sexually active females, the role of contraception and sterilisation in reducing this risk, and the part played by abortion in preventing the occurrence of births as a consequence. Before we can do this, however, we need to look at why couples in a society choose to restrict their child-bearing, starting with the question of what social pressures exist towards having children. This will be the aim of the next chapter which is concerned with motivation in human reproductive behaviour.

SELECTED REFERENCES AND BIBLIOGRAPHY

Arensberg, C. M. and Kimball, S. T. *Family and Community in Ireland*. Harvard University Press, Cambridge, Mass. 1948

Blake, J. *Family Structure in Jamaica: The Social Context of Reproduction*. Free Press, New York 1961

Brass, W. *et al*. *The Demography of Tropical Africa*. Princeton University Press, Princeton 1968

Cartwright, A. *Parents and Family Planning Services*. Routledge, London 1970

Davis, K. and Blake, J. "Social Structure and Fertility: An Analytical Framework." *Economic Development and Cultural Change*. 4, 211 1956

Delvin, D. *Carefree Love*. New English Library 1976

Dorjahn, V. "Fertility, Polygyny and their Interrelations in Temne Society." *American Anthropologist*. 60, 836 1958

Driver, E. D. *Differential Fertility in Central India*. Princeton University Press, Princeton 1963

Ford, C. S. *A Comparative Study of Human Reproduction*. Yale University Publications in Anthropology, no. 32 1955

Ford, C. S. and Beach, F. A. *Patterns of Sexual Behaviour*. Harper, New York 1951

Goody, J. *Production and Reproduction: A Comparative Study of the Domestic Domain*. Cambridge University Press, Cambridge 1976

Hajnal, J. "European Marriage Patterns in Perspective." in Glass, D. and Eversley, D. *Population in History*. Edward Arnold, London 1965

Hartley, S. F. *Illegitimacy*. University of California Press, Berkeley 1975

Hawthorn, G. *The Sociology of Fertility*. Collier-MacMillan, London 1970

Mead, M. *Sex and Temperament in Three Primitive Groups*. Routledge, London 1935

Molnos, A. *Cultural Source Materials for Population Planning in East Africa, vol. 3: Beliefs and Practices*. University of Nairobi, Nairobi 1973

Nag, M. *Factors Affecting Human Fertility in Non-industrial Societies: a Cross-cultural Study*. Yale University Publications in Anthropology, no. 66 New Haven, 1962

Nag, M. "The Influence of Conjugal Behaviour, Migration and Contraception on Natality in Barbados." Polgar, S. (ed) *Culture and Population*. Schenkman, Cambridge, Mass. 1971

Nag, M. "Sex, Culture and Human Fertility: India and the United States." *Current Anthropology*. 13, 231 1972

Robbins, J. *Too Many Asians*. Doubleday, New York 1959

Rodman, H. "The Lower Class Value Stretch." *Social Forces*. 42, 205 1963

Saucier, J. F. "Correlates of the Long Post Partum Taboo: A Cross-cultural Study." *Current Anthropology*. 13, 238 1972

Shorter, E. *The Making of the Modern Family*. Collins, London 1976

Turnbull, C. M. "Demography of Small-scale Societies." Harrison, G. and Boyce, A. (eds) *The Structure of Human Populations*. Clarendon Press, Oxford 1972

Turnbull, C. M. *The Mountain People*. Cape, London 1973

Udry, J. R. "The Effect of the Great Blackout, 1965, on Births in New York City." *Demography*. 7, 325 1970

Chapter 5

Motivation in Fertility Regulation

If we are to understand why the level of fertility varies from society to society—or why within a century the women of Britain, instead of having typically several live births, had only two or three—we need to turn from questions about what mechanisms (biological or social) keep birth rates high or low, to why people want children, how many they want and when they want them. In this chapter, therefore, we consider the social pressures affecting individual decision-making in human reproduction, as a prelude to a discussion in Chapter 6 of the options open for the voluntary control of family size.

It is now universally accepted that the decline in fertility in developed countries over the past hundred years or so has been the result of deliberate regulation of births, reflecting a desire amongst an increasing number of married couples for a relatively small number of children. In current debates about world population, it is often suggested that fertility levels in developing countries remain high because couples want many children. In this case, family planning programmes are doomed to failure because the best that they can do is to reduce the number of unwanted births, which would still leave fertility high enough to ensure rapid population growth. Many observers insist, therefore, that an adequate population policy must concentrate on changing motivation towards child-bearing as an essential prerequisite of family planning, while others argue that only social and economic development can bring about any substantial changes in fertility levels.

WHY HAVE CHILDREN?

In all societies, whether industrial or non-industrial, a large majority of women become mothers. Marriage is the common experience of women in all societies and parenthood is usually an essential aspect of marriage. Most married women engage in regular sexual intercourse and, in the absence of contraception, this nearly always leads to frequent pregnancy and child-bearing. Near universal parenthood remains the pattern even in societies where birth-control is widely practised, and where sex and reproduction are to a large extent separated. There is, therefore, an almost universal expectation that women will become mothers and that they will bear children within some sort of recognised sexual union. The questions we now seek to answer are: why this should be, how parents perceive such expectations and what factors influence their decision to have at least some children.

Adequate reproduction is essential to the survival of human societies, whatever their level of mortality. For much of his history, man has been engaged in a struggle to find enough food for his own survival and to ensure that some members of society live long enough to produce children to take over when they die. To achieve this in the face of high and fluctuating mortality, institutions were developed to ensure potential for adequate child-bearing and child nurture, even at times of exceptional mortality. There was, therefore, a universal pressure to see that women who survived to adulthood produced children. Such pressures continue today in societies where mortality is low and far fewer births are needed to ensure a balance with deaths.

In all human societies women are socialised from an early age into an expectation of marriage and parenthood, and in many instances entrance into marriage is arranged by the woman's family. Once married, the social pressures to become pregnant are great and it is parenthood, rather than marriage or physical maturity, that marks the final attainment of adult status in society. Evans-Pritchard describes marriage amongst the Nuer as involving four steps from betrothal, wedding and consummation ceremonies to the birth of the first child. In modern Western society, children are often described as "making a family". The married couple with children are seen as constituting a proper, natural and complete family and the childless couple is seen as excluded from the joys of family life.

Nearly all married couples share such attitudes (for a discussion of voluntary childlessness *see* Chapter 9), but most will also give more specific reasons for wanting to have children. Firstly, there is a clear sense of personal achievement in parenthood, both in having physically produced a child and in meeting creatively the challenge of rearing children. Having children involves a new range of experiences not available by any other means. Children are seen as a source of emotional satisfaction and of interest and variety in life. Youngsters provide fun and laughter in the home, and the birth of a new baby (even where the conception has been treated with many misgivings) provides a sense of occasion in which the mother is for once the centre of attention in the family. The particular satisfactions derived from having children will vary, but most parents will mention the pleasures of handling babies, the companionship they bring, the joy of watching them grow up and teaching them. For some mothers, children may provide the affection they find missing in their marriage, whereas for fathers they may offer one of the few relationships in which they feel free to express warmth and tenderness.

Most parents derive satisfaction from what they can do for their children. A child provides purpose in life, by being someone who needs attention and care, and in return gives unquestioning affection. Children offer to parents an opportunity to achieve vicariously what they missed in their own youth, so that doing things for a child can bring an immediate personal reward. For many mothers, being a "good parent" justifies existence and provides a socially approved role, whereas for the father, the need to work may be justified by the demands of the family, which in turn provides a haven from the strains of the outside world. Children thus provide a meaning for many every-day activities.

Children are also subject to parental expectations. Satisfactions derive not just from doing things for children, but from what the children themselves do—seen often as at least in part a result of what the parents have done. They bring status to the parents by their success in the wider community—"My son, the doctor"—and likewise can bring shame if they fail. They provide parents not only with someone to love, but with someone who will offer love in return. Hence the tensions when a child's search for independence is seen as ingratitude, or the tragedy of unrealistic expectations of what a very young child can offer; tensions which seem to lie behind many cases of child abuse.

Children may also be seen as a form of self-preservation, even as offering a kind of immortality. Here is someone, sharing with the parents certain physical and personality characteristics, who may be expected to outlive the parents and, in the mean time, provide memories of a youth that is past. When the parents die, they can live on through their children. On a more practical level, it is the child who continues the family line by inheriting the name, the property and the status of his parents, and this has traditionally been a major factor in childless couples (especially those with property) seeking an heir (*see* p. 253). Such a process is not without its tensions as it conflicts with the expectation that parents will seek to live on through their own flesh and blood, so that childless couples uncertain of their infecundity may choose to adopt a girl in the hope that they may yet give birth to a son. In many societies, however, adoption is only permitted once a wife has passed through her childbearing years.

The satisfactions derived from having children change as they grow older. They are most immediate when the children are young and always present and dependent, but it is usually anticipated that they will continue to offer pleasure after they have grown up and left home, not least through the provision of grandchildren. In many developing countries children are a very important, often the only, source of security to the parents in old age. Sons especially may be essential to survival, or at least the difference between poverty and well-being. In developed countries there is usually less expectation that children will be a source of major financial support in old age, as society builds up its own means of provision through social security systems, but it remains true that for a majority of old people children are a major source of comfort and care. Institutions for the aged are often filled largely by those who have no children, or whose children have gone away or failed to meet parental expectations.

More direct economic advantages of children, as a source of family income as they grow up, are now largely confined to developing countries, and especially to rural areas, where children can help on the land from an early age. In many such areas, the economic benefits of children are seen as outweighing the costs of rearing them, and economists have talked of children as "production goods" in many Third World countries. In industrial societies this is seldom true and the utilities derived from children are mainly non-economic, so that they seem rather to represent a form of "consumption" good. However, in practically all societies there is a real sense in which children are seen as "investments", ultimately repaying the efforts involved in bearing and rearing them. As such, they are subject to a parent's assessment of the cost in parental time and effort in producing and bringing up a family, so that decisions about having children may be constrained by perceptions of alternative and "better" investments of the mother's human capital.

HOW MANY CHILDREN?

The existence in most societies of strong pressures for a majority of women to become mothers does not mean that such pressures demand that women have as many children as possible. For most women the crucial question is not whether to have children, but how many to have and when to have them. It is to these issues that we must now turn.

The question of how many children people want is central to any understanding of fertility and the need for fertility regulation. If a woman is to have only two children over her lifetime, she will need to practise some form of fertility regulation for much of her life. If, on the other hand, she wants several children, and infant mortality is high so that many children die, the need for family planning may seem minimal.

In most societies today, human fertility falls well below its maximum potential, while still being high enough to produce rapid rates of population increase. The importance of considering family size norms is to help determine the extent to which existing levels of fertility reflect the needs and desires of adult members of a society. In other words, are birth rates high because fertility is restrained only by factors such as age at marriage and ritual abstinence, which may be unrelated to individual ideas of limiting family size? Are they high because couples accept many births, not knowing how to avoid them? Or does the high fertility of many developing countries result from societal values about having children which lead to a majority of parents choosing to have more children than would be necessary to replace the existing generation of parents?

Freedman has argued that human fertility, whether at a high or low level, is so important to the family and to society everywhere that its level is more or less controlled by cultural norms about family size, and related matters such as marriage, abortion and contraception. He argues that a majority of societies today have ideas about the right number of children to have. In the various social surveys on family size carried out since the end of the Second World War, most respondents have felt able to give answers to questions about their ideal family size, or whether they wanted more children. Freedman believes that where fertility is high, this is generally the result of norms supporting a high average family size. These norms can in turn be seen as arising from the need of society to adjust to high and variable mortality, and from the central importance of familial and kinship ties.

The typical experience of six or seven live births amongst women in developing countries reflects a desire for at least three or four children and the need to have more if such a number is to survive adulthood. To want three or four is compatible with having more, and if there is a need to have several children to ensure the desired family size, then motivation to use family planning will be weak. Even if mortality falls and fewer children die, it will take time before couples are confident enough that their children will survive.

But this does not explain why the desired number of children is still relatively large. Why do most women in Asia want at least three or four children and most African women as many as five or six? Freedman asserts that the family size norms will tend to correspond to a number which maximises the net utility to be derived from having children in any society; this in turn will depend on the economic structure and family organisation patterns in that society. Large numbers of children are desired if the values considered worthwhile are obtained through familial ties rather than social institutions; these numbers will tend to be highest where there is a corporate kinship system, involving a clan organisation, permeating all aspects of life. They will be moderately high where there is a joint family system, and lowest where there is a nuclear neolocal family unit, with fewer routine functions carried out within the family. It is argued that fertility decline can only be expected when there are fundamental changes in such institutions and in the economic value attached to children. In this case, family planning programmes alone can achieve little and certainly cannot bring the level of fertility down to that needed to halt population growth. To achieve this there is need to increase education and literacy and to change those institutions which reward the parents of relatively large families.

Acceptance of such views led to assumptions that family planning programmes could only succeed amongst those women who already had the children they needed, ignoring the other sources of motivation towards family planning which we shall discuss later in this chapter. It also led many to argue that such programmes would only have a limited impact in most developing countries, being able at most to eliminate excess and unwanted fertility; this would, however, still leave parents with at least three or four children, enough to ensure a continuing high population growth rate, especially where the age-structure exerted a further upward pressure.

Furthermore, some writers have asserted that any decline in fertility rates must rely on social and economic developments which will reduce the number of children wanted, arguing that this was the pattern in developed countries and that in such cases fertility will fall no matter what the structure of family planning provision is (*see* p. 218). This we shall discuss in more detail in a later chapter.

Others have argued that family planning programmes should be replaced by genuine "population control" policies, which would concentrate on countering ingrained desires to have large numbers of children. This would be done by educating people into wanting fewer children, by attempting to change institutions which support high fertility and by providing disincentives to having many children. One advocate of such an approach is Kingsley Davis, who, in a famous article entitled "Population Policy: Will Current Programs Succeed?", foresaw that family planning programmes, while of value in their own right, could not achieve population control. Davis argued that family planning as currently presented could not even be seen as a first step towards such control, but was rather an escape from the real issues involved. As such it became an obstacle to the development of population control, which required more attention to the underlying issue of "wanted" births and the social institutions that determined desired family size.

The weakness of such arguments is that they ignore the manifest achievements of family planning programmes in accelerating the rate of fertility decline when couples do not want more children—although in fairness it may be said that many supporters tend to overrate the extent to which such declines are the direct result of the programmes. They also neglect the possibility that widespread

TABLE 12: PROPORTION OF WOMEN WANTING NO MORE CHILDREN, BY NUMBER OF LIVING CHILDREN

		Number of Living Children			
Country	*Year*	*2*	*3*	*4*	*6+*
Hungary	1960	*85*	92	95	93
United States	1965	*72*	81	87	94
Hong Kong	1967	*68*	87	96	99
Argentina	1963	*52*	79	83	90
Thailand (rural)	1969–70	47	*65*	75	92
Philippines	1963	42	*56*	68	85
Taiwan	1970	30	*68*	84	97
South Korea	1968	24	*54*	74	94
Mexico City	1963	32	49	*65*	79
Indonesia	1968	30	42	*57*	66
Pakistan (Lahore)	1960	29	45	*66*	75
Tunisia	1964	26	44	*68*	92
W. Malaysia	1966–7	17	30	43	*55*
Upper Volta (rural)	1969	7	10	13	35
Kenya (rural)	1966–7	4	19	30	*60*

(*Source:* K.A.P. surveys quoted in *Population and Family Planning Programs: A Factbook*. Population Council, New York 1973)

NOTE: *See also* Fig. 20. **Numbers in italics indicate majority wanting no more.**

acceptance and use of family planning may lead in turn to changes in norms concerning family size, as couples begin to realise the possibility of limiting their fertility effectively. Finally they often make generalisations about high fertility norms in the Third World which are not borne out by the facts.

Replies to questions about desired or ideal family size are notoriously unreliable, but they do provide some idea about attitudes; some credence can be given to replies given by women with varying numbers of children about whether they want any more. Table 12 gives data on such questions from various countries, indicating the wide range of responses found. In developing countries, the stage at which a majority of women want no more children varies from two (for Hong Kong), three (for Taiwan, Philippines and Thailand), to six or more for many African countries. To say of the former countries that the women want large families is clearly misleading.

It can of course be argued that the meaningfulness of answers to questions about family size preferences is limited in countries where means of achieving small families are not easily available, and that in such cases we should rather be asking questions about who should have children, when child-bearing should commence and cease, and what intervals are desired between children. It is to these and other alternative motivations for the use of family planning that we turn later in the chapter.

All this does not deny the validity of Freedman's argument that there are strong social pressures towards having large families in many countries, and that these are rooted in the perceptions of women about their own role and their needs. This can best be illustrated by looking at the pressures towards a moderately large family in a country such as India, where the impact of a long-standing family planning programme remains limited.

FAMILY SIZE IN INDIA

We saw in Chapter 4 that marriage is universal in India and that the typical young girl in an Indian village is likely to find herself married in her mid-teens. Once married and past puberty, there will be strong expectations from her husband and his family, with whom she will probably be living, as well as from her own family, that she will become pregnant as soon as possible, and have more children after her first. With no alternative roles for her in the society, there is little chance of her thinking in terms of delaying such a pregnancy or limiting her family to a particular number, but a very real fear lest she prove barren. Prior to the birth of her first child, life in her mother-in-law's home may be little more than the misery of slavery. She is likely to be the first to get up and the last to go to bed and to be loaded with the hardest daily chores. Her status as a wife will largely depend on bearing and rearing healthy children and her success in doing so will be rewarded by the treatment she receives once she is pregnant. For many years her life in the village will centre round her children and her participation in social life will be dependent on her position as the mother of a growing family.

But there are other fundamental reasons for wanting children. The young wife will have seen the importance of children to the older women in the village; particularly for widows for whom sons are a major source of security as they grow old. She will also have seen that many children die and so realise that it is not easy to ensure that there is a son to care for her in later years. In many villages, a third or more of the children die before their first birthday. If a child she bears does die, it becomes important to become pregnant again soon; if only daughters are born, further pregnancies are needed to ensure that she has a maximum chance of getting a boy, thus simultaneously proving her worth and ensuring her own future. If asked how many children she wants, she may well reply "three or four", but this means that she wants to have at least two sons who grow to adulthood, and a daughter who will in time make a good marriage. To be certain of achieving this, she will need to bear many more. If all of these happen to live, she will count herself fortunate for the sons she has, even if the burden of raising many children is a great one.

For her husband, too, there are reasons to want many children. They, especially sons, will bring him full adult status and as they grow up will provide help for him, especially if he works on the land. Against such potential benefits the cost of rearing the children is seen as small. The economic advantages are well portrayed in Mamdani's *The Myth of Population Control*, in which he criticises the famous "Khanna" study of six Indian villages. Mamdani argues that the reluctance of many villagers to adopt modern methods of birth-control was due to their desire for many children. He cites the need for a farmer with little land to rely on family labour, with the hope that if he had more sons than were needed for this he might be able to spare one from the land to work away in the nearest town, and bring back money to purchase more land, or to provide opportunity for education for himself or others.

The work of Mamdani and others has led many critics of family planning programmes to attack these for their emphasis on pushing contraception or trying to change motivation by educating women in the realities of mortality decline when, in Mamdani's own words "they have large families because they want them and they want them because they need them". It has been argued that this is true throughout the Third World and that accordingly family planning programmes are not meeting the needs of women in such countries.

The data given in Table 12 shows that this is far from being true in any simple way and there are clearly many countries where women have many more children than they want and are desperately in need of family planning help. A classic example of this is Puerto Rico, where as early as the 1950s a majority of women said they wanted only two children, but the mean family size was nearer to six.

FAMILY SIZE PREFERENCES IN DEVELOPED NATIONS

In most Western countries, the vast majority of married couples want children, but favour a family of only two to four children. with an increasing concentration on two children as the preferred number. Such preferences for a small family are usually couched in economic terms and reflect the high perceived costs of children in relation to the benefits derived from them. For most couples the satisfactions gained from parenthood are adequately met by having relatively few offspring. Nevertheless, many couples talk about having children in a way that reflects pressures towards both higher and lower figures within the two to four range. To have no children is seen as unnatural and undesirable; in addition there is still a widespread feeling that the only child is disadvantaged, and that it is selfish to produce just one child without providing at least one sibling for him or her. Few couples, therefore, express preferences for having one child or none at all, and two is seen as the minimum number for a "proper" family. Indeed three or four is often considered to be "ideal" but for economic difficulties, and a larger family is seen as offering greater companionship for children, greater parental satisfaction and a happier family atmosphere. There is also a tension between "quantity" and "quality", so that decisions about how many children to have are not simply a matter of resources.

In his study of American fertility in the early 1960s, Lee Rainwater suggested that the central norm prevailing at that time was that "one should not have more children than one can support, but one should have as many as one can afford". Since then, other considerations have come in, which may lead many couples to question the right, let alone obligation, to have "as many as one can afford". There is growing awareness of world population growth and of the disproportionate demands on scarce world resources by those in more affluent nations. At the same time, increases in the non-familial role options for women have introduced a new reason for restricting family size for many wives, whilst improved access to birth-control has made the two-child family seem not only desirable but attainable. This latter factor should be put in context by recalling that in the 1930s many couples in Western nations restricted their families to one or two children, despite the relatively limited means, by current standards, of fertility regulations. One thing is certain, that in the West today marital fertility largely reflects the conscious desires of couples, and that a majority of women who "want" two children can now hope to achieve this number and no more, with a high degree of certainty that both are likely to survive to adulthood. For most of the Third World, neither of these assertions holds true.

EXCESS AND UNWANTED FERTILITY

One use of information on family size preferences is to provide a crude measure of the extent of "excess" and "unwanted" fertility in women who have completed their child-bearing. If most women in a community say they want two to four children, but many actually have five or more, it is reasonable to conclude that many of the later births in larger families will not have been planned or wanted at the point of conception.

Where such a pattern is found, the explanation often lies in the absence of the opportunity to achieve the desired small family. The wish for only a few children is a key source of motivation towards the use of birth-control, and a major requirement of family planning programmes throughout the world is to serve the still unmet demand for effective contraception by those having more children than they really want. The experience of unwanted pregnancies may be thought of as a source of further motivation; it has often been noted that contraceptive practice becomes more effective as desired family size is reached or passed—but often it can work in quite another way, as experience of repeated failures induces resignation and a belief that control over fertility is an unattainable goal. This is often compounded by a general belief, firmly rooted in actual experience, that life is unpredictable and that the future is not open to manipulation by the individual.

It is also important to recognise that effective motivation is not just a matter of wanting a small family, but of how strongly the goal is sought and how committed a person is to the means of achieving it. If the costs of an additional pregnancy are likely to be high and the benefits of having few children clearly outweigh any disadvantages inherent in seeking and using contraception, a couple will be more likely to come close to achieving their desired family size, given access to the means of doing so. But often this is not the case. There may be ambivalence about the number of children wanted, a lack of faith in the realistic possibility of achieving a small family, or an awareness that failure to keep to two or three children will not make that much difference, and that success in so doing will not bring many tangible benefits. If this is the case, the costs involved in contraceptive use may outweigh any expected benefits, especially if access to effective birth-control is difficult or methods are experienced as unpleasant.

Hill, Stycos and Back, in their study of poor couples in Puerto Rico, found that a large majority expressed preferences for only two or three children, but that many of these actually had many more. Concern over family size typically arose only after the desired number had been reached. Commitment to the goal was often ambivalent and unlikely to lead to the achievement of a small family, unless there was easy access to family planning advice and supplies, an ability to discuss contraception with the spouse and an absence of religious doubts about birth-control.

Similarly, a study of high fertility in Britain (carried out by one of the authors) suggested that this was largely due to ineffective contraceptive practice, reflecting a lack of opportunity to obtain effective methods of birth-control. But there was also a weaker motivation, not in the sense of wanting a larger number of children, but in the lack of strength in the desire for a small or moderate family size. This weaker motivation was in turn related to a situation of relative deprivation, in circumstances which were not conducive to long-term planning and in which the relatively high cost of contraceptive use led to a large amount of risk-taking, with inevitable results. The majority of such couples have a genuine desire for fewer children. Improved availability of effective contraception will do much to enable them to achieve their goals, but they are likely to continue to run a higher risk of unwanted pregnancy as long as their social situation makes the practice of birth-control more difficult and the benefits less tangible.

CHILD LOSS

Infant mortality is still high in many developing countries (*see* Fig. 21). One of the most widely discussed influences on motivation to control fertility is the child-survival hypothesis. This states that declining infant and child mortality will contribute to increased family planning motivation and consequent falls in fertility, because parents will no longer need so many pregnancies to ensure a particular family size. In places where up to a third of all children die before the age of five, parents will have many births, both as an insurance against the loss of those children already born and as a response to actual deaths. It is pointed out that low fertility has seldom been achieved in the absence of declining mortality and that achieved family size in many parts of the world is highly rational, in the light of existing mortality rates or at least of those prevailing in earlier years.

Mandelbaum has argued that Indian villagers who say they want three or four children are really seeking at least two grown sons and a married daughter, who can provide support and comfort in their later years. Given the mortality rates and sex ratios prevalent in India, a woman would need to bear six or seven children in order to have a 95 per cent certainty that at least one son would survive

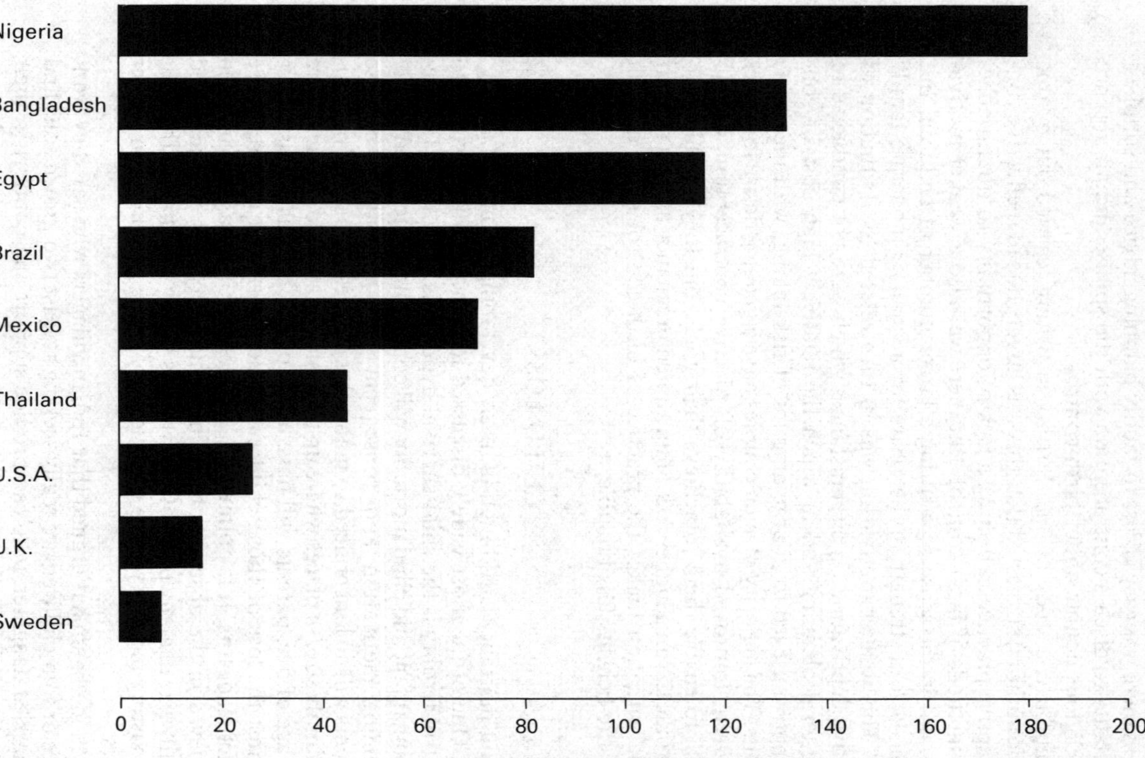

(*Source: 1977 World Population Data Sheet*. Population Reference Bureau Inc. Washington D.C. 1977)

Fig. 21. *Infant mortality rate for selected countries (1974–75).*

to his father's sixty-fifth birthday. Pradervand has put forward similar arguments to explain the high fertility of African countries, arguing that the continued high mortality is the main obstacle to family planning in that continent. He points out that there is no example of a successful, large-scale family planning programme in a country with death rates over 12 per 1,000; and mortality rates throughout Africa are often twice this level.

Certainly it seems unlikely that couples will seek to limit the number of births if they believe that to do so may result in not having sufficient children to provide security in their old age. Where the economic benefits of having children are experienced at a relatively early age, the pressure to restrict births will be even weaker. Any consideration of the relevance to fertility behaviour of family size preferences must, therefore, take into account people's views of the likelihood of survival of those children that are born.

The current high levels of population growth in less developed countries are the result of major declines in mortality, especially in childhood. However, even in countries where mortality levels are relatively high (15–30 per 1,000) growth-rates of 2 or 3 per cent are common, because fertility remains much higher. In such countries, further declines in mortality in the future are to be expected, so that the gap between births and deaths may well widen, as more children survive to become the parents of the next generation. Yet, paradoxically, the main hope for eventually reducing these rates of growth, if the child-survival hypothesis is correct, lies in the intensifying of efforts to reduce infant mortality; even though, in the short term, this may lead to an acceleration of population growth.

Clearly, efforts to reduce infant mortality should be intensified on humanitarian grounds alone. No over-all health plan in the Third World can expect to be well received if it promotes birth-control, while showing insensitivity to the need of the poor to have the children they want, and for these children to grow to adulthood. Moreover, the technology for bringing down infant mortality is simpler, cheaper and quicker to implement than that for reducing births. One can cite many examples, such as the villages in Luristan in Iran, where half the babies used to die in the first five years of life, largely from gastro-enteritis, resulting from contaminated water supplies. When the latrines which used to open into the stream which also supplied drinking water were blocked up, infant mortality fell by one-half in a season.

However, the relationship between infant mortality levels and interest in family planning is a complex one. There are societies where infant mortality has fallen to relatively low levels, but fertility remains high, as in the Philippines. On the other hand, there are other places, such as Bali in Indonesia, where significant declines in fertility have occurred during a period when infant mortality has changed only slowly; likewise, in Calcutta, Northern Thailand and amongst the hill tribes of Burma, there is a demonstrable demand for family planning although infant mortality is still high.

The child-survival hypothesis often refers to the experience of Western nations as possibly being relevant to the situation in less developed countries today. In most developed countries, both fertility and infant mortality levels today are low, whereas those non-Western countries which have achieved similar low levels of births also have very low levels of infant mortality. However, a consideration of the actual trends of births and deaths in nineteenth century Europe shows the relationship between changes in mortality and fertility to be far from straightforward. In some countries, fertility fell before or at the same time as mortality, whereas in those where major declines in fertility occurred at some stage after the beginning of mortality decline, the changes in fertility began at differing levels of infant mortality from country to country.

In England and Wales the birth rate began to fall in the 1870s at a time when life expectancy at birth was 41.4 for men and 44.6 for women. The crude death rate was about 20 per 1,000, and of every 1,000 children born, 150 died before reaching their first birthday—figures comparable to those of many African countries today. Infant mortality was lower than it had been a century earlier at the commencement of increased population growth, but further declines did not occur until the turn of the century, by which time the birth rate was below 30 per 1,000, although child mortality at older ages was declining. By the time the birth rate had come down below 20, in the 1920s, the death rate was 12, but infant mortality was still around 70 per 1,000 live births and life expectancy for males about 56. In 1973 Mexico, with a crude birth rate of 40, had a male life expectancy at birth of 61.3 and an infant mortality rate of 51.4, lower than Britain in the inter-war period although high by current Western standards.

In recent years, attempts have been made to examine the child-survival hypothesis at an individual (or micro) level. Chowdhury and his colleagues have considered the effect of child mortality experience on subsequent fertility in Pakistan and Bangladesh. If a child dies, the next birth is brought forward, but this shortening of the pregnancy interval seems to be not a conscious choice to replace the dead child in the family, but a consequence of the woman not lactating (*see* p. 330). Conversely, any fall in fertility that results from an increase in lactation and longer birth intervals consequent upon a reduction in infant mortality tends to be negated, in terms of population growth rates, by the fall in mortality. Other studies at the micro level, which have been reviewed by Taylor, Newman and Kelly, likewise point to there being no automatic response by couples to reduced infant mortality other than a "biological" one.

There are, then, a number of possible explanations of the apparent link between reductions in infant and child mortality and declining family size.

Firstly, both could be a consequence of primary socio-economic development and not directly linked to each other. In Britain and other Western nations, falling mortality reflected general improvements in social and economic conditions, rather than the impact of medicine, and so can be seen as having arisen from the same forces that influenced later fertility decline. In many developing countries, on the other hand, much of the recent decline in mortality can be attributed to the impact of modern medicine, so that the hidden link may not exist here.

Secondly, we can follow the child-survival hypothesis in arguing that reductions in child loss mean that fewer births are needed to ensure that the desired number of children grow to adulthood; so the need for "insurance" or "replacement" births is reduced. This implies a degree of rationality in fertility decisions by individual couples. Where such a response does not occur, it is often put down to a perceptual lag—couples are said to be unaware of changes in mortality, or to have failed to grasp their implications, so that they act "irrationally" in having similar numbers of births to their parents in times of higher mortality; but this view can overlook the possibility that the couples may welcome the greater number of children surviving because, previously, too few lived.

Thirdly, the lowering of infant and child mortality, in the absence of any immediate offsetting control over births, imposes strains on the family as more children survive; it can be argued that it is to this that parents react, while the increase in household size also produces stress in a social structure which had evolved to accommodate lower rates of survivorship. Beaver gives the example of inheritance systems, where arrangements that were workable for redistributing land in times of high mortality are overloaded when too many children survive to be adults and potential heirs. In this case, individuals come to control their family size, not because of any specific understanding of demographic trends, but rather as a reaction to the burdens of a family size larger than the existing social and economic structure can handle. Lower fertility is thus a response to the consequences of mortality decline, so that a time-lag is inevitable. In contrast, a lack of response, even after a period of years, would have to be explained in terms of the social structure, rather than the blindness of individuals to the consequences.

Finally, we should remember the point made earlier that in any society where prolonged lactation is practised a reduction in early deaths will result in a longer average birth interval, as more mothers will be breast feeding for some months or years after birth. Fertility decline can thus be simply a biological reaction to reduced infant mortality.

Although we may agree that replacement level fertility is only likely to be achieved in a situation where most couples can be confident that any child they have will have a very high probability of survival to adulthood, the question of the nature of the relationship between declining infant and child mortality and reductions in the birth rate remains in doubt. We should perhaps not expect to be able to find any magic threshold of infant mortality, below which fertility must begin to fall; we must instead see changes in infant mortality as just one aspect of the total life experience of a people, in which individual, specific adjustments are not the key factor.

Furthermore, if Coale and Hoover are correct in their assertion that "substantial economic improvement may be a sufficient condition for a decline in mortality, but it is not today a necessary condition", we are faced with the problem of how true this is of fertility decline as well. Can the reduction in mortality achieved by modern public health measures, in advance of socio-economic changes—which is the basis of the population explosion in the Third World—be paralleled by a reduction in fertility, in advance of achieving standards of affluence approaching those of the West? The experience of the one-fifth of mankind who live in China, and of isolated, but not insignificant, areas in the rest of Asia, suggest that this is indeed possible (*see* p. 312).

A BOY OR A GIRL?

Most couples have fairly clear ideas not only about how many children they want, but also about the number of boys and girls they would like, ideas which are influenced by both personal preferences and social pressures. In many societies it is seen as particularly important to have male children and for these to reach adulthood and fulfil certain social, economic and religious functions for the parents. Indeed, in nearly every society parents, and especially fathers, seem to prefer sons (*see* Table 13); there are, however, a few societies, such as parts of Sumatra, where land inheritance is through women, or there is a high brideprice (i.e. the wealth transferred by the kin of a groom to the kin of his bride, in compensation for the release of claim to the children that are produced in the marriage), and the preference is for girls. As no-one yet knows how to predetermine the sex of a child, such preferences for one sex can create an upward pressure on total child-bearing amongst couples who have sons or daughters only. Negative feelings about children of one sex can be dealt with rather differently, as in the female infanticide of the Netsilik Eskimos or the relative neglect of female babies which may account for the higher infant mortality amongst females in India and Egypt.

In countries like the Sudan, where there is a very strong preference for male children, this is undoubtedly a major barrier to the accept-

TABLE 13: SEX PREFERENCES OF MEN

Country	*Percentage preferring*		
	Boy	*Girl*	*Either*
Bangladesh	91	2	8
India	78	5	17
Nigeria	67	2	31
Chile	56	5	39
Argentina	33	3	63

(*Source:* Inkeles, A. and Smith, D. M. *Becoming Modern: Individual Change in Six Developing Countries*. Harvard University Press 1974)

ance of birth-control, and it would be possible to cite many examples of other developing societies where sons are still a dire economic necessity, as we saw earlier in the case of India (*see* p. 93), where the need to ensure the survival of at least one son in the face of high infant and child mortality leads to women having on average six or seven births.

In Singapore, Hong Kong and Japan, the traditional preference for sons seems to have waned sufficiently to allow for the emergence of a two child norm in family size, but in other societies where birth rates have been falling and infant mortality is low, a continuing preference for sons presents a barrier to the achievement of replacement fertility. This seems to be the case for Korea where Williamson reports that "daughters are scarcely considered to be a part of the family" and Taiwan, where recent surveys have shown that 80 per cent or more of couples want at least two sons. In 1973, women in their twenties wanted on average 1.8 sons and 1.2 daughters, and contraceptive practice was found to be related to the existing sex composition of the family. Among couples with two children, the proportion who wanted no more rose from 29 per cent of those with two daughters, to 63 per cent of those with two sons, with similar differences in the proportion currently using birth-control.

In some traditional societies, preference for sons can lead to the divorce or ill-treatment of a wife unlucky enough to bear a succession of daughters. As the sex of a child is the only genetic constituent which is not equally divided between parents, but is solely determined by the father, such practices are not only socially unjust but also biologically indefensible. Perhaps as an intermediate way of helping women, it might be an idea to educate men in the view that the sex of their child is so important that nature has given the choice entirely to them.

Sex preferences are also relevant to patterns of fertility, when there is no strong desire for one sex in preference to the other, if a balance of the sexes is required. Indeed it has been argued that the desire for equal numbers of each sex has a stronger upward effect on fertility than a preference for sons alone, because in the latter case mothers of several sons will be happy to stop, especially if the possible birth of an additional girl is viewed negatively. In many African societies, there is a preference for equal numbers of sons and daughters, so that the former can marry with the brideprice brought into the family by their sisters. Both boys and girls are needed to perform different tasks within the family and couples with children of one sex only, or an imbalance of sexes, may tend to have an additional child in an attempt to equalise numbers.

The impact of sex preferences on fertility behaviour in developed countries has been widely documented. The 1973 National Fertility Survey indicated that American wives are still more likely to show a basic preference for sons rather than daughters. An earlier study of women with two children showed that those who had a boy and a girl wanted an eventual completed family size that averaged 3.2 children, while those with two sons or two daughters wanted 3.7 and 3.9 respectively. In a follow-up to this study, it was discovered that more additional pregnancies had occurred to those couples who had previously had single sex families. British studies have indicated that a large majority of couples expressing any strong preferences about sex composition—and about a third say that they do not mind—opt for a boy and a girl, with single-sex families rarely sought. A recent survey of couples with at least one child, found that those with single-sex families were more likely to say that they hoped to have another child and that two-thirds of these wanted the next child to be of the opposite sex.

One area for speculation concerning sex preferences is the implications of an ability to predetermine the sex of a child, if any of the techniques discussed in the next chapter become a practical possibility. The advantages in countries like the Sudan where boys are strongly preferred, and where mothers of girls are subject to condemnation, lie in the possibility of reduced fertility and women no longer being blamed for producing too many girls. The consequent imbalance of the sexes, however, would clearly create new social problems in the area of sexual activity and mate selection. Such a change in the "market situation" of women could well increase the perceived value of daughters and so reduce preferences for sons only.

At the moment, the only situation where couples do have some degree of control over the sex of their children is when they adopt. Here, however, those couples who do express preferences seem to act in a way that differs strikingly from natural parents. The majority of would-be adopters express a preference for a girl, especially for their first child. The reasons for this remain uncertain, but may be associated with a concern over the possibility of the later birth of a son, and with fears of conflict concerning who is to become the male heir and perpetuate the family name. For other couples the choice of a girl may be made on the assumption that girls present less risk and will adapt better to adoptive families than boys of unknown heritage.

THE TIMING AND SPACING OF BIRTHS

Motivation to use birth-control does not arise only from a desire to limit family size. Even in a society where large families are considered desirable and infant mortality is high, there may be a demand for birth-control to avoid extra-marital pregnancies and to space children within marriage. There may also be societal pressures to avoid child-bearing at too young or too advanced an age. Indeed, it can be argued that for developing countries, we should pay less attention to the norms about family size and more to those governing who should have children, when child-bearing should start and end and what intervals are seen as desirable between children. The question which is rarely asked, but which may be more meaningful to many women than "How many children do you want?", is "Do you want to menstruate this month?" By doing this, we may become less ready to make assumptions about birth-control only being acceptable to older women who have had all the children they want, less concerned to "motivate" people to want fewer children, and more willing to meet the existing demand for family planning services. Motivation towards the use of birth-control can and does exist in women who still want children and any resultant postponement of child-bearing can be of considerable demographic significance. Period fertility rates will be reduced and the length of generations extended. For the individual woman potential exposure to reproduction decreases, and motivation to limit child-bearing at a later stage may be strengthened as she becomes aware of the possibility of controlling her fertility and the advantages of doing so.

The spacing of children within marriage may have been of particular importance in primitive hunting and gathering communities. Where a mother has to carry a dependent child with her in a nomadic society, there are great difficulties facing any woman who has more than one such child. The existence of long periods of post partum abstinence in these societies (and in contemporary Africa) suggests that there is more concern for birth spacing than for family limitation, and that this could be an important source of motivation to use modern methods of contraception. A major reason for wishing to space births is to maximise the chances of a child surviving his first few years. A major killer in less developed countries is the protein deficiency disease *kwashiorkor*, which is a West African word meaning "the illness a child develops when the second baby comes too soon". There are many local African terms of abuse for the "sex-crazed" behaviour of those who have children too close together. Similarly, many Indian women see the spacing of births as a means of protecting their own health and that of their youngest child. Often an interval as long as three or four years is seen as desirable, but this is seldom achieved, as post partum abstinence tends to be much shorter. Further evidence for a potential interest in contraception as a means of achieving such birth intervals comes from a study in Calcutta, which found that over a third of induced abortions involved second pregnancies.

A further example of the existence of interest in child spacing in a high fertility society is the study by Barnett, Jackson and Cann of a highland Guatemala community, where, in response to a question about the best number of children for a family, 40 per cent of the women replied that it was up to God (*Lo que me manda Dios*); the remaining 60 per cent named five or more children as ideal. When asked what was the ideal interval between children, only 7 per cent said that this should be left to God; 40 per cent advocated an interval of at least three years and the remaining 53 per cent said two years or more. There was little interest in limiting family size as such, but much awareness of the advantages of a lengthened interval between births.

The importance of family spacing as a motivating factor in the use of birth-control is by no means limited to less developed societies. Recent studies of the history of fertility decline in Britain suggest that the initial decline derived as much from the use of contraception to postpone births as from any conscious desire to limit family size. The initial impetus was a desire to delay the wife's next pregnancy rather than a feeling that any particular number of children was appropriate, but the effect was striking. Period birth rates began to fall and an increasing number of couples became aware of the possibility of controlling child-bearing, which in turn led to a formulation of specific goals of only a few children. Likewise, the very small families of couples marrying in the late 1920s and early 1930s can be seen as the result of a postponement of child-bearing during the years when a woman was most likely to conceive, followed by an inability or disinclination to "catch up" later, rather than a clear decision to have only one child. If couples delay child-bearing, they may develop tastes and patterns of leisure which are not compatible with having many children, and so reduce family size preferences. If, in contrast, they have children early in marriage and at short intervals, they may limit their alternative activities and face more years of potential child-bearing, intended or otherwise, and may not be able to reduce their family size if the economic situation worsens. As Ryder succinctly puts it, "Parity is elastic upwards but not downwards." Today, many recently-married couples in developed societies are choosing to defer starting a family so that the wife can continue to work and they can enjoy a period of marriage without children.

Postponement of child-bearing within marriage is one example of "child-spacing" before reproduction commences. Another important feature of motivation that relates to the "tempo" rather than the "quantity" of births is the desire to avoid pregnancy before marriage. The need to avoid the unwanted results of extra-marital sexual activity provides a source of motivation towards birth-control, which is independent of any ideas concerning the number of children eventually wanted. It is possible, therefore, that motivation to control fertility before marriage may exist in a society, even when there is little desire to limit family size after.

Sexual practices which stop short of full intercourse are common amongst unmarried adolescents (*see* p. 72) and if a pregnancy does result from an illicit union, abortion or infanticide is widespread and has nothing to do with the birth of too many children. It has been argued that in Africa one source of growing interest in contraception may be the increase in pre-marital sexual activity, associated with a rising age at marriage and the availability of new educational opportunities for young people (*see* p. 184). Motivation to practise birth-control may, therefore, be strongest amongst those who have never had children. The encouragement of "contraceptive innovation" amongst such groups may lead to a greater interest in the later use of birth-control within marriage, either to space births or to avoid traditional patterns of post partum abstinence.

We have already discussed (*see* p. 71) the pattern of declining fertility at older ages in many Asian communities, associated with sexual abstinence in the later years of marriage. This avoidance of late child-bearing seems to be motivated as much by feelings of shame as by any desire simply to terminate child-bearing; so it may be seen in part as an example of motivation arising from a concern over the timing of births. In this case, the key factors are the age of the woman and, especially, the birth of a grandchild. So Mandelbaum, in his study of Indian fertility, refers to the "pregnant grandmother complex". Many villagers in India believe that a woman whose children are old enough to become parents themselves is demeaned if she becomes pregnant again, especially if a daughter-in-law is present in the home. She is, therefore, expected to abandon sexual relations—or at least to reduce their frequency—as the need for procreation is no longer present. Similar beliefs have been reported amongst the Yoruba in Nigeria (*see* p. 183). The strength of such motivation will vary according to whether a woman already has several children, or at least a certain number of surviving sons, but its roots clearly lie in more than just considerations about family size.

Finally, we should perhaps stress that motivation to space or limit births is often influenced by personal considerations which go far beyond any feelings about the ideal size and spacing of a family. A woman may seek to avoid further pregnancies for such reasons as previous adverse child-bearing experience, because she wishes to preserve her figure or pursue a career or further education, or because of doubts about her marriage. Some couples who want children may decide not to produce their own, through fear of the possible transmission of a known hereditary disease. Furthermore, motivation to use modern methods of contraception may be influenced as much by a desire to improve sexual relationships as a wish to avoid further conceptions. Indeed, a woman may opt for a method such as the I.U.D., in the knowledge that it is less effective than the Pill, because she has experienced loss of libido on oral contraception, or fears possible side-effects. Where illegal abortion is widely practised, as in much of Latin America, the initial spread of contraception may partly replace this, without having any impact on the actual number of live births a woman experiences. Such moves to more acceptable methods of contraception may nevertheless be of considerable significance in changing the balance of costs and benefits in contraceptive practice, and so may strengthen the motivation to avoid further pregnancy.

RISK-TAKING IN CONTRACEPTIVE PRACTICE

The motivational factors we have been discussing have a strong bearing on the readiness of couples to practise birth-control, but successful use of family planning will also be dependent on the opportunities available to obtain and use effective means of contraception. The use of contraception, and to some extent the sex act itself, is a learned skill, similar in many ways to learning to drive a car or type a letter. The failure rate for all reversible methods of contraception declines with each step in family building, being less between first and second child than between marriage and first pregnancy, and lower still after the second and subsequent children (*see* Table 14). One reason for this is increased motivation, as the desired number of children is approached or passed; another reason is undoubtedly a growing capacity to control fertility.

TABLE 14: FAILURE RATES (PREGNANCIES PER 100 WOMAN-YEARS) FOR CONTRACEPTION (U.S.A. 1960)

Pregnancy Interval	*Number of children desired*		
	2	*3*	*4*
1	30	37	60
2	13	23	32
3+	4	15	22

(*Source:* Whelpton, P., Campbell, A., and Patterson, J. *Fertility and Family Planning in the United States*. Princeton University Press, Princeton 1966)

As is well known, the insurance on a young driver is higher than that on a man of fifty, who has been driving for twenty-five years. Similarly, one would expect to find most contraceptive mistakes among the young, where lack of practice combines with impetuousness to encourage risk-taking. To pursue the analogy with driving, contraceptive risk-taking is not always associated with pregnancy, just as careless drivers are not necessarily involved in road accidents. Contraceptive risk-taking involves the added problems that you do not know for some while whether you have failed or not; the penalty for mistakes is postponed for at least nine months, and the main costs do not fall on the risk-taker for several years.

In developing countries, driving is often poor and the traffic conditions found in Nigeria or Iran have to be experienced to be understood. In contrast, driving in the U.S.A. is in some ways more disciplined than in Europe; and it seems as if second and third generation users of a technology often do better than their parents at the time of adopting the skill. The same may apply to contraceptive use and could be one of the reasons why abortion is most common at the beginning of the demographic transition.

There is a profound difference in the way fertility regulation is learnt between those who are married and those who are unmarried. Where pre-marital intercourse is rare, nearly all couples are going to learn the skills of contraception as they build up their desired family. Here mistakes will appear as mistimed pregnancies, which carry relatively little penalty. However, in a society where pre-marital intercourse is common, risk-taking and contraceptive failure usually lead to unwanted pregnancies which in turn give rise to abortion, a shotgun wedding or an illegitimate child, either kept by the mother or offered for adoption.

The occurrence of apparently unwanted extra-marital pregnancies may reflect ambivalent motivation rather than psychiatric disturbance, or lack of knowledge of and access to birth-control. The latter has been vividly demonstrated by Kristin Luker in a recent study of applicants for legal abortion in California. Luker suggests that many such pregnancies may be best understood in a framework of contraceptive risk-taking based on decision-making theory. She argues that women often take chances, not through ignorance or irrationality, but as a result of weighing-up the costs of acquiring and maintaining contraceptive use, against the perceived likelihood of falling pregnant and the possible costs and benefits of pregnancy. The costs of contraception are not so much monetary as social and cultural. In addition to the perceived disadvantages of many methods and the difficulty experienced in obtaining them, there are problems associated with acknowledging sexual activity or availability for it, and the associated lack of spontaneity. Intercourse is natural, but rational use of birth-control unnatural, and to prepare for possible intercourse by being on the Pill, or purchasing a diaphragm or sheath, is seen as morally worse than being swept into bed unprepared. At the same time, views on the risk of pregnancy associated with unprotected intercourse may not correspond with the biological reality of the situation, and good luck in avoiding conception in early sexual experience can reinforce such false perceptions.

For many women there may also be feelings about possible benefits from pregnancy, most of which disappear once the pregnancy is confirmed. Pregnancy can demonstrate her fecundity, offer the prospect of a baby to love, test the commitment of a partner, or attract attention from parents or a lover. For some women the risk of possible conception may even increase enjoyment of the sexual act. Finally, it may improve her bargaining position for marriage, at a time when in many developed countries the previous rewards of marriage (from sanctioned sexuality to the provision of household services) seem less attractive as they become attainable by other means.

In the developing world, particularly in the poverty and misery of the shanty-towns, risk-taking in relation to pregnancy can also have positive advantages. Prostitution is exceptionally common and cheaply available in most shanty-towns. Even an unemployed man can afford to buy his sexual satisfaction, or to acquire it from a variety of women with little social or economic cost. Within such a situation, the only bargaining power possessed by a woman who develops a common-law relationship with a man relates to the bearing of his children. Often, with relatively little effort, the man can acquire a mate who is younger and in conventional terms more exciting sexually. Therefore, in an effort to maintain the links she has built up, a woman may risk pregnancy repeatedly, even though she knows in economic and emotional terms that she may find it difficult to make provision for any child that is conceived.

CONCLUSION

The study of motivation in human reproductive behaviour is of central importance to any attempt to understand fertility patterns and in the design and implementation of family planning services. A great many factors are involved in determining a couple's desired family size and their preferences for the timing and spacing of births. We have tried to review some of these, including perceptions about the chances of infant mortality and preferences for children of a particular sex. Against this background of beliefs set by their society, men and women meet, marry, have intercourse and in the process use contraception, take many chances and resolve some resultant pregnancies through abortion. Risk-taking, combined with difficulty of access to the means of controlling fertility, which is still found over much of the world, leads to many unplanned or unwanted births. Even in the U.S.A., many births are still said to be unplanned (*see* Fig. 22), while in poorer countries the problem is as great or greater. In the next chapter, we shall turn to look at the means available to mankind to space and regulate pregnancies, and at some of the difficulties involved in using these.

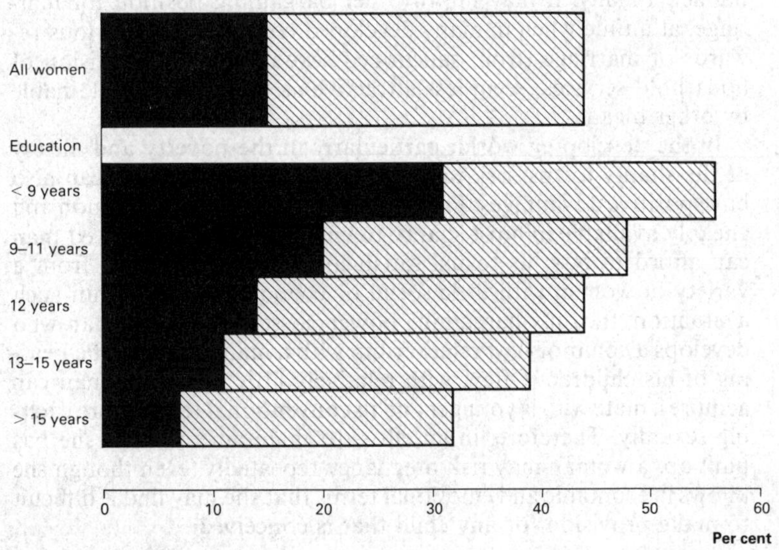

(*Source:* Based on data from the *U.S. National Fertility Survey* (married women under the age of 45)

Fig. 22. *Unplanned* (=*hatched*) *and unwanted* (= *black*) *births in the U.S.A.* (*1966–70*).

SELECTED REFERENCES AND BIBLIOGRAPHY

Barnett, C. R., Jackson, J. and Cann, H. "Child-spacing in a Highland Guatemala Community." in Polgar, S. (ed) *Culture and Population*. Schenkman, Cambridge, Mass. 1971

Beaver, D. *Demographic Transition Theory Reinterpreted*. Lexington Books, London 1975

Busfield, J. "Ideologies and Reproduction." in Richards, M. P. M. (ed) *The Integration of the Child into a Social World*. Cambridge University Press, Cambridge 1974

Chowdhury, A., Khan, A. and Chen, L. "The Effect of Child Mortality Experience on Subsequent Fertility in Pakistan and Bangladesh." *Population Studies*. 30, 249 1976

Coale, A. J. and Hoover, E. M. *Population Growth and Economic*

Development in Low Income Countries. Princeton University Press, Princeton 1958

Davis, K. "Population Policy: Will Current Programs Succeed?" *Science*. 158, 730 1969

Evans-Pritchard, E. *Kinship and Marriage among the Nuer*. Oxford University Press, London 1951

Freedman, R. "Norms for Family Size in Underdeveloped Areas." *Proceedings of the Royal Society*. 159, 220 1963

Hill, R., Stycos, J. M. and Back, K. *The Family and Population Control*. University of North Carolina Press, Chapel Hill, 1959

Hinshaw, R., Pyeatt, P. and Habicht, J. P. "Environmental Effects on Child-spacing and Population Increase in Highland Guatemala." *Current Anthropology*. 13, 216 1972

Luker, K. *Taking Chances: Abortion and the Decision not to Contracept*. University of California Press, Berkeley, 1975

Mamdani, M. *The Myth of Population Control*. Monthly Review Press, New York 1972

Mandelbaum, D. G. *Human Fertility in India*. University of California Press, Berkeley, 1974

May, D. A. and Heer, D. M. "Son Survivorship, Motivation and Family Size in India: A Computer Simulation." *Population Studies*. 22, 199 1968

Polgar, S. "Population History and Population Policies from an Anthropological Perspective." *Current Anthropology*. 13, 203 1972

Population Reports, Series 1, no. 2. *Sex Preselection—not yet Practical*. George Washington University, 1975

Pradervand, P. *Family Planning Programmes in Africa*. O.E.C.D., Paris 1970

Rainwater, L. *Family Design: Marital Sexuality, Family Size and Contraception*. Aldine, Chicago 1965

Ryder, N. "The Time Series of Fertility in the United States." in *International Population Conference, London 1969*. I.U.S.S.P., Liege 1971

Taylor, C., Newman, J. and Kelly, N. "The Child Survival Hypothesis." *Population Studies* 30, 263 1976

Williamson, N. E. *Sons and Daughters: A Cross-cultural Survey of Parental Preferences*. Sage Library of a Social Research, Beverley Hills, California 1976

Chapter 6

Methods of Fertility Regulation

During most of human evolution, lactation was the sole factor governing the spacing of conceptions. Today in traditional societies it remains the prime factor, but can be supplemented by varying periods of abstinence, the practice of coitus interruptus and sometimes abortion.

In developed countries, contraceptive practice is increasingly replacing lactation as the major factor in the spacing of pregnancies. However, it is interesting to note that the interval between pregnancies is often not markedly different in a rural society such as the villages of Bangladesh from that in a modern urban environment in North America or Europe.

For a married couple building their family, conceptions due to the failures that occur with most methods of contraception and those due to the difficulties caused by the undefined limit to the period of lactation amenorrhoea as a birth-control method are acceptable. This is the case especially when the woman's role is mainly directed to home-making. Accidents of pregnancy-timing are more serious when women wish to postpone the first pregnancy in marriage because they are involved in outside employment, or when they wish to return to work between deliveries, or in the case of pre-marital intercourse. In these cases pregnancies may end in abortion.

Perhaps the main difference between a traditional society with moderate to high fertility, and a community where the birth rate is falling (or has reached low level) lies in the steps that are taken in the latter to terminate child-bearing prior to the menopause. In a high fertility society child-bearing continues until the menopause; it is slowed, but not halted by, the process of ageing (*see* Fig. 9). The time taken to conceive is somewhat extended in an older couple and lactation may exert an even stronger delay on the return of fertility post partum; nevertheless women in their thirties and forties continue to add to their families.

It is in the area of fertility termination that the limitations of modern methods of contraception are most apparent. In industrialised nations, couples commonly achieve their desired family size in the later twenties or early thirties. A woman may then have ten to fifteen years or more of potential fertile life ahead of her. Unhappily, even in the closing decades of the twentieth century, no reversible method of contraception (with the possible exception of the conscientious use of oral contraceptives) is sufficiently predictable to be used as a control over fertility during this long period of a woman's life. Hulka has used a computer model to calculate the number of accidental pregnancies likely with different methods of contraception (*see* Table 15). Observational data on the widespread use of I.U.D.s

TABLE 15: LIMITATIONS OF REVERSIBLE METHODS OF CONTRACEPTION

Theoretical model

Percentage of women who exceed goal of three children in a fertile lifetime of 20 years using I.U.D., diaphragm or condom.

	Percentage
Women achieving goal of three children	16.0
Women with one additional pregnancy	33.5
Women with two additional pregnancies	30.0
Women with three or more additional pregnancies	20.5
Total exceeding fertility goal	80.0

(*Source:* Hulka, J. "A Mathematical Study of Contraceptive Efficiency and Unplanned Pregnancy." *American Journal of Obstetrics and Gynecology*. 104, 443 1969)

in Taiwan confirms the reality of Hulka's hypothetical findings for at least one method of reversible contraception (*see* Table 16).

Relatively few administrators, clinicians, policy makers, or enthusiasts in family planning fully appreciate the limitations of contraceptives in terminating fertility as opposed to spacing wanted pregnancies. Most family planning programmes are based on a use of contraceptives which has yet to be achieved in community practice. To this extent family planning programmes are built on false hypotheses. When the recipients of these programmes are the poor of the Third World, struggling to adapt to and take advantage of the new economic changes that characterise a modern way of life, then implicit or explicit claims for a contraceptive effectiveness, which will not in practice be achieved, border on the fraudulent.

Contraceptives are best viewed as mechanisms for extending the time taken to conceive (*see* Fig. 5). Although some individuals may be lucky, there is no way in which a society can achieve a low birth rate by the use of contraception alone. If most women need to terminate their fertility some significant time before the menopause, then

TABLE 16: LIMITATIONS OF REVERSIBLE METHODS OF CONTRACEPTION

Observational data

Additional births observed among I.U.D. users and non-users in Taiwan (1960s)

Age of woman (years)	*Additional births observed*		
	No family planning	*I.U.D user*	*Difference*
22.5	7.14	6.48	0.66
32.5	3.10	2.24	0.86
42.5	0.38	0.13	0.25

(*Source:* Potter, R. G. "Inadequacy of a One-method Family Planning Program. *Social Biology*. 18, 1 1971)

they must have access to abortion and/or sterilisation. A family planning programme that excludes the surgical methods of fertility regulation is not a realistic programme.

The following chapter reviews the individual methods of fertility regulation. The advantages and disadvantages of each method should always be seen in the wider context of the problem of lifelong fertility regulation and not, as is all too often the case, as concerns merely the time between visits to the clinic.

METHODS

The frequently asked question, "What is the best method of family planning?" is neither useful nor valid. Family planning, like transport, benefits from a number of options, each one of which may fulfil a particular need for a particular couple for a particular interval of that couple's life.

FAILURE RATES

Unexpected pregnancies have occurred even after a hysterectomy. Pregnancy after sterilisation is sufficiently common that married women having the operation should be informed of the risk. All the reversible methods of contraceptives have significant failure rates.

Failure rates are usually compared according to the "Pearl Formula", which is calculated by dividing the number of accidental pregnancies occurring to a defined group of women using the method by the total months of exposure to risk of conception, and multiplying by 1,200 to give a failure rate in relation to 100 woman-years of use (i.e. 100 women using a method for one year, or fifty women for two years). Rates are usually calculated on relatively large numbers of women over only a few years of use. More sophisticated "life table" analyses of contraceptive failures are possible. These can show, for example, the number of users who have become pregnant after six, twelve and twenty-four months, but also how many gave up contraception after a certain period of use and other events such as expulsions and removals in the case of the I.U.D.

Some reviews attempt to distinguish between "method failures", e.g. a conception that may occur when a condom tears, and "user failures", e.g. a conception that may occur when a previously regular condom user decides to take a risk. User failure rates for most methods vary with the economic background of the user and the stage of family building when the method is used (*see* Table 14). It is rare for authorities to calculate statistical confidence limits for each method and if they did there might be a considerable overlap between separate studies. Whereas such a distinction might provide impressive statistics in a piece of manufacturer's sales literature, or salve the conscience of a physician faced with a tearful patient, it is not a useful distinction from the point of view of the potential user making a choice from a selection of methods. Furthermore, on closer analysis even the apparently simple division into method and user failure becomes blurred. There are certainly "provider failures" as well as user failures. Some family planning workers are more likely to obtain good usage and a low failure rate through the conviction and care they put into the provision of a method, than others who may well transmit to the client their own sexual problems or their fears for the method. Snowden has shown that both the length of time for which women continue to retain an I.U.D. and their chances of becoming pregnant while doing so vary according to the clinic at which the device was inserted.

The many factors affecting contraceptive failure rates make it impossible to provide universal "measures of failure" for each method. The diaphragm, when used by a well-educated woman who has completed her family and selects this method for positive reasons, may well have a lower failure rate than the oral contraceptive used by a young, newly married woman who partially wants to give up a poorly paid job and whose sister has just won family admiration with new-born twins. In this chapter, exact "measures" will be avoided and only ranking orders and broad ranges will be given (*see* Fig. 23).

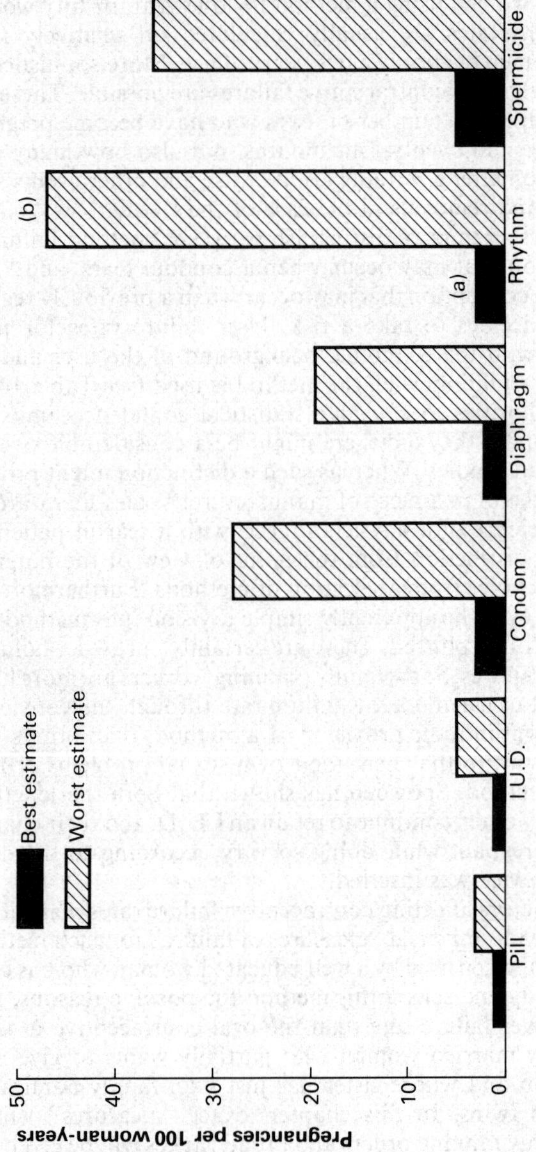

(*Source*: *Population Reports*. George Washington University)

Fig. 23. *Failure rates for contraceptive methods*. (a) rhythm using basal body temperature methods; (b) calendar rhythm.

SIDE-EFFECTS

All methods have at least a few undesirable side-effects. The hormonal methods are unique in having good as well as bad side-effects.

Side-effects may be trivial (the supposed messiness of spermicides), serious (increased blood loss leading to anaemia with I.U.D.s) or life-threatening (thrombotic episodes on the Pill). Understandably, the potentially important life-threatening side-effects are also the most unusual, but rare adverse side-effects pose complex problems of evaluation.

Briefly, two techniques are available for studying rare side-effects, each of which carries with it certain epidemiological problems. The most obvious, but technically most laborious, is to mount a "prospective study". This has been done in the case of the important oral contraceptive study organised by the Royal College of General Practitioners (R.C.G.P.) in Britain. A matched series of women using the method and women not using it is assembled and followed for several years and the outcome of a variety of events is monitored. Prospective studies require large numbers of patients to be studied over many years. This is expensive and difficult. For example, it has not been possible to follow young unmarried Pill users, because they are a mobile group in society.

The exact number of users and controls required for a prospective study is determined by the incidence of the disease under consideration in control groups, the assumed change in incidence consequent on the use of contraceptives, the length of time for which the study is planned and the degree of statistical significance sought. For example, if an attempt is to be made to test the hypothesis that oral contraceptives double the incidence of cancer of the breast, meaning that a statistical significance of 0.05 is wanted after one year, then 85,000 users and 85,000 controls would be needed. In the case of cancer of the uterus (which is a less common disease) 600,000 users and 600,000 controls would be required. A study which ran for ten years would only involve one-third of this number of pairs, but the difficulties of keeping thousands of women under review for many years would be immense.

The R.C.G.P. study began in 1968 and recruited 23,600 married women using oral contraceptives and 22,700 married controls matched for age. The two groups were chosen for reasons of similarity of social class and other factors. By the time the first report was published in 1972, 6–7,000 users and controls had been lost from each group, but the study has produced, and continues to produce, important information. Prospective studies are also taking place in the U.S.A., although no significant study is yet planned or seems likely in any developing country.

"Retrospective studies", using the case-control method, are simpler and cheaper to conduct and most of the available information about rare adverse contraceptive side-effects has come first through this route. The number of cases needed to achieve a statistical significant result is determined by the proportion of women in the population using the method of contraception under study, and this number is independent of the incidence of the disease under investigation. Thus, for a statistical significance of 0.05, if a quarter of all women in a population has ever used the method, only 120 cases of the disease and 120 controls are needed to detect a doubling of the disease rate due to contraceptive use. Where half the population used the method, only 110 controls and 110 users with the disease in question would be needed.

Retrospective studies, however, have their own problems. If the doctor making the diagnosis suspects a relationship between the disease and the method, he may be biased in his judgment. It is not always easy to know the proportion of users in the population at risk. Nevertheless, retrospective studies have proved invaluable in the study of thrombotic disease among Pill users and early findings with this method have been confirmed in later prospective studies. The methodology has also been applied to breast disease among Pill users and to problems with I.U.D. use. It is likely to remain the most rapid and straightforward method of analysing rare contraceptive side-effects.

COITUS INTERRUPTUS (WITHDRAWAL)

Withdrawal is the oldest method of contraception. It is still widely used and in some countries of increasing importance, yet it remains the most misunderstood of methods.

In Genesis there is a verse which runs: "Then Judah said to Onan, 'Go to your brother's wife, perform your duty as brother-in-law and raise up seed for your brother.' Onan knew that the descendants would not be his own, so whenever he had relations with his brother's wife he let the seed be lost on the ground." It is a text which has been subject to volumes of exegesis, but it remains unclear whether Onan's sin was to have practised coitus interruptus, to have disobeyed his father, or to have failed in his family duty.

The later Jewish 'Talmudic" writing refers to coitus interruptus with the charming phrase, "threshing inside and winnowing outside." St. Augustine, whose thinking is pivotal in the Christian theology of contraception, may well have used the method himself, achieving a low failure rate and good continuation—he lived as a Manichean for eleven years faithful to the same woman and had only one child. In the sixteenth century, St. Bernadine wrote of the city of Sienna, "Of 1,000 marriages, I believe 999 are the devil's"—by which she meant the couple used coitus interruptus. Although St. Bernadine's knowledge, attitude and practice survey may have been rather inaccurate, there is no doubt that the method was well known in pre-industrial Europe and became more common during the nineteenth century in all industrialising nations.

Coitus interruptus is omitted from many contemporary K.A.P. (Knowledge, Attitude and Practice) surveys and in others use may be underestimated, as couples do not always classify it as an explicit contraceptive method. In Cartwright's study from the late 1960s, 39 per cent of men and 46 per cent of women claimed the method was being used—this may be due to the fact that the men were embarrassed to report the method, or that the wives thought or hoped that it was being used when it was not. Whatever the irregularities of use, coitus interruptus was for long the commonest method in Western Europe, only giving way to the combined use of Pills and condoms in the 1950s and 1960s. Even in 1967–8 in England 27 per cent of professional couples and 52 per cent of unskilled workers had used the method at some time and 4 per cent and 12 per cent respectively were current users. In Eastern Europe withdrawal remains the commonest single method of birth-control and is associated with some of the lowest birth rates in the world.

In many developing countries the use of coitus interruptus is increasing, especially in Islamic societies. The Prophet Muhammad was the only great religious leader to mention birth-control specifically and a number of remarks concerning coitus interruptus are recorded in the *Hadith* (a record of the traditions or sayings of the prophet). "A man said, 'Oh Prophet of God! I have a slave girl and I practise withdrawal with her. I dislike her becoming pregnant, yet I have the desires of men. The Jews believe that withdrawal constitutes killing a life in miniature form.' The Prophet replied, 'The Jews are liars. If God wishes to create it, you can never change it.'" Elsewhere, commenting on side-effects, the Prophet said, "Had this practice been injurious it would have harmed the Romans and Persians."

Today, Islam still feels comfortable with withdrawal and in Turkey, for example, use of the method rose from 14.5 per cent of couples claiming use at some time in a 1963 survey, to 22.5 per cent in 1969. As at the time of the latter survey, use of the Pill was only reported by 2.3 per cent of couples and use of the condom by 10.3 per cent, it seems reasonable to conclude that coitus interruptus averts more births in Turkey than all the modern methods of family planning. Yet almost without exception, family planning teaching in developing countries either ignores the method or dismisses it as ineffective and dangerous.

Like other coitally related methods of fertility regulation, the failure rate for withdrawal varies widely, but it can be low. In the 1949 Royal Commission on Population in Britain, no difference had been found between the users of appliances and the users of non-appliance methods (mainly coitus interruptus) as regards the average number of children. In the U.S. Indianapolis study in 1941, coitus interruptus users had 10 pregnancies per 100 woman-years of use, compared to 12 for other methods. In high income groups the failure rate was 3.

The main reason for failure with withdrawal is probably failure to withdraw, although nearly every textbook of family planning repeats the myth that viable sperm from the pre-ejaculatory fluid may cause conception. It is a story that goes back to the American birth-controller Abraham Stone who in the 1930s posed the very reasonable question as to why coitus interruptus should ever fail at all. He asked "several of (his) medical friends who have microscopes" to examine the pre-orgasm secretion for sperm. In 24 slides from 18 friends, sperm were seen in 5, which he concluded was "insignificant for any definite conclusions". Today, the physiology of male reproduction is better understood and whereas it is true that only one sperm is required to fertilise an egg, hundreds of millions must be deposited in the vagina. Any man tested for fertility who had only the number of poorly-motile sperm usually found in the pre-ejaculatory fluid would be given a very disappointing prognosis.

The attitudes and perceptions of the providers of family planning are often as important as the motivation of users. Nowhere is this more clearly shown than in the literature attached to coitus interruptus concerning psychological side-effects. Stopes said it was "harmful to the nerves", which probably meant little more than that she did not like it. A hundred years ago "conjugal onanism" was said to cause "ovarian dropsy", "galloping cancer", nymphomania, mental decay and suicide. Contemporary writers use less florid terms but still imply that the method is emotionally harmful—which would seem unlikely for something which more than half the men in Europe have done. Coitus interruptus, like any other method of family planning, is satisfactory for those who choose to use it and when the couple are happy with each other, and probably causes misery when the couple dislike each other.

Use of withdrawal costs nothing, it has no known side-effects, it cannot be forgotten if the couple go away at the weekend and, among practised couples who have completed their families, it has a low failure rate. The neglect of the method in the programmes of contemporary developing countries is unfortunate. The attitude of many professional workers in family planning towards the method is rather like people denigrating primary education because children who leave school early cannot do calculus. There is nothing contradictory in being realistic about the usefulness of withdrawl and assuming it will give way to other methods with the passage of time.

CONDOMS (SHEATHS)

The sheath is a versatile common-sense method of contraception, without any significant side-effects. Nevertheless it has a failure rate that varies widely according to the pressure to control fertility and the familiarity of the couple with the method.

The condom is an excellent method of spacing pregnancies and can be a fair limiting factor in fertility. Combined with legal abortion, as is common in Japan, it is a powerful fertility regulator, acceptable, safe and predictable.

Manufacturers usually run their own wet or dry electronic tests for holes in the condoms. Most manufacturing nations, such as Britain, Japan and the U.S.A., and some importing nations (for example Sweden) have national tests to check the standard of condoms. Such tests involve filling the condom with water and looking for leaks, inflating with air to bursting point or tests of tensile strength on cut strips of condoms. Currently, an effort is being made to establish an agreed international condom test, but like all efforts of international co-operation, from ballet to airlines, even condoms bring out the worst in nationalism and progress is slow.

Tietze and Gamble (Gamble of Proctor and Gamble, who launched the Pathfinder Fund out of Boston, U.S.A. as one of the first international family planning agencies) studied condom use in the U.S.A. in 1966 and found a failure rate that varied from 6–10 per 100 woman-years. Some more recent studies have given still better results, but in developing countries failure rates tend to be higher.

Modern condom manufacture is capital intensive and it is best concentrated in a few places; but packaging can involve up to half the wholesale price, requires little capital and no adherence to standards. This makes it an appropriate local industry. The lubrication and colouring of the modern condom has made it into an attractive and acceptable method. A spermicidally lubricated condom is now marketed. A plastic condom suitable for labour intensive manufacture has been developed, but never widely used.

SPERMICIDES

It is logical to attempt to kill the sperm in their passage from the man to the woman, but as pointed out the anatomy of the cervix makes it a difficult task to accomplish. In general terms, spermicides can be a way to extend the pregnancy interval, having a useful function, for example, as lactation ends. Spermicides are prepared as pessaries (e.g. Rendell's), aerosol foams (e.g. Emko), tablets (e.g. Sampoon) and, in an ingenious presentation, as part of a water soluble plastic film (C-film). Where it is essential to avoid pregnancy and the Pill is not acceptable, the use of a spermicide in mid-cycle to supplement an I.U.D. forms a very safe combination.

Laboratory testing of spermicides with masturbation specimens of sperm dates back to the mid-nineteenth century. A variety of individual tests have been devised, but the only internationally accepted one is the I.P.P.F. agreed test for total spermicide power. Clinical trials give failure rates varying from less than 5 to almost 50. Personal factors and pressures are probably even more significant for spermicides than for most contraceptives.

Spermicides carry no serious side-effects—although anything which kills sperm (and spermicides are often cell poisons containing mercury compounds or detergents) can cause vaginal and penile irritation.

VAGINAL BARRIER METHODS (DIAPHRAGM/CAP)

The limitation in the use of spermicides lies in the anatomy of the cervix, which protrudes into the vagina. Most spermicide is displaced into the *posterior fornix*—the blind cul-de-sac behind the cervix—and the entrance to the womb itself is wiped clean of spermicide during intercourse. The way round this problem is to apply the spermicide to a barrier which holds it over the cervix. This is what the diaphragm (or Dutch Cap) does: it is not a sperm-tight barrier, but a mechanism for exposing sperm to a chemical which kills them. It is a dome-shaped piece of flexible rubber with a wire ring embedded in the periphery to hold it in the vagina; it is lodged behind the pubic bone at the front and reaches up into the *posterior fornix* at the back. Diaphragms must be inserted before intercourse and remain in place for six to eight hours afterwards.

Cervical caps are smaller and thicker rubber barriers which adhere to the cervix itself. A disposable sponge impregnated with a spermicide is under trial.

The diaphragm was the first method which placed a reliable method of birth-control in the hands of women and it was the mainstay of family planning clinics in the Western world, before the invention of the Pill and rediscovery of the I.U.D. Today it is losing out to these two methods, although it has occasional resurgences whenever the Pill comes in for adverse criticism.

PERIODIC ABSTINENCE (RHYTHM METHOD/SAFE PERIOD)

The rhythm method has accumulated a significant and a partisan literature, both promoting and condemning it, for the reason that it has been sanctioned as a licit method by the Vatican. The method works on the principle that ova and sperm have a limited life prior to fertilisation and if abstinence is practised on the days preceding and succeeding ovulation fertilisation will not occur.

It is essential to distinguish between calendar techniques, which attempt to predict ovulation on the basis of previous menstrual records, and methods which involve the attempt to identify some physiological correlate of ovulation, restricting coitus until forty-eight hours or more after the time when reasonable evidence of ovulation has been detected. Sub-categories of the method are at least as likely to be significant determinants of effectiveness as variations in the shape of an inert I.U.D. The following variations are in use:

(*a*) temperature only: restricting coitus to post-ovulatory interval;

(*b*) combined temperature and calendar;

(*c*) sympto-thermic: recognition of ovulation depending upon changes in the amount and consistency of the cervical mucus, combined with temperature recording;

(*d*) mucus recognition alone;

(*e*) the Groden method combines hormone tablets, as in the routine oral contraceptive, but these are only given for half the cycle. The method has been welcomed by some Roman Catholic leaders and is distributed by nuns in at least one country. To the cynical, it seems as if the only criterion for theological acceptability is a high degree of risk; to the pragmatic, it can be a potentially acceptable way to recruit sincere, if somewhat odd, assistance in the continual battle to control human fertility.

The more predictable variants of rhythm tend to be more difficult to teach and to follow. The day of ovulation can be assessed by estimates of basal body temperature, ovulation pain, cervical mucorrhoea and vaginal smears. For the most part, the physiological basis of these changes is understood. However, the translation of laboratory tests into the sort of self-observation necessary to use these clues as adjuncts to the practice of periodic abstinence is only developing and is still subject to partisan interpretation. Most variants of rhythm are useless in predicting the first post partum ovulation after delivery.

It is uncertain if ovulation can be induced by external stimuli in the human female. Does pregnancy follow rape, or do more normal physiological stimuli lead to conception more often than might be predicted from the analysis of cyclical spontaneous ovulation?

Several authors have considered the statistical basis of the rhythm method. Tietze and Potter suggested that calendar rhythm offers a 90 per cent chance of avoiding pregnancy for five to ten years. James pooled data from various types of menstrual records and found that within an individual, and within groups of women, variance estimates of the post-ovulatory phases usually exceeds those of pre-ovulatory phases of the cycle. On theoretical grounds, James has calculated expected pregnancy rates per 100 years of exposure by coital rate and a system of rhythm calculation (*see* Table 17).

In the Philippines, a national study of contraceptive users through the family planning programme showed that rhythm users had approximately the same failure and continuation rates as the condom users in that particular country.

There is strong evidence from animal experiments that when fertilisation takes place with old gametes (ova or sperm) there is a rise

TABLE 17: PERIODIC ABSTINENCE: THEORETICAL CONSIDERATIONS

Coital per cycle	*Method (Pregnancies per 100 w.y.)*	
	Ogino	*Knaus*
4	4.6	10.4
6	6.4	14.8
8	7.7	18.5

(*Source:* James, W. "Parameters of the Menstrual Cycle and the Efficiency of Rhythm Methods of Contraception." *Population Studies*. 19, 45 1965)

in the foetal abnormality rate. When unplanned conceptions take place during use of the periodic abstinence, then there will be a more than usual chance that fertilisation will involve an aged egg or sperm that has been in the female tract for many hours.

A small number of observations exist which suggest that the problem be examined more systematically than it has been to date. An observed high incidence of anencephaly and spina bifida among Roman Catholics has been attributed to the use of periodic abstinence, although genetic or dietary difference variables are probably more likely explanations. One small case-control retrospective study suggests a higher than usual incidence of congenital abnormality in children born to women using a rhythm method.

Another possible biological consequence of the use of periodic abstinence could be a rise in the incidence of abnormal implantation. A hypothesis has been put forward that tubal ectopic pregnancies (where the conceptus attaches itself in the uterine tubes) and *placenta praevia* (where the conceptus attaches itself to the lower part of the uterine cavity and the placenta grows over the cervical opening) might be due to fertilisation occurring late in the cycle, with failure to inhibit menstruation and consequent displacement of the ovum to an abnormal site.

One thing that can be said about the rhythm method is that it is anything but natural. The ultimate paradox of the rhythm method, in view of its history, is that in no Catholic country has it ever become a major, or even a significant, method of family planning, while in Japan (which has few Catholics) it has become one of the commonest reversible methods. It does, of course, work well as a method of extending the pregnancy interval and, when linked with abortion, makes a powerful combination for fertility-control. There is some evidence, for example from Brazil and Switzerland, that Catholics who use the rhythm method have more illegal abortions than those who use no method, or those using alternative mechanical and pharmacological techniques of birth-control.

HORMONAL CONTRACEPTIVES (PILL AND INJECTABLES)

The Pill is the only twentieth century method of birth-control, but everything about it—its history, its interpretation, its evaluation and its use—illustrate the tensions that still exist in family planning.

Biologically, there are two reasons why a Pill for women has become available before one for men. One of the first physiological events in pregnancy is the suppression of the next ovulation. There is no analogous turning off in the male reproductive system. Secondly, in the female, all the ova that are going to be used during the reproductive life are complete and set aside by the time of birth. In the male, sperm production continues throughout life and any compound that might suppress it could also damage sperm (with the risk of causing abnormal babies). In the long term, both these problems will probably be overcome and then the world may enjoy a male pill.

The female Pill has a long history. The biological possibility of imitating early pregnancy was well understood by the Austrian physiologist, Ludwig Haberlandt, when he published a series of papers on the possibility of what he called "hormonal sterilisation" beginning in 1921. Ovaries from pregnant does were transplanted into non-pregnant rabbits, rendering them infertile for several months. By 1927, Haberlandt was exploring the possibility of oral contraception and he collaborated with a pharmaceutical firm in Budapest to produce a preparation called *Infecundin*.

"It needs no amplificaton", wrote Haberlandt in 1931, "that of all methods available, hormonal sterilisation based on biological principles, if it can be applied unobjectionably in the human, is an ideal method for practical medicine and its future task of birth-control." A few months earlier, in a more widely reported statement, Pope Pius XI said in his Encyclical *Casti Connubii*, "assuredly no reason, even the most serious, can make congruent with nature and decent what is intrinsically against nature".

When oral contraceptives were eventually produced, the natural way in which they controlled fertility was recognised by many Catholics, and most especially by their clinical inventor, the Catholic obstetrician John Rock, from Boston, U.S.A. In 1963 he published *The Time Has Come*, which argued for the theological as well as the clinical acceptance of oral contraception. Clearly, from its first development, the Pill was destined to be like no other drug.

The laboratory work that led to the Pill was headed by the late Gregory Pincus, a physiologist at the Worcester Foundation, also in Boston. The Foundation was given a specific donation by the Planned Parenthood of America to launch contraceptive research. Oral contraceptives became a possibility when ovarian hormones became cheap and when such chemical modifications were made as to render them active through the mouth. This part of the story occurred in California and Mexico, with the brilliant inventions of Russell Marker who, in the 1930s and 1940s, found it was possible to make ovarian steroids from plant sources. His first effort was to manufacture enough progesterone to fill two jam-jars, then an amount worth $160,000 at market prices. The Pill was first marketed in 1957 and approved by the U.S. Food and Drug Administration in 1960. By 1959 steroid costs were one-hundredth of what they were a decade previously.

Today, approximately 60,000,000 women take oral contraceptives. A great deal is known about the action and side-effects of the Pill. The exogenous hormones oestrogen and progesterone act on the brain which, in turn, influences the pituitary gland. The secretion of gonadotrophin hormones, which control ovulation, is suppressed. The hormones in the Pill control the growth of the lining of the womb and in the commonly used "combined" oral contraceptive, when active tablets are taken for twenty-one days, and placebos (or iron or vitamin tablets) taken for another week, then uterine bleeding occurs shortly after hormone withdrawal.

The Pill has fulfilled the first requirement of a contraceptive—it has given an unprecedented ability to control fertility. The changes which the Pill induces in the body are widespread, as are those of the menstrual cycle, lactation, and pregnancy itself. Animal trials and carefully supervised small scale human studies have necessarily been of limited value. The adverse side-effects which have turned out to be most important in relation to oral contraceptives were truly unpredictable. There is no way of proving the safety of any pharmacological compound in advance of its widespread use. In the case of the Pill, most of the useful information has come from the type of prospective and retrospective epidemiological studies discussed earlier. Each new discovery has given rise to a social battle, with one group feeling that the Pill is the invention of the devil, eroding the moral fibre of society and therefore overemphasising adverse effects, whereas others, welcoming the freedom given by the Pill, may on occasion have been over-optimistic. Knowledge of the Pill's side-effects has also issued a particular challenge to the medical profession and some doctors have felt it their responsibility to pass on

TABLE 18: MORTALITY ASSOCIATED WITH VASCULAR DISEASE AND ORAL CONTRACEPTIVE USE

Age (years)	*Deaths per 100,000 users per year*	
	Non-smokers	*Smokers*
15–19	1.2	1.4
20–24	1.2	1.4
25–29	1.4	1.4
30–34	1.8	10.4
35–39	3.9	12.8
40–44	6.6	58.4

(*Source:* Tietze, C. and Lewis, S. "Mortality and Fertility Control." *International Journal of Gynaecology and Obstetrics.* 15, 100 1977)

NOTE: After Tietze and Lewit, 1977. Note the analysis involves the work of several authors attempting to derive the maximum information from limited observations. The trends and orders of magnitude are generally agreed but the detailed figures may require revising as more information is accumulated.

objective information enabling women to make informed choices, whereas others have felt it is the doctor's responsibility to decide for the woman and have fought to retain the Pill on prescription.

Oral contraceptives affect blood-clotting mechanisms and may also alter the walls of blood vessels. Women on the Pill are at a greater risk for thrombosis of the veins (with the risk that a clot may pass to the lungs), stroke and cardiovascular disease. The degree of risk rises with age and, in a particularly marked way, after about the age of forty. It is significantly greater in women who smoke (*see* Table 18). The risks of blood-clotting disease are less in those Pills which contain least oestrogen (50 micrograms) and may also be lower in Asian than in Caucasian women.

For the older woman, the risk of heart disease is significant and common practice is to inform the women over forty of the dangers, and to advise on alternative methods. On the whole, the Pill, like pregnancy, is best for younger women. It is not certain if there is any cumulative effect over a period of time. Due to misinterpretation of the initial food and drug regulations in the U.S.A. concerning oral contraceptives, there are still doctors who recommend that a woman should "have a break" from the Pill every two years. There is no scientific basis for this and, indeed, it is bad advice, because the body takes a few months to adapt to Pill-taking.

Pill-use is also associated with some other diseases, although they are more uncommon and in certain cases very rare indeed. There is a measurable increase in the risk of gall-bladder disease and rare benign, but potentially dangerous, liver tumours reported. The blood pressure can rise with oral contraceptive use.

The Pill confers some advantages on users as well as presenting risks. Uterine blood loss is approximately halved and women using the Pill are less anaemic than others. In Western women this may not seem a great boon, but in the developing world, where diets are poor, it is a change which contributes greatly to well-being. Once a woman takes the Pill, there is no biological reason for inducing a uterine withdrawal bleed once a month and recently some experiments have been conducted on so-called "Tricycle Pills". The Pill was given in such a way that a woman had four periods a year instead of thirteen. Many of the users appreciated the partial elimination of a somewhat messy process of menstruation. In some developing countries, menstruation is perceived as an unclean process and Buddhists and Muslims cannot enter a temple or mosque at this time. Some pilot studies are taking place to see if Muslim women may wish to postpone menstruation during the fast of Ramadan. Some Muslim women of the upper classes already use oral contraceptives to alter patterns of menstruation if they go on pilgrimage to Mecca.

Potentially, another important beneficial effect of the Pill may concern breast disease. Breast cancer is more common in women who postpone their first pregnancy (*see* Fig. 43). Biologically, it is not unreasonable to suggest that the Pill, which imitates pregnancy, could have a protective effect against breast cancer, although it is a hypothesis which it would be exceedingly difficult to prove or refute, because the most important effects may take ten or twenty years to develop. Nevertheless, it is encouraging that users of the Pill are less likely to be admitted to hospital with a lump in the breast than those who have never used oral contraceptives (*see* Fig. 24). Current studies involve a pooling of benign and malignant disease. Women who have benign lumps in the breast are more likely to

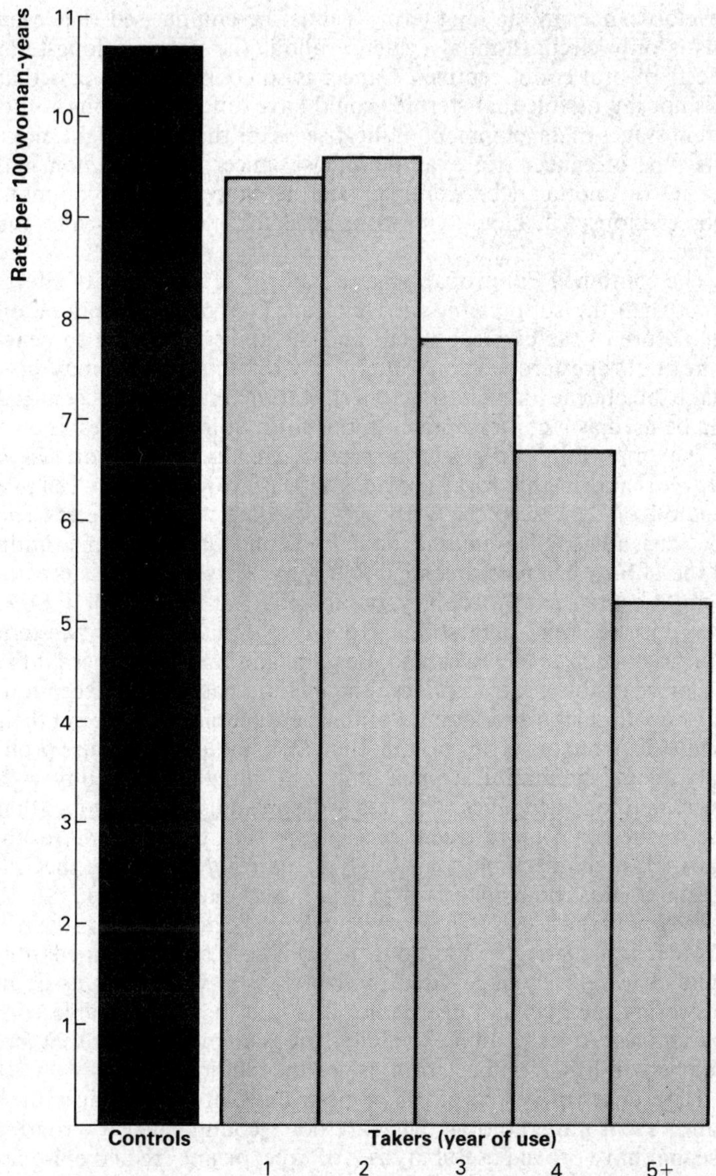

(*Source:* Royal College of General Practitioners, Oral Contraceptives and Health. Pitman, London)

Fig. 24. *Breast lumps and oral contraceptive use.*

develop cancer in the long term. It must be emphasised that even this is only circumstantial evidence about the possible long-term effects of oral contraceptives. Cancer is so complex a process that it is not impossible that steroids could have different actions at different stages of development of the disease, or that they might make one type of cancer (for example breast cancer) less common and yet make another (for example, uterine cancer) more common. Observations will have to be continued for many years into the future.

The combined Pill probably has a number of anti-fertility effects other than the suppressing of ovulation. One of these may be on the nature of the cervical mucus and the ability of sperm to penetrate it. Progesterone alone alters cervical mucus and may also make the uterine lining hostile to fertilisation if it should occur, and can be used as a contraceptive. In this form, it is sometimes known as the "mini-Pill." Progesterone can be given as an injection (*Depo Provera*) and in this form provides an easy-to-use, highly reliable method of contraception with very few known side-effects. The specialist advisory committee to the Food and Drug Administration of the U.S.A. has recommended that *Depo Provera* be registered as a contraceptive in that country, but for political reasons the F.D.A. has rejected this suggestion. However, a number of western countries, such as New Zealand, Belgium and Britain, do permit the use of injectable contraceptives. The method has proved exceptionally popular in the developing world, where people expect to get their medicines from the syringe rather than from tablets. There are probably about one million women now controlling their fertility with injectable contraceptives. This less widespread use, and the fact that the method is a more recent one, means that there are more unknowns about injectable contraceptives than there are about the Pill. Again, it must be emphasised that the valid questions that can be asked about the use of *Depo Provera* will not be answered in advance of wider human use. No additional information can be obtained from animals, or closely supervised human studies, which will assist in answering the question of whether it is safe to use injectable contraceptives. At least, unlike the Pill, there is no proof so far that any one person has ever died from use of the method.

High doses of oestrogens have been used after fertilisation and will prevent implantation. They are not recommended for routine use, but have proved useful in cases of rape, or unexpected episodes of unprotected intercourse. However, if the procedure fails, an abortion should be advised. High doses of hormones can damage an embryo and oestrogens, which were once quite widely used in the supposition that they might prevent threatened abortion, can cause cancer of the vagina in the next generation. Fortunately, there is no evidence whatever that the Pill in normal doses, even if taken by pregnant women in error, will damage the embryo.

INTRA-UTERINE DEVICES (COIL)

The presence of a foreign body in the uterus prevents pregnancy in a great many cases. This fact seems to have been discovered empirically in the nineteenth century, when attempts were made to block the cervix with metal pessaries. These required an intra-uterine portion to hold them in place and sometimes they broke, when it was noted that they still acted as successful contraceptives. In 1909 Richard Richter, in a German medical journal, described a flexible ring made of silk which he placed in the uteri of women seeking contraceptive help. As in the case of the Pill, the scientific and medical community looked the other way for a generation. Then, in 1929, Ernst Grafenberg began making I.U.D.s of silk and later of silver wire. However, interest in his devices was also short-lived and they were condemned by most gynaecologists as sources of infection. Between 1934 and 1959, only one publication appeared in the English language concerning use of I.U.D.s, but a few brave doctors, such as Hall in America, Margaret Jackson in England and Knock in Indonesia continued to use the devices.

In Japan, Dr. Tenrei Ota, who knew of the European work on I.U.D.s, developed his own device, publishing his first results in 1934. He was one of the few Japanese of high intellectual calibre to oppose his country's entry into the Second World War. For this, as well as for his enthusiasms in birth-control, he spent a number of years in prison. At the very time when tens of millions of individuals were suffering private agonies attempting to control family size and when thousands were dying from illegal abortions, society as a whole was unable to handle even the simplest scientific developments in contraception.

Modern I.U.D.s are made out of flexible plastic and can be introduced through a small sterile tube about the size of a drinking straw. A variety of shapes have been devised and some fortunes made (and lost) by the commercial promotion of what turned out to be relatively trivial differences between the performance of devices. On the whole, intra-uterine devices obey a particularly awkward form of Murphy's law! The greater the surface area of the device, the lower the pregnancy rate, but the higher the probability that the device will have to be removed because of excessive uterine bleeding (*see* Fig. 25).

Removals for bleeding and spontaneous expulsion of devices are their main drawbacks, but infection can also occur. If pregnancy

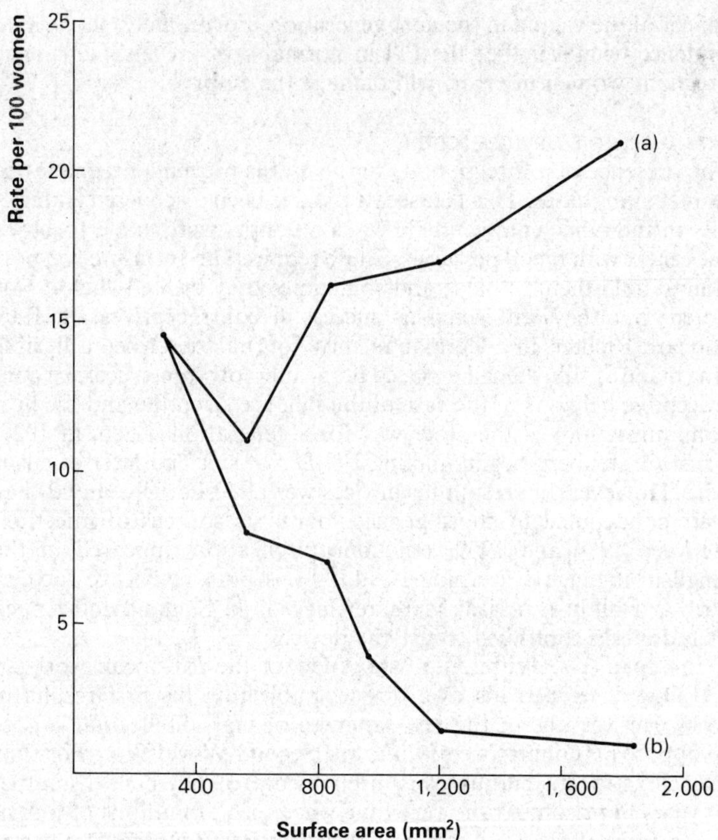

(*Source:* Kessel. E., Bernard, R. and Thomas, M. *I.U.D. Performance and Hypothesis Testing in International Clinical Trials.* I.F.R.P. Chapel Hill)

Fig. 25. *Effectiveness and complications of I.U.D.s.* (a) removal (pain/bleeding); (b) pregnancy.

takes place, a device should be removed, as there is a danger that if it remains in place, an infected abortion may occur in the second trimester of pregnancy. An I.U.D. does not prevent tubal (ectopic) pregnancy, so in a population of users this condition becomes relatively more common that uterine pregnancy.

Like the Pill, I.U.D.s may have a number of anti-fertility effects. They may interfere with the passage of sperm, but it is also clear that fertilisation can occur with an I.U.D. in place and yet pregnancy is usually prevented. If an I.U.D. is inserted after unprotected coitus it prevents pregnancy occurring. The post-coital use of I.U.D.s is much more acceptable than the post-coital use of hormones and is likely to become more common. Conversely, if a device is removed in the middle of a cycle, even if a woman takes contraceptive precautions afterwards, an already fertilised egg may still implant. Biologically, intra-uterine devices may work partially as abortifacients. No doctor is going to stop using them because of this possibility and no reasonable woman is going to be disturbed by this fact, both of which observations emphasise the very genuine difference between the destruction of a newly fertilised egg and an abortion later in pregnancy.

In the 1970s in the U.S.A., an unusual syndrome of infected, spontaneous, second-trimester abortions occurring in women with I.U.D.s in place was recognised. There was a rapid onset of septicaemia which could lead to sudden death. The complication was first observed in relation to the then widely used "Dalkon Shield". This device was subsequently withdrawn and the recommendation tentatively put forward that all devices should be removed in cases where pregnancy was diagnosed. A full analysis of the American experience became available through the Centre for Disease Control, using nationwide data. Between 1972 and 1974, a total of fifty spontaneous abortion deaths occurred in the U.S.A. and it was shown that seventeen were associated with an I.U.D. If a woman had an I.U.D. in place at the time of a spontaneous abortion, she had fifty times the risk of death compared with a woman having a spontaneous abortion without an I.U.D. in place. Most of the deaths involved Dalkon Shields but also a few other devices. At the time of the withdrawal of the Dalkon Shield it was suggested that infection might have descended the multifilament tail, but the epidemiological data suggested that the deaths were related to the size of the device. Thus the wisdom of withdrawing it was confirmed. More important, the removal of a device from a woman if pregnancy is diagnosed, or to offer an abortion if she wishes it, must now be obligatory.

STERILISATION (VASECTOMY AND TUBAL LIGATION)

Sterilisation is the most straightforward, cost-effective and, for many couples, acceptable method of terminating human fertility. Every couple knows the menopause will put an end to child-bearing and the acceptance of sterilisation by one or other partner merely brings this natural process forward by a number of years.

The first vasectomies were not done for fertility regulation but for a mixture of an ill-understood physiology of the prostate gland and ideas of sexual rejuvenation. In 1899, an American surgeon, supposedly at his patient's request, vasectomised a nineteen-year-old man in an attempt to cure his guilt over masturbation. The surgeon said, "Several weeks afterwards he reported he was still masturbating and saw no change in his feelings."

Sterilisation has proved acceptable in all communities at all stages of socio-economic development (*see* Table 19): it is more common in Puerto Rico than in Sweden; a third of couples on the west coast of the U.S.A. have had some form of sterilising operation by the later thirties; the demand for sterilisation in Bangladesh, Mexico or the Philippines greatly outruns the available services. The balance between male sterilisation (vasectomy) and the female operation (tubal ligation) varies in different cultures, although the attitudes of providers are probably the single most important determinant of

TABLE 19: ESTIMATED NUMBER OF COUPLES CHOOSING SURGICAL STERILISATION BY SELECTED LOCALITY

Country or Continent	*Number (millions)*
Peoples' Republic of China	35
India	23
U.S.A.	8
Europe and U.S.S.R.	4.5
Latin America	2.5
Asia and Oceania, excluding China and India	2
Canada	1
Africa	0.5
	Total 76.5

(*Source:* United States Agency for International Development (U.S.A.I.D.) 1971)

current levels. Unlike all other methods of fertility regulation, the individual seeking sterilisation is totally dependent upon the skills and attitudes of a second party. There is no reason to suppose that male and female sterilisation could not have been very popular operations in the nineteenth century and it is interesting that a series of more than 6,000 vasectomies was recorded from California in the first three decades of this century.

The evolution of medical attitudes follows a predictable course. Initially, the female operation is usually offered and the attitude of doctors is that tubal ligation is a "treatment" for a disease, namely over-fertility. In Britain and the U.S.A. after the Second World War, women over thirty with four or more children could usually obtain the operation, but younger couples of lower parity were refused it. Similar age and parity rules have been introduced in contemporary developing countries. With the passage of time, it is discovered that the possibility of subsequent regret by those who have a sterilising operation is not related to age and parity. Attitudes alter until sterilisation becomes an elective choice by the couple concerned and the role of the surgeon changes from one of paternalism to that of ensuring that the individual is correctly informed about the nature and consequences of the operation, and that he is making a free and unpressurised choice.

As the choice element in offering vasectomy is paramount and the operation can never be considered a "treatment", it tends to be offered later in the history of society than tubal ligation. But even so, the attitudes of providers often influence the type of people coming forward for vasectomy. For example, when Pai in Bombay offered the operation in a hospital service, only a small number of middle-class men came forward: but when the same operation was made available in booths on railway station platforms and on street corners, then hundreds of thousands of men from the poorest sections of society came forward to have the operation. As one man said, "In India you only go to hospital to die and if the operation is as safe as the doctors say, why must it be performed in a hospital?"

It is rare for vasectomy to be instantly popular in a country, but it is common for numbers to build up with community experience of its use. Deys has suggested that the operation appeals most to male-dominant groups who, within marriage, have a clear segregation of sexual roles. She observed that men coming for vasectomy had commonly used condoms or coitus interruptus, had strongly masculine jobs, such as firemen, policemen, members of the armed forces, fishermen, long-distance lorry drivers and coal miners. They often gave their wives "house-keeping money" and most objected to their wives working outside the home and to being "mucked about with" in relation to female methods of contraception, such as the Pill. It is interesting that vasectomy has proved popular in some Muslim countries and in Korea, which has a strongly dominated male culture.

In Latin America, the quality of "machismo"—the need to demonstrate masculinity and sexual prowess—is well known. As Goldsmith (1972) has pointed out, "It would be easy to conclude that there could be little reason to open vasectomy clinics in Latin America because few men there would be interested in the operation." However, when made available in a culturally meaningful way, the operation is acceptable. The social class distribution of nearly 500 men surveyed in Colombia and Costa Rica demonstrates that most acceptors, as in other countries, come from among skilled (36.5 per cent) and unskilled (20.5 per cent) manual workers.

Technically, vasectomy is an easier operation than tubal ligation because the *vas deferens*, carrying the sperm from the testicle to the prostate at the base of the bladder, courses directly under the skin of the scrotum. It is easy to palpate prior to the operation and it can be cut through a skin incision only a few millimetres long which requires a very small amount of local anaesthetic. The complications of the operation are rather like having a tooth removed, the possibility of infection and haemorrhage, but in practised hands, these should be relatively rare. The man is not immediately sterile, as sperm will be stored in the *vas* on the prostatic side of the cut and up to twelve ejaculations are necessary before the man is secure against the risk of causing an unwanted pregnancy. There is no discernable difference in the volume of ejaculate, as most of the fluid comes from the accessory glands, such as the prostate. The testes continue to function and to produce both hormones (which pass directly into the blood-stream) and sperm after the operation. It is not entirely clear what happens to the sperm that are produced and in some men there is a rise in antibodies against sperm following the operation, but this change has not been demonstrated to have any adverse effect. Some men have congenital abnormalities of their reproductive tract and have what is a natural vasectomy from birth. Occasionally, these have been repaired and fertility restored, demonstrating that it is possible to block the *vas* for many decades without ill effects. Many millions of vasectomy operations have now been performed and it is likely that numbers will increase further in the coming decades.

There is no totally satisfactory way of approaching the fallopian tubes. Greater skill, better facilities and more costly equipment are required to carry out the female operation. The tubes can be exposed through an abdominal incision and so-called "minilaparotomy" is an increasingly popular method. This can be done under local, spinal or general anaesthesia and requires an incision no longer than the last joint of one's thumb. An instrument is inserted into the uterus via the vagina, prior to operation, so that this rather mobile organ and the attached tubes can be brought under the small incision. A variety of endoscopic methods of tubal occlusion are possible. The laparoscope is the one most commonly used and, although it costs up to $10,000 to equip and train a surgeon, it has been possible to make this procedure available in developing as well as developed countries. From the woman's point of view, it provides a rapid, convenient operation, with a small scar which usually becomes invisible in the rim of the umbilicus. In the long term, it may be possible to devise some method of blocking the fallopian tubes by injecting a liquid or paste into the uterus, but until such a method is devised, it seems that minilaparotomy (and also tubal ligation im[illegible] after delivery, which is especially simple) will be performed [illegible] areas and primary health centres in the developing world, [illegible] laparoscopy will probably be reserved to high turnover urban c[illegible] with a particularly skilled specialist team. In Thailand, female s[illegible]lisation has been performed at an average cost of $12.50 per case and as it often gives ten or more years of protection against pregnancy, there need be no limitation about making it available to women who choose it, even in very poor situations.

The *vas* is a thick-walled, long tube and a practised surgeon has a reasonable chance of restoring continuity in men who may have reasons for attempting to reverse the operation. The majority will get sperm back in the semen and an encouraging number will be able to father children. The fallopian tube has thin walls and is comparatively short and attempts at repair are disappointing. In selected cases they may be worthwhile, but they also have the added hazard that, if pregnancy does occur, it may take place in the tubes and not in the uterus.

ABORTION

Abortion is known in all cultures, but the hazards to the woman depend upon two important variables: whether the operation is legal or not and at what stage it is carried out.

The woman seeking an illegal abortion may either attempt to use drugs to "bring on a later period" or seek a mechanical abortion. Wherever abortion is illegal, there is a vigorous trade in supposed abortifacients. Having attempted to terminate a pregnancy with these, many women will turn to operative procedures. The commonest method used by illegal abortionists is to insert a urinary catheter (*sonda*, as it is called in Latin America) and leave this in place for twenty-four hours. Almost always it results in the initiation of labour, although there is a risk of infection, especially if the method is used in unsanitary conditions. Haemorrhage can accompany the actual abortion itself. Like any person in a risk-taking situation, the woman assumes that she will be the one to get away with it—which indeed many do. And the topic is one that arouses such passion that it is almost impossible to comment upon it. Certainly, many women do die from illegal abortions and there can be no justification whatsoever for laws which do nothing to modify the number of abortions taking place, but do subject women to unnecessarily hazardous procedures, humiliation and financial exploitation.

One of the few incontrovertible facts about abortion is that the legal operation is of spectacular straightforwardness and simplicity when compared with most illegal procedures. Up to six weeks after the last period, the products of conception are so small that they can be removed through a 4–6 mm tube or cannula (*see* Fig. 26), rather like an I.U.D. introducer, without any artificial stretching of the cervix—a procedure sometimes called "menstrual regulation". Any source of vacuum can be used to extract the placental and embryonic material, but the most convenient is a cheap, hand-held 50 ml plastic syringe which can be used again many times, because the cervix is not dilated; general or local anaesthetics are not obligatory. The woman may feel nothing, or may suffer menstrual-like cramps of varying severity. The whole procedure takes three to four minutes and can be done in any clean room by a single operator, who must be trained, but need not be medically qualified. Early in pregnancy, the conceptus is so small that it can be missed and then the operation must be repeated. Menstrual delay is not always due to pregnancy, but commercially available pregnancy tests can give false negatives at this time. Where abortion is legal, then the risk of performing a redundant procedure worries some doctors. However, if one waits to be more sure of dealing with a proven pregnancy,

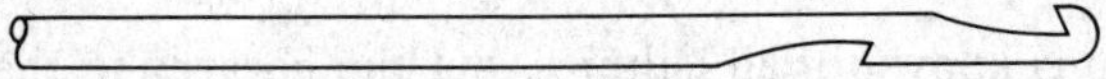

Fig. 26. *The Karman Cannula used in menstrual regulation.*

there will be a slight rise in complications (*see* Fig. 27). Where abortion is illegal, the inability to prove pregnancy can be an advantage and in the Philippines, Malaysia, Taiwan and Latin America doctors are taking creative advantage of the ambiguous nature of menstrual regulation to extend this choice to women.

Vacuum aspiration in the first twelve weeks of pregnancy is an extension of menstrual regulation. As the foetal parts enlarge, a bigger cannula is needed to remove them and the cervix must be stretched. Stretching the cervix is painful and more forceful manipulation increases the risk of perforating the uterus with the operating instruments. As a consequence, the operator needs to be more qualified. A local anaesthetic becomes increasingly necessary and some surgeons use rapid, light, general anaesthetic. The vacuum source for operations in the first twelve weeks needs to be more robust, but can still be hand-powered and need not cost more than $50–100.

The alternative to vacuum aspiration involves scraping the uterus. It is slightly more dangerous than vacuum aspiration, although in the hands of experienced operators it can also be very safe, and it remains the predominant method in countries such as Japan and Hungary.

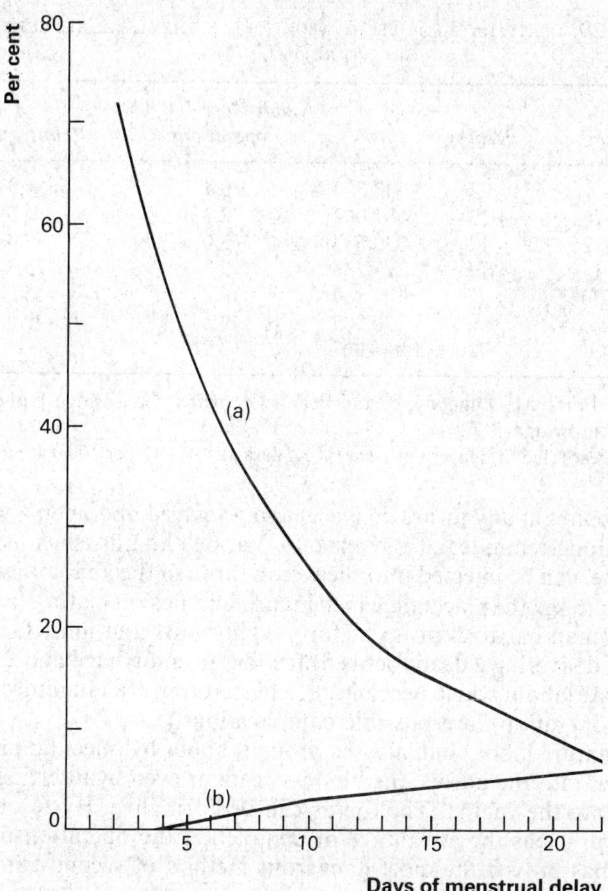

(*Source:* Fortney, J. A., Miller, E. A. and Kessel, E. "Competing Risks of Unnecessary Procedures and Complications (of Menstrual Regulation)." *Studies in Family Planning*. 8, 257 1977)

Fig. 27. *Menstrual regulation: redundant operations versus complications.* (a) unnecessary operations; (b) significant complications.

There is no satisfactory way of performing a second-trimester abortion, which is why a number of apparently dissimilar methods are in use side by side. Most second-trimester operations (up to the sixth month of pregnancy) either require two stages (the first of which initiates premature labour and the second expels the foetus) or involve cutting the uterus and removing the foetus in one operation. One-stage operations leave a scarred womb (a fact to be taken

TABLE 20: DEATH RATE FOR LEGAL ABORTIONS IN THE U.S.A., BY WEEK OF GESTATION (1972–74)

Menstrual age	*Deaths*	*Cases*	*Number per 100,000 operations*	*Relative risk*
8	3	747,550	0.4	1.0
9–10	13	581,002	2.2	5.5
11–12	12	330,537	3.6	9.0
13–15	12	129,536	9.3	23.3
16–20	27	147,160	18.3	45.8
21	6	30,282	19.8	49.5
Total	73	1,966,067	3.7*	—

(*Source:* Potts, M., Diggory, P. and Peel, J. *Abortion*. Cambridge University Press, Cambridge 1977)

NOTE: *Death due to delivery at term (U.K. data 1970s)—12 per 100,000 births.

into account at any future delivery) and a scarred abdomen—which is a lifelong reminder of the episode. Various liquids, such as urea or saline, can be injected into the womb through the abdominal wall in order to kill the placenta, which in turn initiates premature labour. The woman has to wait up to forty-eight hours and must face the pain of delivering a dead foetus. Infection, haemorrhage and failure to initiate labour which necessitates a hysterotomy (a miniature Caesarian operation), are possible complications.

Premature labour can also be brought about by injecting prostaglandins into the uterus, the blood-stream or even by inserting pessaries into the vagina. The foetus can be born alive. Hysterotomy, although it has the advantage of completing the operation in one stage, has proved the most dangerous method of second-trimester options.

It is almost an affront to language to call operations as different as menstrual regulation at six weeks and a hysterotomy at sixteen weeks by the same name of abortion. They vary up to fifty-fold in their risks (*see* Table 20) and by as much, or more, in their emotional costs to the woman and in the burden on those who must operate. Many would argue they also vary greatly in their ethical implications.

RANGE OF METHODS

Where all options of family planning are available each proves acceptable to some people, although the proportion of couples using different methods varies in different societies (*see* Fig. 28).

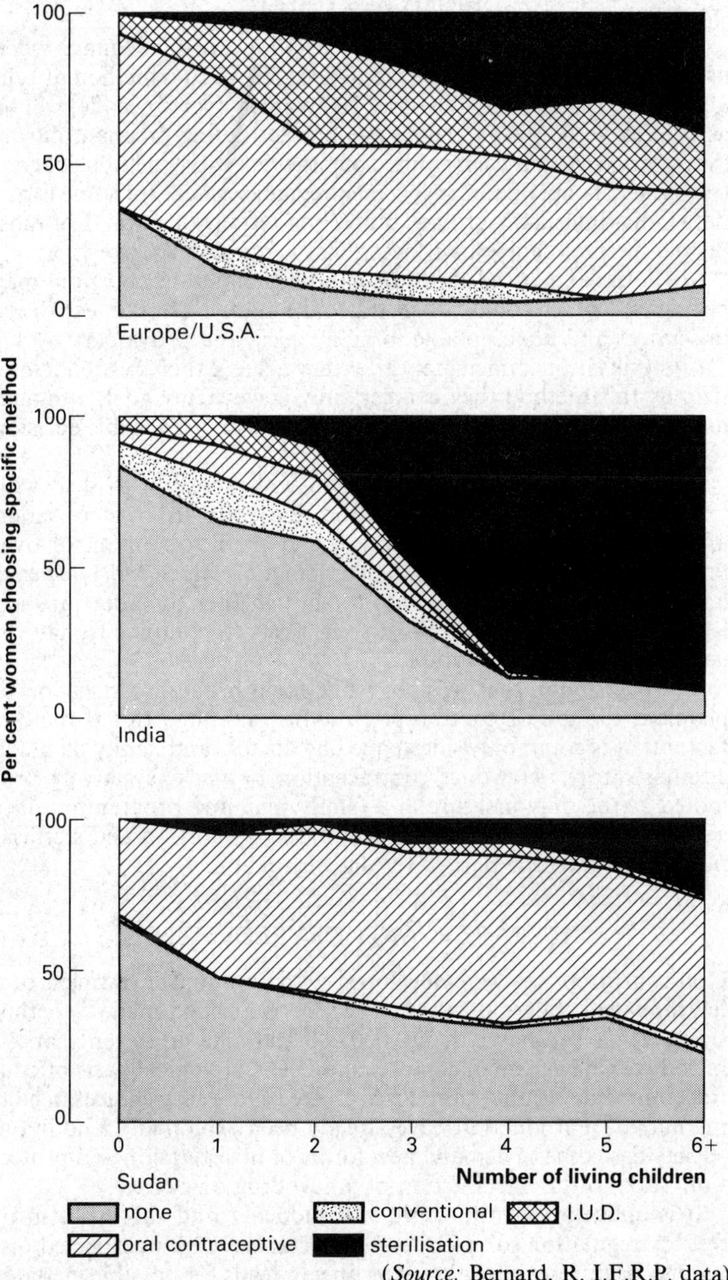

(*Source:* Bernard, R. I.F.R.P. data)

Fig. 28. *Family Planning practices in selected countries (maternity hospital data).*

The reversible methods of contraception are inadequate when used to control fertility over several decades. Even a method as reliable as the I.U.D., when used by 100 women over a decade, will be associated with approximately one-quarter falling pregnant during that interval. As has been pointed out, the reversible methods of contraception are adequate for spacing pregnancies and, for some fortunate individuals, may provide more long-term protection. For most people the real choice that faces them is one of the following:

(*a*) the use of induced abortion, although numerous abortions may be required which could be harmful to the mother's health, expensive in services and unacceptable to many users and providers;

(*b*) sterilisation immediately after they achieve their desired family size. By this method they can certainly achieve any goal, although many parents may not wish to be hurried into an irrevocable decision so quickly;

(*c*) a combination of contraception with abortion to deal with failures, or of contraception (and abortion) followed by sterilisation after some interval, permits secure and predictable control over family size. It is, in practice, the combination which most societies have used in the past, most use today (whether the abortions are legal or illegal) and which most seem likely to continue to have to use for the short-term future.

The one option that will not work for a broad cross section of people is the use of contraception alone, although this is the one factor that is commonly sidestepped by doctors and family planning administrators. At worst, contraception by itself is actively promoted as the only measure in a family planning programme: it is a recurrent theme of this book that induced abortion and sterilisation are an intrinsic part of fertility regulation.

RESEARCH AND DEVELOPMENT

Oral contraceptives were developed with an initial investment of a few thousand dollars and the first I.U.D.s were hand-made by enthusiasts. Today, it may cost $10,000,000 and take up to ten years to introduce a new form of contraception. The biological basis of contraception has become more sophisticated as the easy choices in halting human reproduction have already been exploited. In addition, society has come to demand new forms of investigation and protection prior to the introduction of a new drug or device.

It is unlikely that the world will suddenly find the problem of fertility regulation solved by some spectacular and unexpected discovery. Basic research is throwing up new leads for possible methods of birth-control, but progress is necessarily slow and relatively easy to predict. Current work on hypothalamic-releasing hormones and work on the brain itself may eventually lead to new methods of contraception. In recent years, there has been a burst of work on prostaglandins. These are long-chain fatty acids found in many organs of the body, but in particularly high concentration in the uterus at menstruation, spontaneous abortion and delivery. Given vaginally, by injection or directly into the blood-stream or the uterus itself, prostaglandins will imitate these three processes. Unfortunately, higher doses are required to bring on menstruation than to send a woman into labour and, with the compounds currently in use, side-effects of diarrhoea, vomiting and asthma-like syndromes make the method impractical for routine use. However, as in the development of the Pill, there is a search for prostaglandins which will have the required effect without distressing side-effects and there does remain a possibility that a medical method of "menstrual regulation" will become available within the next decade.

For almost seventy years reproductive scientists have wondered whether it would be possible to immunise women against pregnancy in the way that individuals can be vaccinated against cholera or polio. The human body makes antibodies to most foreign tissues and one of the puzzles of mammalian reproduction is why the mother does not make antibodies against her own foetus, which is in many ways like a skin graft or organ transplant. Despite the special and ill-understood machinery which prevents the embryo and afterbirth making antibodies in the mother, if placental tissue is ground up and injected into an already pregnant animal it will cause abortion. It has not been possible to apply this discovery to the human situation because the antibodies are not specific and they badly damage other tissues such as the kidneys, so that the animals die as well as undergoing the process of abortion.

Human chorionic gonadotrophin (H.C.G.) is a protein hormone formed by the pituitary gland and it is essential to the reproductive cycle. It is also made by the placenta of the embryo and is essential to the maintenance of pregnancy. The placental hormone has the same effect in the mother as the pituitary hormone, but differs structurally. In 1975, Talwar in India used the placental part of the hormone to raise antibodies which might prevent a pregnancy, but without damaging the mother's organs. Immunology is in some ways more like cookery than science and Talwar did the trick of combining immunisation against H.C.G. with immunisation against tetanus, as this improves the strength of the response. The method has been used in some Indian women and by Stevens in post-menopausal women in the U.S.A. It seems likely that the method would need repeating every few years and, while reversibility might be attractive, there is also the possibility that as the effect wore off women would fall pregnant and then abort at relatively late stages of pregnancy. The method is an intriguing one, but it will be some years before it can be fully evaluated.

BARRIERS TO PROGRESS

In the last decade, the support of research relevant to contraceptive development has undergone two set-backs. The pharmaceutical companies have withdrawn more and more from the field. This is because the major profits for innovation come from the developed world. Here the cost of introducing new drugs and the possibility of litigation in relation to rare, adverse side-effects, are so great that directors of companies are likely to encourage research in entirely different fields. Secondly, the amount of money going into universities and specialist institutions has declined in absolute terms. There has been an increase in the amount of money available internationally, particularly within the W.H.O. system, but this represents the least useful resource. International agencies of this type (with their committee structure and expert panels) can literally spend half the money deciding how to invest the other half. Such diffuse and cautious decision-making is not likely to produce backing for the more adventurous areas of research. It is true that considerable investment has been put into prostaglandin research and into the immunological aspects of fertility regulation in recent years, but both followed up leads that had been developed elsewhere. In the case of immunological research the pattern of testing and introduction of possible new technology has been unjustifiably cautious. Currently, it is suggested that fertility control vaccine should be tested for seven years in baboons. While primate testing is prudent, the likelihood of discovering previously unsuspected reaction over seven years of use, compared with two years, is not significant.

GENETIC ENGINEERING

Genetic engineering implies an ability to alter the chromosomal structure of a man or animal, thereby possibly eliminating a harmful genetic trait. In the laboratory it is possible to alter genetic material at the level of bacteria. However, the possibility of doing this in mammals presents almost insurmountable technical problems and, even if there was a strong desire to do it, it is unlikely that any type of genetic engineering of this type would be achieved before well into the next century.

Once conception has taken place and the egg begins to divide, many thousands of individual cells are produced within a few days. Both eggs and sperm can be taken from the body and handled in test-tubes and then replaced in the reproductive tract. There is nothing whatever remarkable about this. After all, fertilisation in fishes and frogs takes place entirely externally and in a dirty pool of water. In fact, it is perhaps surprising how long it took to achieve the successful test-tube fertilisation of the human egg. Using a laparoscope (that is, an optical instrument which can be inserted through a thumbnail-sized incision in the woman's abdomen) the egg is collected immediately prior to ovulation. Since most men masturbate, specimens of semen can be obtained at any time. However, it does seem that sperm need to mature in a special environment in the uterus or outside before they achieve their full fertilising capacity; and the egg, even if it is fertilised outside the woman's body, needs to be returned to a woman in the correct phase of the menstrual cycle.

Theoretically, some manipulative procedures can be carried out in the five days before the blastocyst attaches to the uterus. In experimental animals, a number of remarkable experiments have already been conducted. It is possible to induce twinning or to take two genetically different embryos and mould them into a single entity, or so-called "chimera". It is possible to take the egg and transfer it from the uterus to some other environment, such as under the tissue which surrounds the kidney, or even to the eye, or the brain. Surprisingly, in the new environment, the egg grows more rapidly than it does within the uterus. Indeed, if the free-living egg is removed from the experimental animal and placed in the testes of a male of the same species, it grows particularly rapidly. It seems that the invading cells of the embryo, which will form the placenta (or afterbirth) are rather like cancer cells and have an ability to destroy other cells with which they come into contact. The womb, rather than being a place to receive and nurture a delicate embryo, seems rather to be one of the few places in the body that can adequately resist the remarkable invasive properties of early embryonic tissue.

It is possible to take the egg of one species, for example, a mouse, and transfer it successfully to a related species, possibly a rat. The eggs grow and survive for a number of days, but in no case have gone on to produce a liveborn embryo. These same manipulations could of necessity be conducted with human eggs. There already exists the technology to transfer a fertilised egg from one woman to the womb of another. This does not raise any unique ethical issues, as most societies already have the legal and social machinery for the adoption of children from one family to another (*see* p. 252). And, certainly, the influences which are exerted on a developing human being by its family after birth are much greater than the variation which it would be likely to meet between one intra-uterine environment and another. One could visualise a situation where a woman might, for example, have had a hysterectomy and yet still have her ovaries intact; her egg might be fertilised with her husband's sperm and transplanted into the womb of another woman who might agree to bear this child and return it to the mother at birth. The obvious emotional trauma of the woman who carried the child and then gave it back to its genetic parents would have to be considered carefully by the individuals involved, but it would not be a unique situation. It is common, at least in Western society, to remove children from unmarried mothers and give them to adoptive parents. At least in the biological engineering envisaged, any choices would be mature and informed.

The most extreme manipulation that might be brought about would be to take a dividing egg, separate the cells and allow each to grow into separate embryos, giving rise to a large number (ten or twenty) identical individuals.

It is unlikely that embryos would be transferred between species, and the idea of an ape giving birth to a human baby is not feasible; if not for biological reasons then for straight population reasons. There are not many apes left in the world!

In summary, the application of contemporary or foreseeable biological technologies to human reproduction does not create a serious and uncontrollable threat to society. It does not present any unique choices; but as it does relate to the profound and central facts of human reproduction and of the love and responsibility of bringing up children, these are choices which will have to be handled in the same context as those of maternity, adoption, abortion and sterilisation.

The common newspaper headlines about "test-tube babies" are misleading. The mammalian egg floats free in the tubes and uterine cavity during the first five days of development and can be transferred at this stage from one female to another, or from one organ to another, or even between species. However, once the egg attaches or implants in the uterus it sets up exceedingly complex anatomical relationships between the embryo and the mother, which it is impossible to reproduce in the laboratory. The idea of a test-tube baby developed entirely outside the womb, placed in an incubator and leading to a full term infant screaming on some laboratory bench is an exercise confined to science fiction.

SEX DETERMINATION

In both sexes the cells which will give rise to the next generation are identifiable early in embryonic development. Each ovum and sperm cell has half the complement of chromosomes of a normal body cell. If this were not not the case, every generation would double the number of chromosomes carrying genetic material at the time of fertilisation. Every egg and every sperm cell has an individual and different combination of genetic material set aside as its contribution to the embryo of the next generation.

A normal human body cell contains 46 chromosomes in 23 pairs. In each pair one is derived from the father and one from the mother. In all cases but one, the chromosomes are identical; the genetic information they carry, however, is unique and individual and consists of a sharing of the genetic information which the parents have received from their parents at the time of their conception. In the case of eggs, each one contains 22 body chromosomes and a so-called X chromosome. In the case of sperm there are 22 autosomes or body chromosomes and either an X or Y sperm. If an X sperm meets an egg the result of fertilisation produces an individual with 2 X chromosomes, which is a female. If the sperm fertilising the egg contains a Y chromosome, the resulting individual has an X and Y chromosome and this is a genetic male.

Chromosomes differ in size, X chromosomes are relatively large, whereas the Y chromosome is especially small. Therefore, a sperm carrying a Y chromosome is marginally lighter than one carrying an X chromosome. There is evidence that Y-bearing chromosomes can move slightly more rapidly than X-bearing chromosomes and may be they can survive slightly longer in the female reproductive tract. There are several ways in which sperm could be manipulated so as to increase the probability of one or other sperm surviving and therefore changing the sex ratio. If sperm are taken and placed in a medium of varying density, male sperm can be separated from the female. It may also be possible to do this by centrifugation. There is also some evidence that if unprotected coitus is either timed to be very close to ovulation or to be forty-eight hours or more removed from it, then the sex ratio may be altered.

From the veterinary point of view there is an obvious economic incentive to conducting research aimed at the separation of X and Y sperm. Once it has been achieved in domestic animals, it is likely that the techniques will be applicable to the human situation.

Existing evidence in the human situation suggests it may be possible to change the sex ratio by altering patterns of coitus (*see* Fig. 29), although the change is not sufficiently large to make it a very predictable way of determining a baby's sex.

It is likely that any potential developments in physical separation of sperm would be moderately complicated and possibly sufficiently expensive to put them beyond the reach of the poor of the Third

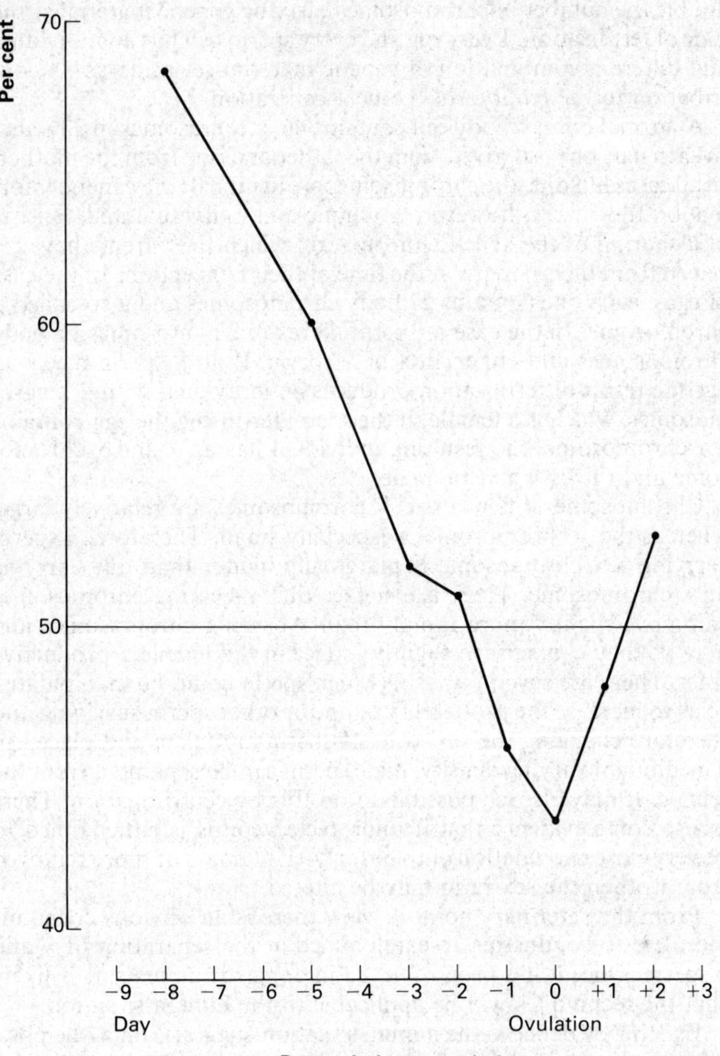

(*Source:* Guerrero, R. "Association of the Type and Time of Insemination within the Menstrual Cycle with the Human Sex Ratio at Birth." *New England Journal of Medicine*. 291, 1056 1974)

Fig. 29. *Percentage of male children born by day of coitus.*

World. However, it is in many of the Third World countries that the desire for boys is powerful. In Korea there are particularly strong social pressures in favour of boys; in most Muslim countries boys are desired and a woman who has a sequence of girl children will lose social status, may be ill-treated and can be divorced. In India the family of the bride is expected to donate a considerable sum of money, property, jewellery or goods as a dowry. Although the system is formally outlawed in India, it is still almost universally applied. It can be economically crippling for a man to have a number of daughters and have to part with his very limited wealth each time he arranges a marriage. It is said that the first thought of a man when told that his wife has delivered another child is to ask what sex it is and if it is a girl to plan how he can raise her dowry. It is not uncommon in Indian newspapers to see court cases when young brides have been mentally or physically ill-treated, even to the point of death, because the in-laws consider they did not bring a big enough dowry with them.

If the ability to determine the sex of one's offspring became a technology that was cheap enough and simple enough to use in the Third World, then in a number of cultures it would be taken up and perhaps would lead to a significant excess of boys in the succeeding generation. If this happened, it would occur most markedly in societies where women currently have a very low social status. We might hope that when an excessive number of boys had been selected, the reduced number of women in the following generation would find themselves in the situation where society valued them more than usual. The ability to undertake biological engineering of this type could effect a welcome social change in the long run.

CONCLUSION

Over the past century contraception has been a controversial subject and the truth has often been obscured.

Undoubtedly, a great many scientists and doctors were frightened away from any objective investigation of fertility control. Yet the few who dared were remarkedly inventive; sound descriptions of the clinical use of I.U.D.s, menstrual regulation, and the potential of the Pill date from the first two decades of the twentieth century. Yet at a time when hundreds of millions of individuals were suffering the private agonies of attempting to control their family size and when thousands of individuals were dying from illegal abortions, society was unable to handle these discoveries. It looked the other way. When clinical use of the I.U.D. did begin on any significant scale it was short-lived.

All methods of fertility control, from coitus interruptus onwards, were condemned as dangerous. When moral sanctions against contraceptive use proved to be ineffective, then threats of cancer were brought in. In this cheap game, the medical profession had a particularly disreputable record.

By the time oral contraceptives became a reality the world was beginning to mature, although old attitudes still influenced many decisions. This new and remarkable drug became the focal point of an emotional whirlpool, the centre of a social storm; the problems posed by clinical use were often obscured by a scientific fog. The

TABLE 21: MORTALITY ASSOCIATED WITH CHILD-BEARING AND WITH FERTILITY REGULATION

	*Deaths per 100,000 women per year**		
	Age		
	20–24	30–34	40–44
No birth-control	6.1	13.9	22.6
Legal abortion only	1.6	1.7	1.2
Pill (non-smokers)	1.4	2.2	7.1
(smokers)	1.6	10.8	58.9
I.U.D.s	1.0	1.4	1.9
Condoms (and other traditional methods)	1.6	3.6	4.2
Condom plus legal abortion	0.2	0.3	0.2

(*Source: Modified from Tietze and Lewit 1977*)

NOTE: * For each method birth related deaths due to method failures are included as well as method related deaths. The calculation is based on maternal mortality, measured Pill, I.U.D. and abortion risks and known failure rates for Western women.

basic questions about side-effects were not clearly enunciated. The public wanted proof of safety when none was possible. Even today, the major biological questions surrounding the use of oral contraceptives, such as any possible adverse or beneficial effect on the incidence of cancer, remain unanswered. Certain side-effects are unpredictable in advance of widespread and prolonged use. This generalisation applies not only to the Pill but to any other pharmacologically active method of contraception which may be introduced in the future.

The world has moved from a stage when any method of contraception is condemned to a stage of alternating enthusiasms. In the case of both the Pill and the I.U.D., adverse effects have been proved which were not initially suspected. However, in both cases, for potential users the benefits outweigh the known risks and the methods continue to be popular. Their use is also likely to increase in developing countries (*see* Table 22). Injectable methods of contraception are newer than the Pill but already have a substantial usage in the developing world. New methods of contraception are likely to arrive slowly and each one will provide as many unknown factors and problems as those already in use.

Abortion and sterilisation are by far the most controversial of fertility regulation methods. However, as surgical procedures, they carry with them less unknown factors than medical methods. One of the tragedies of the contemporary world is that, while the record of the Pill and I.U.D. has been more disappointing than many people hoped, the record of safety for early abortion has been better than

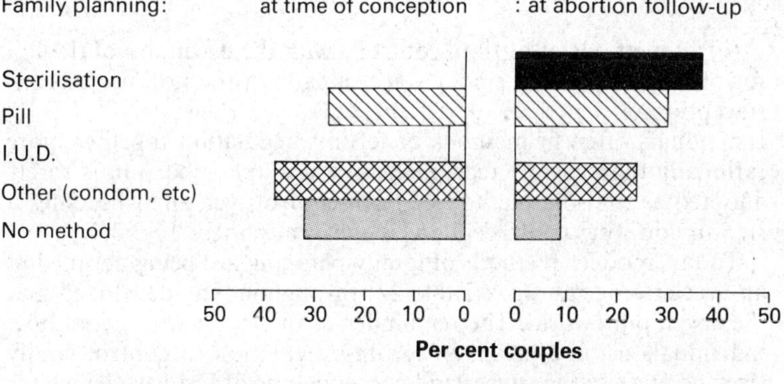

(*Source:* Bernard, R. I.F.P.R. data)

Fig. 30. *Abortion as a turning point in family planning* (*Singapore: 3,152 legal abortion cases*).

anyone would have guessed even a decade ago. But, just as the world refused to use I.U.D.s when they first became a possibility and lost precious years in the development of the Pill through society's collective obscurantism, so the developed and the developing world is still not using abortion and sterilisation as effectively as it might.

The combination of abortion and the reversible methods of contraception is not only a predictable and effective way of controlling human fertility, but it provides the least dangerous choice from the point of view of the user (*see* Table 21). When the risks of all methods, and possible combinations of methods, are reviewed, two major conclusions stand out very clearly:

(*a*) the combination of legal abortion and mechanical methods of contraception is an order of magnitude safer than any other option facing a couple—with the exception of sterilisation;

TABLE 22: ESTIMATED GLOBAL USE OF CONTRACEPTION

	Millions of Users	
	1970	*1977*
Voluntary sterilisation	20	80
Oral contraceptives	30	55
Condom	25	35
I.U.D.	12	15
Other	60	70
Total	147	255
Abortion	30–35	30–55

(*Source:* Ravenholt, R.)

(*b*) all methods of fertility control—with the exception of the Pill for older women who smoke—are safer than the non-use of contraception.

Individuals often fit methods of fertility regulation together more rationally than society recognises. For example, abortion is rarely adopted as the sole method of birth-control, yet often becomes a step in adopting contraception or sterilisation (*see* Fig. 30).

Today, modern methods of family planning are being adopted at an accelerating rate (*see* Table 22) throughout the developed and the developing world. The remainder of this book will review how individuals use the means of fertility regulation to control family size and analyse the causes and consequences of fertility change for the community.

SELECTED REFERENCES AND BIBLIOGRAPHY

Aitken-Swan, J. *Fertility Control and the Medical Profession*. Croom Helm, London 1977

Cartwright, A. *Parents and Family Planning Services*. Routledge & Kegan Paul, London 1970

Henry, L. *Anciennes Familles Genevoises*. Presses Universitaires de France, Paris 1968

Himes, N. E. *A Medical History of Contraception*, Gamut Press, New York 1963

Hulka, J. "A Mathematical Study of Contraceptive Efficiency and Unplanned Pregnancy." *American Journal of Obstetrics and Gynecology*. 104, 443 1969

James, W. "Parameters of the Menstrual Cycle and the Efficiency of the Rhythm Method of Contraception." *Population Studies*. 19, 45 1965

Karim, S. M. M. *Prostaglandins and Reproduction*. M. T. P. Lancaster 1975

Kleinman, R. (ed) *Family Planning Handbook for Doctors*. I.P.P.F., London 1974

Lee, L. T. and Paxman, J. M. *Legal Aspects of Menstrual Regulation*. Law & Population Monographs (No. 19) Tufts University, Boston 1974

Morris, N. & Arthure H. *Sterilization*. Peter Owen, London 1976

Oldershaw, K. L. *Contraception, Abortion and Sterilization in General Practice*. Kimpton, London 1975

Peel, J. and Potts, M. *Textbook of Contraceptive Practice*. Cambridge University Press, Cambridge 1969

Population Reports. Department of Medical Affairs, The George Washington University Medical Center, Washington, D.C. 1973 onwards

Potter, R. G. "Inadequacy of a One-method Family Planning Program." *Social Biology*. 18, 1 1971

Potts, M. "Against Nature." *Biologist*. 17, 143 1970

Potts, M., Diggory, P. and Peel, J. *Abortion*. Cambridge University Press, Cambridge 1977

Rock, J. *The Time Has Come*. Knopf, New York 1963

Royal College of General Practitioners *Oral Contraceptives and Health*. Pitman, London 1974

Short, R. V. and Baird, D. T. (eds.) *Contraceptives of the Future*. The Royal Society, London 1976

Tietze, C. and Lewit, S. "Mortality and Fertility Control." *International Journal of Gynaecology and Obstetrics*. 15, 100 1977

Westoff, C. F., Potter, R. G. and Sagi, P. C. *The Third Child*. Princeton University Press, Princeton 1963

Whelpton, P. K., Campbell, A. A. and Patterson, J. E. *Fertility and Family Planning in the United States*. Princeton University Press, Princeton 1966

Wood, C. *Vasectomy and Sterilization*. Temple Smith, London 1974

Chapter 7

Achieved Fertility

The level of fertility in any society is determined by a wide range of factors. These have been examined in previous chapters. We have noted the importance of cultural norms influencing patterns of marriage, attitudes towards the size and spacing of families, and the use of contraception and abortion. The most concrete realisation of all these influences is the typical range of achieved family size in a society. This varies from the two-child family of most Western nations today, to the average of ten live births found in married women amongst the North American Hutterites.

The aim of this chapter is to look at achieved fertility in various societies and explore the particular combination of factors which determine this. We start by considering two societies in which fertility has come close to a biological maximum and contrast these with the lower levels of fertility found in many of the so-called "primitive" societies. We then look at fertility levels in pre-industrial Europe and in the transition from moderately high to low fertility in developed nations. Finally, we consider fertility in developing countries, taking the examples of Nigeria, Brazil and mainland China.

NATURAL FERTILITY

Louis Henry has suggested the term "natural fertility" as appropriate for societies where births are not subject to any deliberate control and fertility approaches a biological maximum. Two populations which have achieved very high levels of fertility, which have been well documented for half a century or more, are the Hutterites of North America and the Malay population of the Cocos Keeling Islands in the period 1890–1950. In both societies, total fertility rates of 8.0 or higher have been recorded. A brief consideration of these two populations provides us with a yardstick by which to measure the extent of fertility control in most other known societies.

THE HUTTERITES

The Hutterites, or more precisely the members of the Hutterian

Brethren Church, are an Anabaptist religious sect, originating in Zurich in 1525, who now live in North America in small self-contained colonies. They migrated to the U.S.A. in the late nineteenth century and then to Canada, during and after the First World War. Detailed church records of births, marriages and deaths have been kept since their arrival on the American continent, so that it is possible to obtain an accurate picture of the demographic history of this unique population.

Eaton and Mayer show that in the seventy years from 1880 to 1950, the Hutterite population increased nineteen-fold from 443 to 8,542 and at the end of this period was growing at a rate of 4.1 per cent, or doubling every sixteen years. By 1964, the population had reached an estimated 15,000, the majority of whom lived in the provinces of Alberta and Manitoba, on the Canadian prairies.

In the period 1946–50, the total fertility rate was 8.06 live births per woman. The average family size of women who had completed their child-bearing was about ten, two-thirds having between seven and twelve children; only 3 per cent remained childless, but there were no recorded instances of women with more than sixteen live births. A married woman had an average probability of twelve children, if she married in her eighteenth year and lived with her husband to the end of her reproductive period.

Although the Hutterites have a higher level of fertility than most developing countries, their mortality rates are those of a highly developed country. Infant mortality in 1950 was 45 per 1,000 live births. The gross reproduction rate in that year was just over 4.0, but more significantly, the net reproduction rate of 3.66 was uniquely high, due to the low mortality. Thus, the gross reproduction rate of Palestinian Arabs in the same period was 3.81, comparable to that of the Hutterites, but the net reproduction rate was much lower at 2.17. Unlike most other societies, Hutterite men tend to outlive their wives, probably as a result of excess mortality in women, resulting from the burden of child-bearing.

The high fertility is the result of a generally high level of reproduction amongst the whole female population. By the age of thirty-five, only 4 per cent of women remained unmarried and by forty-five this had fallen to 1 per cent. Nevertheless achieved fertility is still below its potential, as a consequence of relatively late age at marriage. Marriage is delayed until a woman has been baptised. As baptism is possible only for mature adults with a good understanding of the Hutterite creed, it is unusual before the age of nineteen. As a result, few women marry under the age of twenty. Illegitimate births are virtually unknown. Hutterites believe that sexual relations prior to marriage are very sinful and there is a strong indoctrination of the young against these, with strict supervision of adolescents and punishment of offenders by ritual excommunication.

After marriage, women are more or less constantly exposed to intercourse. Husbands are seldom absent from home and between 1875 and 1950 only one divorce and four separations were recorded. Widowhood is more frequent and remarriage rare. The only prohibition on intercourse is for a few weeks before childbirth and about six weeks after. Voluntary abstinence for any significant period is not found. Birth-control and abortion are virtually unknown, so that frequent pregnancy inevitably results from this regular exposure to intercourse. The Hutterites see contraception as the equivalent of murder and believe that the worldly will have to face millions of unborn children on Judgment Day. Withdrawal and all mechanical methods are seen as sinful. The rhythm method, while not specifically condemned, seems not to be used. There was, however, evidence as early as 1950 of a growing use of sterilisation on other than strict medical grounds.

The inevitable result of the pattern of behaviour described is that marital fertility is very high indeed. Between the ages twenty-five and twenty-nine, half the married women produce a child each year and even as late as forty-five, one woman in ten becomes pregnant. Late marriage and the absence of illegitimacy mean that fertility is low under the age of twenty and builds up gradually to a peak in the late twenties. However, it remains high through the later reproductive years, when the frequency of births begins to fall sharply in most countries. Figure 31 contrasts the age-specific fertility-rates of the Hutterites in the period 1946–50 with those of England and Wales in 1964, the high point of post-war British fertility. The higher fertility in England for the 15–19 age-group is due to the greater number of early marriages, prenuptial conceptions and illegitimate births.

This high fertility reflects not simply an absence of any effective mechanisms to reduce the level of births, but also the high cultural value placed on children. Couples follow the directive to "be fruitful and multiply". This is in many ways fundamental to the continual expansion of the sect, without recourse to outside recruitment or proselytising. This in turn has helped their way of life to be preserved and their values to persist. Hutterite society is so organised that there are no economic pressures towards planned parenthood. All property is shared and there is no individual pursuit of wealth. Children are cared for communally and no couple is disadvantaged by having a large family. Good medical care has ensured that most children are born live and survive to become parents themselves, while the communal education prepares them for marriage and parenthood along traditional lines.

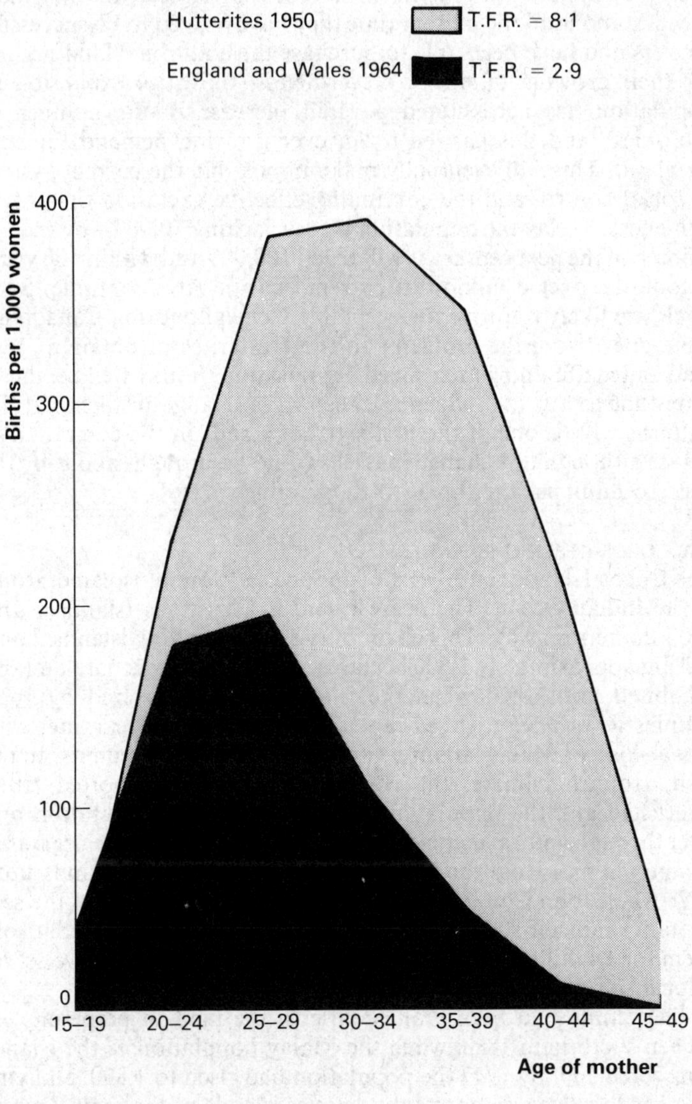

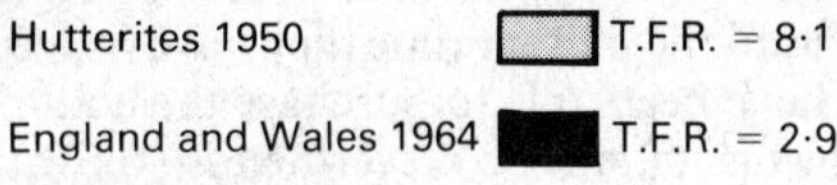

(*Source:* Eaton, J. W. and Mayer, A. J. *Human Biology*. 25, 206 1953; Registrar General's *Statistical Review of England and Wales* for 1964)

Fig. 31. *Age-specific fertility rates for the Hutterites (1950) and England and Wales (1964).*

Unlike many developing countries, there have been no Malthusian checks to population growth (in the form of disease, malnutrition or war), and until the present time they have proved to be successful farmers and have been able to purchase the additional land needed for their growing numbers. Nevertheless, the huge expansion in population has necessitated a rapid increase in the number of "colonies" and this has led to an ever growing demand for new farmland. This will eventually make impossible the current system of social control and the continuing effective exclusion of outside influences. Today the population is approaching 30,000—by the beginning of the next century it will reach 100,000 and within 100 years it could be over a million, if current growth rates continue. Such levels are likely to prove unacceptable to neighbouring Canadians, quite apart from the problems to the Hutterites of obtaining new land and maintaining their social organisation. It may well be, therefore, that as outside influences creep in, a change in their fertility patterns will be one of the first signs of a shift in the community's values although this change in itself would be brought about by the need to minimise the threat to those values.

THE COCOS-KEELING ISLANDERS

The Cocos Islands south-west of Indonesia form an isolated group in the Indian Ocean. The nearest land is Christmas Island, nearly 800 kilometres away. This chain of twenty-seven tiny islands, comprising approximately 1,500 hectares of land area, was bare and uninhabited until 1825 when the islands were discovered by John Clunies-Ross, a Scottish sea captain, who returned a year later with a boat-load of Malay labourers and began planting coconuts. In the lush, tropical climate, the coconuts and other imported fruits flourished and the population grew, initially by immigration and later through natural increase under a paternalistic régime organised by the Clunies-Ross family. This family "ruled" the islands until 1978 when John Clunies-Ross (the great-great-grandson of the sea-captain, and self-styled fifth King or "Tuan" of the islands) sold them for £4 million to the Australian government, who have set up a local self-governing council to run the islands.

The family had been granted title to the land in perpetuity by Queen Victoria in 1888, when the Malay population of the islands numbered 500. By 1947 the population had risen to 1,800, all living in a single village on one of the smaller islands of the atoll. During these sixty years population growth was largely the result of natural increase; the crude birth rate of the Malay population averaged 55 per 1,000, and reached 60 in several years. Overall fertility levels approach those of the Hutterites in the same period, although the growth rate is less spectacular, due to high mortality throughout the period. The crude death rates were well above 30 per 1,000 until 1912 and remained as high as 20 in 1947, while infant mortality was above 300 per 1,000 live births in the earlier period.

The demographic history of the islanders in the period 1888 to 1947 has been studied by T. E. Smith, making use of the virtually complete record of births, marriages and deaths. This enables a detailed reconstruction of the life-histories of individuals from birth through marriage and child-bearing to death. For much of the period the total fertility rate is as high as that of the Hutterites, but there are important differences in the timing of births, which reflect different values concerning marriage and the existence of some mechanisms for limiting fertility at later ages.

During the period with which we are concerned, most Cocos girls married before reaching the age of twenty and had an average of between eight and nine live births if they survived through the child-bearing period. More than two-thirds had conceived their first child before marriage, so that child-bearing at early ages is much more common than amongst the Hutterites (*see* Fig. 32). For the minority of women who married at the age of twenty or later, mean family size was substantially lower than that of the Hutterite women, who typically marry at such later ages, suggesting that some form of fertility regulation existed amonst the Islanders and that the high level of child-bearing in the group as a whole is largely due to very early exposure to intercourse. Throughout the sixty years studied there were fluctuations in period fertility rates linked to shifts in the age at marriage.

By the ages of twenty-five to twenty-nine, the fertility of the Islanders is at its peak, with practically all the women married; nevertheless the level of marital fertility at these ages is below that found in the Hutterites. From the age of thirty onwards there is a more rapid falling-off in the number of births, so that lower fertility rates at these later ages compensate for the higher fertility before the age of twenty-five.

The high fertility of the Islanders results from early marriage and child-bearing, with no resort to family limitation through contraception; although there is evidence of knowledge of and use of abortion, especially in later years. Spacing of children is evident amongst older women and is probably associated with abstention from intercourse during lactation. Smith reports that the Islanders display a great love of children and that in the period studied they enjoyed a secure and peaceful way of life, isolated from outside contacts, with full employment and guaranteed freedom from real want and hunger. Given this pattern of early exposure to intercourse and marriage,

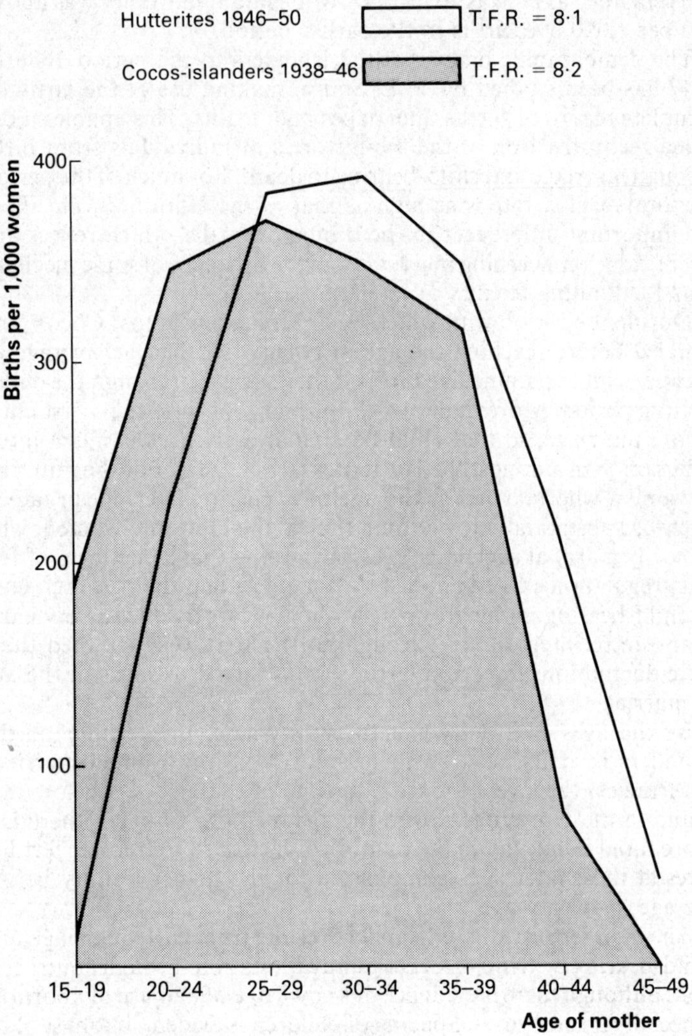

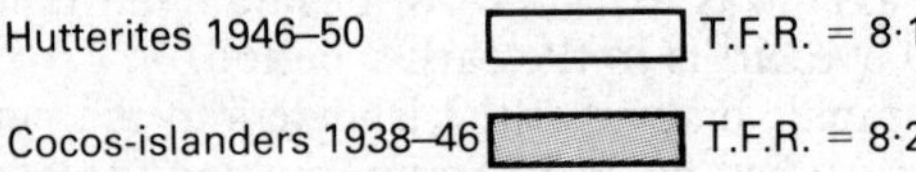

(*Source:* Eaton and Mayer (op. cit.); Smith, T. E. *Population Studies*. 24, 94 1960)

Fig. 32. *Age-specific fertility rates for the Hutterites (1946–50) and the Cocos-islanders (1938–46).*

minimal economic pressures towards family limitation, an absence of contraception and high infant mortality, the exceptional level of fertility is perhaps not unexpected.

By 1947, the population was far greater than was needed to maintain the coconut plantations, and from 1949 onwards the government of Singapore began a scheme of controlled migration which reduced the Malay population of the islands by more than two-thirds in a decade. By the early 1960s the crude birth rate amongst those who remained had fallen to a little over 30 per 1,000 according to the U.N. Demographic Year Book. "Tuan" John is said to have strongly advocated the Pill in an attempt to avert further overpopulation. By 1978, as the old régime wound to its end, the total population of the Islands was estimated at about 700, including the present Clunies-Ross and their six children!

CONCLUSION

The Hutterites and Cocos Islanders are rare examples of a very high level of reproduction which persists over several decades. While both societies share certain common features—a high value on children, the rejection of contraception, a period of economic security in which having many children was not a burden—they differ in respect of factors which limited fertility. Late marriage in the Hutterites and abortion and abstinence at later ages in the Islanders kept fertility below its maximum and resulted in differences in the age-distribution of births (*see* Fig. 32). Population growth in the Cocos Islands was less rapid than in many African or Latin American countries today because of high mortality over many years; in this respect it is the Hutterites who stand out as so exceptional in maintaining very high fertility in the face of low death-rates. This has led to growth-rates of 4 per cent and higher per annum for over fifty years. The pattern of fertility we have described above is often believed to have been the common experience of pre-industrial and primitive societies and it is to an examination of these that we now turn.

HISTORICAL AND ANTHROPOLOGICAL COMMUNITIES

It is often assumed that in pre-industrial societies in the past, fertility was universally high and that the slow rates of population growth experienced over most of mankind's history were the result of high death rates countering this high level of births. Before the Agricultural Revolution of some 10,000 years ago, the average long-term growth rates of human populations must have been very low indeed and it has been argued that at this time unrestricted fertility, at a maximum level, was necessary to avoid the disappearance of the species in the face of very high mortality.

However, several lines of evidence point to a more rigorous control of fertility in many instances. Even if we assume that before industrialisation only 50 per cent of children born survived to reproductive ages, a total fertility rate of 8.0 (such as we described for the Hutterites above) would have led to a net reproduction rate of 2.0 ensuring that the population doubled every generation. Even allowing for a further 15 per cent mortality during the reproductive period, growth rates would be higher than we know to have been demographically possible.

It seems certain, therefore, that population growth was kept in check by other than biological factors and that the balance of population was the result of cultural practices influencing reproduction through delayed marriage, sexual abstinence, abortion or coitus interruptus, together with the deliberate killing off of children soon after birth. Birdsell has suggested that between 15 and 50 per cent of children born were so killed in the Pleistocene Period.

While evidence on the populations of such distant ages is slender, recent studies of contemporary primitive societies indicate that, in many of these, population growth is restricted by cultural practices and historical demographers have likewise shown that rates of natural increase in pre-industrial Europe were restrained by social behaviour which kept fertility well below its biological potential.

Finally, it has been suggested that in animal populations a number of homeostatic mechanisms may exist which keep numbers below the ceiling imposed by resources. Wynne-Edwards provides many examples of otherwise inexplicable animal behaviour, which could have had the effect of limiting reproduction, and seeks an explanation for the development and persistence of these in his theory of "group selection". This latter has been challenged by Lack and others, who argue that he presents nowhere any clear examples of this process occurring. If, however, similar mechanisms are suggested for human populations, there seem to be fewer difficulties in offering explanations in terms of cultural adaptation.

FERTILITY RESTRAINT IN SMALL-SCALE SOCIETIES

Alexander Carr-Saunders concluded from a review of population patterns in a wide range of primitive societies that they all included customs whose prime function was to restrict population to a certain optimum size, in relation to resources. He argues convincingly that the assertion that all societies practise some form of fertility regulation is much more valid as a generalisation than the Darwinian view that slow population growth has been the result of high mortality and that fertility has been necessarily high to ensure survival.

More recently, Devereux, in a study of 350 primitive societies, points to abortion as a near universal practice, often carried out in late pregnancy, which, together with infanticide, was the basic means of spacing children. These two measures, together with post partum abstinence, associated with prolonged lactation, seem to be the essential mechanisms for population control in small-scale societies. This does not mean that they arise out of individual perceptions of population pressure. It is more likely that those who follow such practices do so from a belief that the spacing out of surviving children in a family is personally advantageous, or because the burden of too many dependent children is incompatible with the adequate functioning of the group. However, cultural practices which serve to minimise population increase, and so avoid overexploitation of scarce resources, are likely also to have enough adaptive advantage to be further reinforced. Recent studies of modern hunting and gathering populations support such a view.

The !Kung bushmen One such people are the !Kung bushmen (The exclamation point in !Kung refers to an alveolar-palatal click. In speech, the tongue tip is pressed against the roof of the mouth and drawn sharply away producing a hollow popping sound—Kolata 1975). This tribe lives in the Kalahari Desert of Southern Africa and, until the rapid changes that have overtaken them in the past decade, they reflected a way of life that can have changed little over 11,000 years since their ancestors had lived out their lives in the late Pleistocene period. Indeed, late stone age artefacts have recently been discovered at the same watering holes where the modern !Kung set up camp, which suggests that much the same techniques were used then for hunting animals.

When first studied in 1950, the !Kung bushmen had a life expectancy at birth of only thirty-two years, lower than that of any major developing country today, with only 60 per cent of the population surviving past the age of fifteen. Even with mortality at this level, fertility as high as that of the Hutterites would have ensured a steady expansion of numbers. In fact, there seemed to have been little population growth, and the mean number of children born to women who survived to the end of their child-bearing years was no more than five. The estimated age-specific fertility rates for married women are substantially below those of the Hutterites at all ages (*see* Table 23).

The reason for the low fertility of the !Kung—and indeed of other hunters and gatherers—lies in the need to space births, not with a view to limiting total family size, but in order to accommodate the pattern of child-bearing to their nomadic way of life. The consequent containment of population growth would prevent over-exploitation of resources and thus have further adaptive value.

At the root of the problem is the simple inability of a mother to carry more than one child around with her normal baggage, the importance of her role in the collection of food, and her inability to nurse more than one child at a time. The !Kung mother has to travel over 4,000 kilometres a year with her child and the burden of additional births too soon after a previous child would be an impossible one; at the same time the absence of suitable food for young infants makes prolonged lactation essential to their survival. A minimum of three years between births is essential and a typical birth interval seems in fact to have been closer to four.

TABLE 23: AGE-SPECIFIC MARITAL FERTILITY RATES HUTTERITES AND !KUNG BUSHMEN

Age of Woman	*Hutterites (1946–50)*	*Dobe !Kung*
15–19	92	47
20–24	336	261
25–29	498	205
30–34	442	174
35–39	370	120
40–44	215	64

(*Source:* Eaton, J. and Mayer, A. *Social Biology*. 25, 206. 1953; Dumond, D. *Science*. 187, 713 1975)

The likely mechanism for achieving such intervals—remembering that a Hutterite wife aged twenty-five to twenty-nine is having on average one child every two years—is the effect of prolonged lactation on fecundity, probably combined with a significant period of post partum abstinence. Abortion seems not to have been practised on a scale likely to explain the intervals. Some women admitted to resorting to infanticide when births followed too closely on one another, but this seems to have been comparatively rare, as closely-spaced births were exceptional. Whatever the mechanism, their success is undoubted and of great adaptive importance in that the pattern of mobility, vital to hunters and gatherers, is maintained, population growth is minimised and survival is ensured as reproduction is kept well below potential and so can rise in the face of increased deaths. In times of high mortality, many more children will die in infancy, so that the need for birth-spacing is reduced and the fertility rate will rise in compensation.

Today, 95 per cent of the !Kung live in agricultural villages. This dramatic change has affected their whole way of life. Women have lost a certain amount of their status as their economic role as gatherers has gone. Instead they remain in their villages, preparing food and looking after the shelters, while the men raise crops and take on all the roles with the neighbouring Bantu. In this way they are emulating their traditional pattern of male dominance.

The nomadic !Kung seem to have been free of many of the diseases associated with the diet of more complex societies and also to have suffered less from degenerative disease, but recent studies show that diet has changed in their new settled life: they are taller, fatter, heavier, and more prone to illness. There have also been important demographic changes. Age at menarche has fallen, birth intervals have shortened and the population has begun to grow rapidly due to the resultant increase in fertility. The shortening of birth intervals seems to be due to reduced lactation and increased body fat which enables ovulation to occur earlier. The need for long birth intervals has been reduced now that the society is sedentary, the women unproductive and alternative foods are available for young children.

Such changes do not necessarily reflect those that took place when other hunting and gathering societies became agrarian, but there is a growing recognition that the demographic changes occurring in the Agricultural Revolution may have involved increases in both birth and death rates, with a slight widening of the gap between the two, rather than a fall in mortality with fertility unchanged at a high level. The studies of the !Kung remind us too, as with later industrialisation, that "progress" is bought at a price. The increased population growth can be sustained because of the new systems of food production, but the standard of life for members of the society may fall in certain ways. The association between increased fertility and an abandonment of the women's economic role indicate the importance of examining the status of women in seeking explanations for various fertility patterns.

The Australian Aborigines There is strong evidence for the practice of infanticide as a means of population control in many primitive societies. (Rasmussen reported thirty-eight cases of female infanticide out of ninety-six births amongst the Netsilik Eskimos of Pelly Bay.) This not only limited population increase in a people faced with a life of great hardship and a battle for survival in a particularly hostile environment, but also helped to balance the adult sex ratio in the face of high male mortality associated with hunting accidents, drowning and fighting.

High rates of infanticide have also been noted amongst the Australian Aborigines, some estimates being as high as 30–50 per cent of all children born alive. The reason given for the practice was the need to keep down the number of children, because if numbers increased too rapidly there would not be enough food for everybody. If some children were not killed at birth, many others, both adults and children, would face greater risks of starvation.

When Europeans first made contact with Aboriginal groups, the average family size seems to have been typically two or three, and rarely more than five. Infanticide was especially common where there was an older child still in need of nourishment by his mother, suckling frequently being continued to the age of three or beyond. Today, infanticide is certainly rare, although it may survive in more remote areas, and family size has probably grown as a result of the breakdown of traditional restraints and a fall in natural mortality.

A surgical procedure amongst Australian Aborigines which has puzzled both anthropologists and those interested in family planning is the ritual subincision of the penis. In this the urethra is either opened from the tip of the penis to the base of the scrotum or a second channel is made from the base of the penis to the urethra. This radical surgery is carried out at puberty using a stone knife and subsequently the man must squat like a woman when urinating. Another consequence is that most or all of the ejaculate is deposited outside the vagina when intercourse takes place. Aboriginal informants believe that one act of intercourse is unlikely to lead to pregnancy and that coitus must be repeated frequently if conception is to take place. Perhaps the most attractive of the many theories put forward to explain the origins of subincision is the suggestion that it arose from a desire to imitate the bifurcate penis of the kangaroo, and so to emulate that animal's renowned capacity for repeated acts of intercourse.

The simpler of the two procedures described above gives an anatomical situation rather like a one-holed flute. More imaginative commentators have suggested that the man simply covers the artificial opening if he wishes conception to take place. If this were the case, it would be unique amongst contraceptive methods in rendering the male infertile in all isolated cases, with conscious effort necessary to ensure impregnation; whereas all other techniques either involve permanent sterility or the temporary "turning off" of the potential for fertilisation. However, it remains unclear whether the Aboriginal population does see the ritual as related to contraception. It may have grown up as a result of social evolution and possibly have been sustained because of its adaptive advantage to a population living under harsh conditions. Whatever the view of subincision, it is certain that the Australian Aborigine is as clear in his mind as the rest of the human race that sexual intercourse leads to pregnancy. The well-known controversy that has surrounded Aboriginal insight into copulation, may well reflect that most anthropologists have been more gullible than most Aborigines.

Other small-scale societies To the Aborigines and Eskimos, concern over population control seems to arise from the hardship of their lives and the constant struggle for survival. In other societies the key factor seems rather to be the desire to maintain standards of life and conserve "status" goods. Mary Douglas, citing the examples of the Rendille in Kenya (with their concern over limited camel stocks) and the Tikopia (fearing shortages of ceremonial food such as coconut cream), has argued that "it is the demand for oysters and champagne, not for basic bread and butter, that triggers off social conventions which hold human populations down". She argues from this standpoint that, in studying the developing countries of the world today, more attention should be paid to the gains experienced by the mass of population from controlled fertility. She also asks questions about what hope for advance the masses have, and what valued goods depend on limiting family size, suggesting that the earlier adoption of birth-control by upper socio-economic groups in stratified societies reflects their greater access to prestige goods and greater concern over maintaining living standards.

The Tikopia are outstanding amongst primitive groups in that there exists among them strong social disapproval for couples who have had more than two or three children. They are also outstanding in their use of coitus interruptus alongside abortion, infanticide and celibacy in order to minimise population growth. This pattern, vividly described by Firth on the basis of observations in 1929, later broke down under the influence of Christian missionaries, resulting in a steady expansion of numbers and an apparent worsening of the subsistence situation, leading many to seek work outside the island.

Studies of primitive societies show that many have practices which serve to limit fertility and so reduce rates of population growth. Such practices arise for a variety of reasons and do not all have a direct demographic intent; many do, however, and it can be argued that in the others the value of the resulting population equilibrium would be one reason for the persistence of the practices. When the pattern of life in such communities changes, whether through outside influences, or a shift from hunting and gathering to agriculture, the existing mechanisms of population control tend to break down, leading to an increase in growth rates. What becomes clear is that in such societies there are good reasons for people to want to limit child-bearing, and that measures are available to enable them to do so, even if the chosen means seem unsatisfactory, or even immoral, to Western eyes. The "survival" of the society is much more to do with this search for ecological equilibrium, than a pursuit of maximum fertility to prevent extinction through high mortality. We can argue, therefore, that man's "natural" state is one of balance between deaths and births, but that this has been achieved as much by the control of fertility as through the Malthusian checks of disease, famine and war.

PRE-INDUSTRIAL SOCIETIES

Slow rates of population growth in pre-industrial Europe have traditionally been attributed to generally high mortality, with some periods of exceptionally high death rates associated with famine, epidemic and war. These high death rates countered the prevailing high level of fertility (which was assumed to be largely unrestricted and to vary little from year to year). While over-all population increase was slight in the long run, it was accepted that there would have been both periods of more rapid growth, when mortality levels were relatively low, and periods of population decline following years of plague or harvest failure. The increase in population growth rates during the eighteenth century resulted from declining mortality, while the level of births remained high.

This picture has now been strongly questioned as a result of the work done over the past twenty years or so by historical demographers who have patiently sifted the evidence provided by European parish registers and other local records, in order to build up a more accurate picture of population in the days before census and vital registration. We can now see that European fertility patterns of this period were well below the biological potential and also subject to considerable fluctuation. This suggests that some of the mechanisms of fertility control discussed in previous chapters may have been operating.

The importance of the West European pattern of delayed marriage was recognised at an early stage, as a result of the work of Hajnal (*see* p. 58). Because women typically married in their mid- and late twenties, their potential for child-bearing was limited, so that birth rates were well below those found in developing countries today and mean family size substantially smaller than the ten or so live births associated with unrestricted fertility and earlier marriage.

Evidence supporting the existence of factors regulating fertility within marriage came later through three channels. These were:

(*a*) studies of parish registers;

(*b*) records of births, marriages and deaths for particular groups like the British peerage, especially where these were sufficiently detailed to permit a reconstruction of age-specific birth (baptism) and death (burial) rates;

(*c*) the tracing of defined "cohorts" of women by the technique of family reconstitution, pioneered by Louis Henry and developed in Britain by E. A. Wrigley. This involves bringing together various bits of demographic data from registers, using the names of individuals as a linking device, and enables the computation of age at marriage, completed family size and even birth intervals.

The marital fertility of the French aristocracy in the eighteenth century was well below that of the peasants of the time, especially at later ages (*see* Table 24); this is a pattern which indicates effective family limitation, most probably through the use of coitus interruptus (*see* p. 116). Further support for such practices in less aristocratic groups is to be found in Meuvret's documentation of a sharp

TABLE 24: LEGITIMATE FERTILITY RATE—
EIGHTEENTH CENTURY FRANCE

Wife's age	*Aristocracy*	*Peasantry*
20–24	0.226	0.420
25–29	0.167	0.412
30–34	0.063	0.369
35–39	0.018	0.282
40–44	0.006	0.144
45–49	0.000	0.013

(*Source:* Goubert, P. *Beauvais et le Beauvaisis.* S.E.U.P.E.M. 1960)

fall in marital fertility in parts of France in 1694–5 following a bad harvest. Hollingsworth's detailed reconstruction of the population history of the British peerage likewise indicates a major decline in fertility in the seventeenth century, suggesting a similar resort to birth-control.

Colyton In Britain, the main published work on family reconstitution has come from the Cambridge Group for the Historical Study of Population, and especially from Wrigley's detailed exploration of the parish of Colyton in Devon which possesses an exceptionally complete register (providing an uninterrupted record of baptisms, burials and marriages from 1538 to 1837). Colyton is a large parish of more than 2,800 hectares, with a recorded population of 1,641 at the time of the first census in 1801. During the three preceding centuries, the population fluctuated considerably, reaching a peak of just over 2,000 in the 1640s and falling back to a low point in the early eighteenth century.

During the first hundred years up to 1640 there was in most years a substantial surplus of baptisms over burials leading to the steady rise in population. From 1646 to 1740 burials usually exceeded baptisms and the population declined from its peak. After a period of about forty years in which numbers were approximately equal, there was again a surplus of baptisms over burials which gradually became larger and the total numbers rose towards the level of the mid-seventeenth century.

The major reversal in population growth occurred in 1645, when Colyton experienced its last plague outbreak, which (in the twelve months from November 1645 to October 1646), resulted in the death of about one-fifth of the whole population. The second major shift is also a dramatic one. In the decade 1776–1785, the average surplus of baptisms over burials is 0.5 per annum, a level typical of the previous forty or so years, but in the next ten years this rises to 7.8, and continues to increase thereafter.

TABLE 25: MARRIAGES, BIRTHS AND DEATHS COLYTON 1560–1837

Years	*Age at Marriage M*	*F*	*Completed Family Size (under 30 marriages)*	*Expectation of Life*	
1560–1646	27.2	27.0	6.4	1538–1624	43
1647–1719	27.7	29.6	4.2	1625–1699	37
1720–1769	25.7	26.8	4.4	1700–1774	42
1770–1837	26.5	25.1	5.9		

(*Source:* Wrigley, E. A. "Family Limitation in Pre-industrial England." *Economic History Review*. 29, 82 1966)

If we look at changes in the pattern of marriage, fertility and mortality over these three centuries, the shifting trends are equally striking (*see* Table 25). Expectation of life falls and rises again. Age at marriage for women rises and then declines to a lower level than at the start of the period. Fertility, measured by the mean number of baptisms per woman married before the age of thirty, falls sharply, remains at a low point for over a century and then rises dramatically at the end of the eighteenth century. The proportion of childless marriages rises from 7 per cent to 18 per cent and then falls back to 8 per cent. The fall and rise of marital fertility can be seen at all ages, suggesting the influence of some mechanism of fertility regulation throughout marriage.

Wrigley also provides data on birth intervals, the most striking feature of which is the increase in the interval between the penultimate and last birth in the period spanning the late seventeenth and early eighteenth centuries. He sees this as typical of a community beginning to practise family limitation, where a decision to limit family size is often followed by an unplanned pregnancy or a change of mind, in both cases the resultant birth tends to occur at a later date than would have been the case if normal spacing had occurred. In the same period women marrying under the age of thirty had their last child at an earlier age, thirty-eight rather than forty, which shows success in family limitation in later marriage.

Wrigley sees the fall in marital fertility in the middle years of the period studied as indicating a pattern of deliberate family limitation, in the sense that "social or individual action caused fewer children to be born, or at all events to survive long enough to be baptised, than would have been the case without such restraints". He considers various possible explanations. One is that a change in suckling habits led to longer birth intervals, but this could not account for the more striking lengthening of such intervals at later ages. Another is that there was a decline in fecundity due to undernourishment (at a time of economic reverse), which would fit in with the observed rise in child mortality, but he feels that the change is too sudden to be explained in this way. He doubts whether the lower fertility at older ages of those marrying before thirty can be explained by exhaustion from child-bearing, a more plausible explanation being that they were more likely to have had all the children they wanted and so wished to limit their family size.

On the other hand, deliberate family limitation seems not to fit in with the increase in child mortality, as one would expect mothers to have compensated for this with more births—or, alternatively, that reduced family size would have increased chances of survival. However, Wrigley reminds us that "the early hours of a child's life provide many occasions when it is easy to follow the maxim 'thou shalt not kill, but needst not strive officiously to keep alive'" and suggests that, if we see the fall in fertility as a reaction to population pressure, it might well be expected that women would simultaneously delay marriage, reduce the number of births and permit more children to die, just as we saw that many primitive groups have practised both birth spacing and explicit infanticide.

Wrigley also points to evidence, provided by Gautier and Henry, and Ganiage, that late eighteenth century rural populations in France began to limit their fertility, in the absence of modern methods of contraception, by means of coitus interruptus or reservatus, abortion and possibly infanticide, commenting that any means which were available to French peasants at the end of the eighteenth century were equally possible for English communities a century and a half earlier. Likewise, our review of primitive populations showed

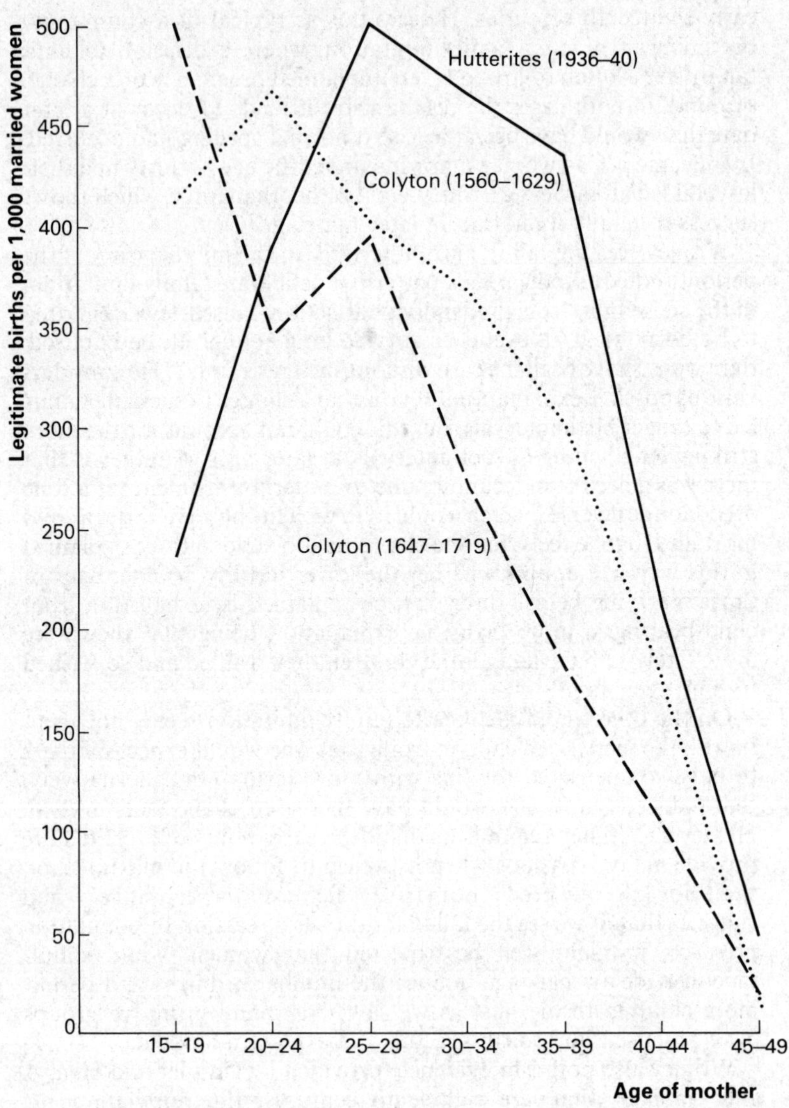

(*Source:* Eaton and Mayer (op. cit.); Wrigley, E. A. "Family Limitation in Pre-Industrial England." *Economic History Review*. 30, 82 1966)

Fig. 33. *Age-specific marital fertility rates for Colyton and the Hutterites*. NOTE: the data in this diagram refers to births to married women only, not to total female population at each age, as in the fertility "silhouettes".

that fertility control was possible by a number of readily available means.

Once we accept that pre-industrial societies have the ability to control their fertility, it is plausible to argue that they will do so, if certain social changes create the need. Plague and hardship in seventeenth century Colyton may well have provided such a trigger for delayed marriage and a reduced number of births after marriage. Certainly, the demographic patterns delineated by Wrigley point to the existence of striking fluctuations in the level of births as well as deaths in at least one pre-industrial community. Even in the earlier "high fertility" period, the level of marital fertility in Colyton fell below that of the Hutterites at all but the youngest ages, when the British figures are kept high by the effect of prenuptial conceptions (*see* Fig. 33).

INDUSTRIALISED SOCIETIES

The achieved fertility of industrialised nations is remarkably similar across the globe. All have experienced major declines in fertility during the last century and during the economic depression between the two World Wars birth rates fell to low levels in many countries, from Australia to Scandanavia, and from Austria to Uruguay. After the Second World War, there was a baby boom in most countries as families were reunited. In the boom years of the later 1950s and 1960s fertility rose to a relatively high level, particularly in the U.S.A. From the mid-1960s, birth rates have been falling in North America and Western Europe and are approaching, or falling below, replacement level, in the mid-1970s.

Two countries, the United Kingdom and Japan, make a particularly interesting comparison because both have experienced a similar secular decline in fertility, although the timing of the decline and the chosen means of achieving this have been very different. It is one of the themes of this book that different societies will struggle to use whatever arbitrary selection of fertility regulation methods happen to be open to them, in order to achieve comparable goals in terms of family size.

ENGLAND AND WALES

At the time of the first census in 1801, the population of England and Wales was just below 9 million. In the next fifty years it doubled to nearly 18 million and by 1910 it had doubled again to reach a total just over 36 million. Since 1910, the rate of growth has slowed considerably, but population increased each year until 1976, when the estimated size was nearly 49¼ million.

The most striking feature of demographic trends over the last hundred years has been the decline in fertility. In the decade 1871–80 the crude birth rate was 35.5 per 1,000 people. By 1901–10 it had fallen to 27, and by 1931–40 it was below 15. Following the Second World War, the birth rate rose briefly to over 20 in 1947, fell back in the 1950s before rising to a second post-war peak of 18.5 in 1964, and has subsequently been falling steadily to reach 11.5 in 1977, the lowest annual figure since civil registration of births commenced in 1838.

From 1870 to 1920 the death rate was also falling, though less rapidly, so that there was a gradual reduction in rates of natural increase. Since 1921, it has been steady at about 12 per 1,000, the increase in life expectancy over the past fifty years being countered by the growing proportion of old people in the population.

The major period of fertility decline lies between 1875 and 1935 (*see* Fig. 34). The birth rate fell for the first time in 1877 and thereafter was reduced in successive years to a low point of 14.4 in 1933. The dramatic nature of this change in reproductive behaviour is well illustrated in the reduced family size of married couples (*see* Table 7). Women marrying in 1860 had an average of about six live-born children and more than a quarter were destined to bear eight or more children. For their great-granddaughters marrying in 1925, the mean family size was just over two and less than 2 per cent had as many as eight children.

It is now generally agreed that this dramatic change was the result of deliberate restriction of fertility by married couples, although many other explanations from sunspots and bicycle-riding to changed diets and the stress of modern living have been put forward at various times. There is no evidence to suggest a reduction in fecundity. Indeed, improved health and a move from normal lactation to artificial feeding in the early twentieth century may have increased the likelihood of conception over the period. The mechanisms involved must, therefore, have been delayed marriage, a decreased exposure to intercourse within marriage, or the deliberate use of abortion or contraception to restrict the number of live births.

The slight increase in mean age at marriage between 1870 and 1910 is not large enough to account for much of the decline in fertility. Nor is there any reason to believe that there was a significant reduction in rates of coitus, although these may have been relatively low. Neither an increase in abstinence by older couples nor a shift to alternative, non-vaginal sexual practices should be ruled out.

The major means by which fertility was controlled probably lay more in the areas of abortion and contraception. There was an increase in resort to illegal abortion (*see* p. 203), the use of coitus inter-

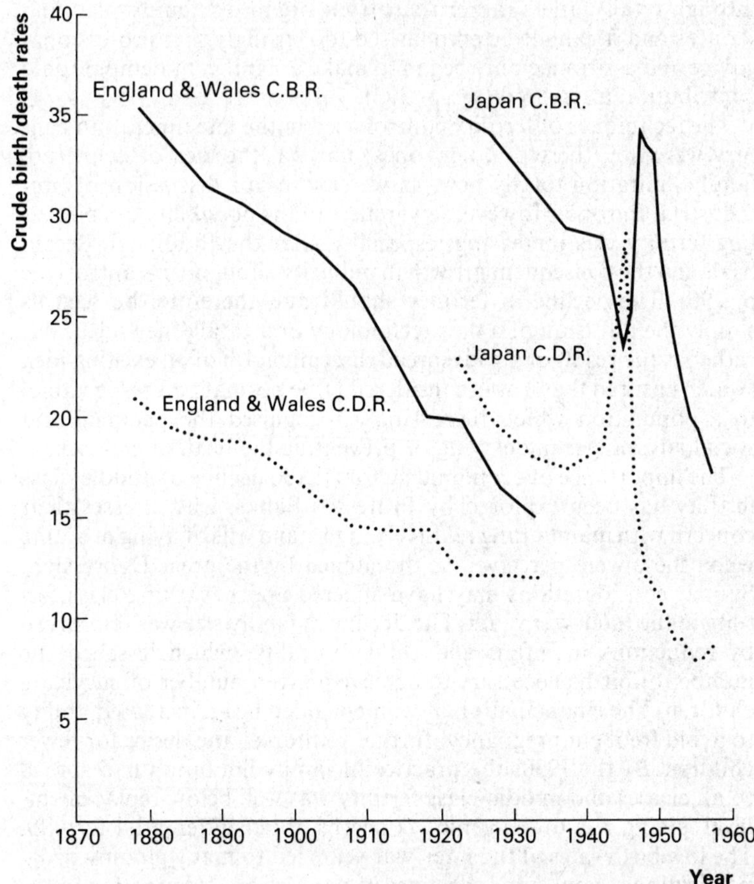

(*Source:* Registrar General's *Statistical Review of England and Wales* for 1965; Muramatsu, M. *Japan*. Country Profile, Population Council, New York 1971)

Fig. 34. *Crude birth and death rates for England and Wales (1875–1935 in five-year averages) and for Japan (1920–1957: in five-year averages from 1920 to 1944).*

ruptus became widespread, and there was a significant trade in rather poor quality condoms. Only 16 per cent of women (marrying before 1910 and using birth-control) adopted appliance methods, with the majority relying on withdrawal. Even for those marrying in the early 1920s, two-thirds still relied on this method and it is not until marriages of the 1940s that appliance methods are chosen by a majority of family planning users. Even then these were largely obtained through retail outlets rather than from organised family planning services and it cannot be emphasised too strongly that professional advice and assistance only began to make a significant demographic contribution after 1960 (*see* p. 293).

The techniques of fertility control used in the late nineteenth century were not, therefore, new ones; nor was the idea of deliberate family limitation totally new, as we saw in our discussion of pre-industrial Europe. However, awareness of the possibility of controlling fertility was increasing, especially after the Bradlaugh-Besant trials and the consequent growth in publicity about birth-control (*see* p. 290). The decline in fertility should not, therefore, be seen as simply the diffusion of a new technology or a totally new idea, but rather as the result of a widespread dissemination of an existing idea (which ensured that it was considered to be normal and respectable) to a population which increasingly recognised the personal and social advantages in delaying or preventing the birth of children.

The importance of economic factors in the decline of middle-class fertility has been explored by Professor Banks, who stresses their concern with maintaining relatively high standards of living at a time when these were perceived as threatened by the great Depression. Similar considerations may have affected upper working class fertility in the inter-war years. The decline in family size was reinforced by reductions in infant and child mortality, which lessened the number of births necessary to achieve a given number of surviving children. The emancipation of women, aided by an increased ability to avoid frequent pregnancy, further reinforced the desire for fewer children. By the 1930s the practice of family limitation had spread to all classes and middle-class fertility was well below replacement-level, giving rise to "eugenic" concerns about differential fertility. The low birth rates of the inter-war years led to many gloomy prognostications about future declines in population, culminating in the appointment of a Royal Commission on Population. From 1922 until 1945, the net reproduction rate was consistently below unity, although in no year did the number of births actually fall below the number of deaths.

After the war, the birth rate rose sharply for a few years, as couples were reunited and started their families, but by the 1950s it had fallen again and most commentators assumed that the pattern of fertility was returning to that of the inter-war years. In fact, a substantially larger proportion of women were marrying, and the post-war cohorts proved more likely to have at least two children. By 1957 the birth rate was rising again and in 1964 the total fertility rate was higher than it had been for fifty years—with the exception of the year 1920, when live births had approached the million mark at the end of the First World War. Fears of a declining population gave way to alarm over possible overpopulation, as projections indicated an increase of 10 million in the population by the end of the century.

In 1965 the birth rate fell and continued to do so for over a decade until, in 1977, it had reached the lowest level since official records were started. The net reproduction rate was back to the level of the 1930s, accompanied this time by an actual decline in population as births fell below annual deaths and net migration continued to be outwards. The *Guardian* newspaper ran a series entitled "Vanishing Britons". Similar falls in fertility had occurred throughout Europe. In West Germany the birth rate fell below the death rate as early as 1973, the total fertility rate falling to 1.47 in 1977.

The precise reasons for this latest fall in fertility remain uncertain. In Britain, changes in abortion legislation, the advent of oral contraception and improved family planning services (*see* p. 295) are all relevant. Certainly, there has been a major change in the pattern of contraceptive usage over the past decade (*see* Fig. 35). However, these changes cannot fully explain the falling birth rates which would probably have occurred even if there had been no Pill, and no family planning on the N.H.S. The basic cause is the decision of increasing numbers of young married couples to postpone child-bearing in marriage, combined with substantial reductions in higher order births and some recent declines in illegitimate and pre-maritally conceived legitimate births. The latter patterns may reflect increased capacity to avoid unwanted births, but equally important is the increase in female work-force participation, growing social and educational opportunities for women, and continuing doubts about the economic future, reflected in uncertainties in the male employment market.

The total size of the population of the United Kingdom is expected to change relatively little over the next forty years. It is projected that the 1976 population of 56 million will decline for a few years, before rising slowly to a level of 56.7 million in 1991. The latest projections for the years 2001 and 2011 are 57.5 and 57.7 million. Anticipated growth rates are, therefore, well below those of the past decade and barely reach one-tenth of the rate of most developing countries. The projected population for London in 1991 shows a decline from its peak in the 1930s to a level comparable to the 6 million of 1900, holding out hope for an improvement in the quality of city life.

Although total numbers may change very little, there will be some important shifts in age structure. The number of children under the age of fifteen, 12.8 million in 1976, is well under 12 million in the projections for 1981 and 1991. There will, however, be an increase

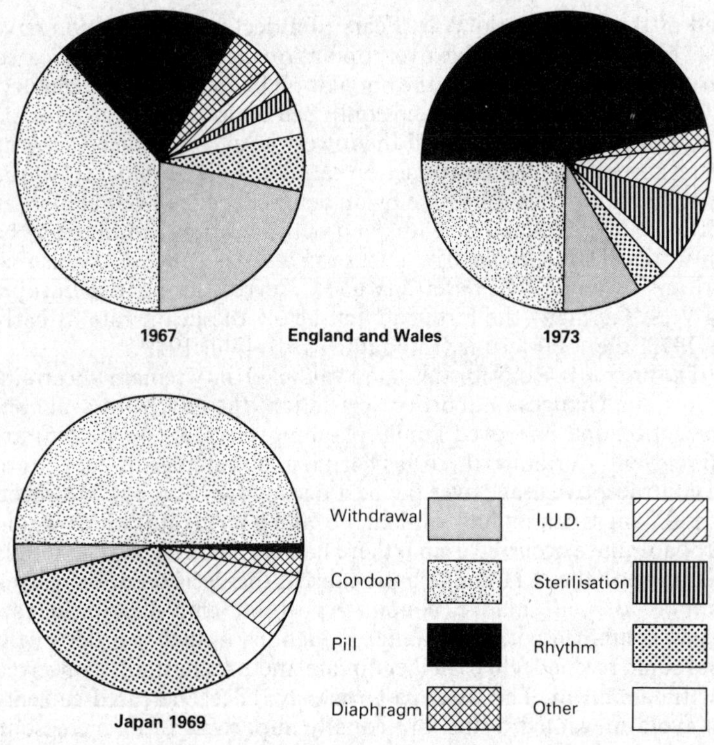

(*Source:* Cartwright, A. *Parents and Family Planning Services* and *How Many Children*? Routledge 1970 and 1976: Public Relations Room, Prime Minister's Office, Japan)

Fig. 35. *Contraceptive methods in current use.*

in the number of people aged seventy-five and over, from 2.8 million in 1976 to 3.6 million by 1991. In this year there would be similar proportions of the population (20 per cent) in the fourteen and under age-group and the sixty and over age-group.

Whether such projections prove accurate will depend largely on the assumptions about future fertility on which they are based. If the current low period fertility rates were to continue and recent marriage cohorts proved to have a completed family size substantially below replacement level, the population of the United Kingdom at the turn of the century could be well below its current level. However, if current rates proved to be reflecting essentially the timing of births, and there were a return to the fertility levels of the 1960s, the population could still reach 60 million by the year 2000.

JAPAN

The story of population growth and fertility regulation in Japan differs in a great many of its details from that of England and Wales, although the over-all pattern of fertility decline has been similar in many respects. The transition from high to low birth rates began later in Japan and was completed in a much shorter period. Japan's experience has been of particular interest to demographers, because it is the clearest example of a non-European nation which has completed this transition.

In 1975, the population was over 110 million, representing a threefold increase in the previous 100 years. As recently as 1920, the birth rate had been 35 per 1,000, similar to that of Britain in the 1870s. From 1925 it declined steadily, rose sharply after the Second World War, and then fell rapidly after 1949 (*see* Fig. 34); a net reproduction rate of unity was reached by the mid-1950s and sustained thereafter in much the same way as Britain in the inter-war period.

Until the later decades of the nineteenth century, Japan's population under the Tokugawa regime had grown only slowly. As in pre-industrial Europe, fertility seems to have been well below its biological potential, as a result of delayed marriage, primitive contraception and infanticide, which was euphemistically termed *mabiki* (literally, "thinning"). The evidence of contemporary reports and the legends of families suggest that infanticide was widely practised, mainly in relation to female children, and reflected in the high sex ratios recorded in the Tokugawa.

After 1870, Japan entered a period of industrialisation and modernisation which was associated, as in Britain, with rapid population growth, the main cause of which seems to have been an increase in fertility. Mortality remained high until the early twentieth century, with dysentery, typhoid, smallpox and malaria all continuing to take their toll. In 1873, anti-abortion legislation, based on Western models, was introduced. The practice of *mabiki* seems to have gradually died out, so that by the end of the century sex ratios were normal and the child–woman ratio increased from 490 per 1,000 in 1888 to 559 per 1,000 in 1913.

Birth rates rose at the end of the nineteenth century and remained moderately high (between 30 and 35 per 1,000) until the Second World War. The peak period for fertility was 1920–24, when the crude birth rate averaged 35.8. Between 1925 and 1937, there was a reduction in both birth and death rates, with an average growth rate of about 1.5 per cent per annum, somewhat higher than in the previous fifty years.

There followed eight years of war during which birth and death rates were inevitably disturbed: in 1945 the death rate rose to 29, while the birth rate fell to an all-time low of 23. After the war came five years of Allied occupation. The Japanese had to withdraw from their overseas empire. Their industry was destroyed and the wounds of defeat ran deep in a nation with a long martial tradition. In the immediate post-war years, 5 million Japanese returned from abroad and with the reuniting of families there was a sharp rise in the rate of conceptions, despite growing pressures to restrict family size. Like other developed countries, Japan experienced a post-war "baby-boom", the birth rate rising to 34.3 per 1,000 in 1947 and remaining high for the next two years. At the same time there was evidence of an increasing number of women turning to illegal abortion. This was one factor which led to the passing of the Eugenic Protection Law which permitted abortion, initially on health and later on wider economic grounds (*see* p. 298 for a discussion of the development of fertility control services in Japan).

Following the passing of the Eugenic Protection Law, the birth rate, which was 32.8 per 1,000 in 1949, fell to under 20 in 1955. In these six years the annual total of births fell from 2,697,000 to 1,727,000, while the total of legal abortions rose by over a million. The dramatic nature of the birth rate decline in these years may give the impression that Japan moved from high to low fertility within a decade using only one method, that of abortion. The true picture is rather more complicated. The post-war level of birth rate was in many respects artificially high and the downward trend in fertility is (perhaps) better seen as commencing in the 1920s and interrupted by the years of war and occupation. Over this longer period, two factors are of importance. Firstly, the age of marriage rose substantially. In 1920, 18 per cent of women aged fifteen to nineteen and 69 per cent of those aged twenty to twenty-four were married. By 1940, this had fallen to 4 per cent and 47 per cent, and by 1955 to 2 per cent and 34 per cent. Secondly, marital fertility fell dramatically at ages above thirty. In 1925, one in four women aged thirty to thirty-four and one in five aged thirty-five to thirty-nine had a live birth each year. Thirty years later the rates were nearer to one in ten and one in twenty. This pattern in typical of a nation moving rapidly towards family limitation.

From 1956 onwards the crude birth rate in Japan has remained below 20 and the death rate has been within one point of 7 per 1,000, with average annual growth rates of about 1 per cent. There was a temporary aberration in 1966, when the birth rate, which had been increasing marginally over the previous five years to a level of 18.7, fell dramatically to 13.8 and then revived to 19.5 in 1967: 1966 was the year of "Fire and Horse" according to the Japanese zodiac signs and a long-standing superstition is that any woman born in this year is doomed to misery and will destroy her husband if she marries. Unable to predetermine the sex of their children, many couples seem to have decided not to have a baby at all that year, resulting in a decrease of about 460,000 births from the 1965 level. There was no change in the reported incidence of legally-induced abortion, so that the mechanism would seem to have been contraception or abstinence.

Crude rates of births and natural increase give a misleading picture of the actual pattern of fertility in Japan today (*see* p. 34). Since 1956, the net reproduction rate has been consistently below unity and the current rapid growth is attributable to the age-structure of the population, which is weighted towards women of reproductive age. Even in the 1970s the number of potential parents remains high, but as the smaller birth cohorts of 1955 onwards reach child-bearing ages, crude birth rates are likely to fall, resulting in a diminishing rate of natural increase. Nevertheless, population projections suggest an increase from 110 million in 1975 to 140 million by 2025, when the proportion of old people in the population will have doubled from 8 per cent to 16 per cent.

The small families of contemporary Japanese couples are achieved by widespread use of contraception, backed up by legal abortion. The most commonly used method is the condom, followed by the safe period, which is practised more extensively in Japan than in any Catholic country (*see* Fig. 35). Coitus interruptus is used by a dwindling minority of couples; I.U.D. use has grown only slowly, the method not being officially approved until 1974, despite its long history in Japan. Oral contraceptives are still not licensed, although they are available for controlling irregular periods, and in 1975 only 3 per cent of women had ever used the Pill. Sterilisation has never been made widely available and currently less than 30,000 female and under a 1,000 male sterilisations are performed annually. The annual number of abortions, which was running at over a million from 1953 to 1962, has been falling and stood at less than 700,000 in 1974, but these numbers may be underestimated, as surgeons have been reluctant, for tax reasons, to declare the numbers of operations performed.

One reason for the more rapid completion of the transition from high to low fertility in Japan undoubtedly lies in the fact that it changed its abortion law at an earlier stage. However, the pattern of rising numbers of abortions as birth rates fell, followed by growing use of contraception, leading eventually to a reduction in the number of abortions, is probably characteristic of all industrialised nations, the picture in most being obscured by lack of data on illegal abortions.

Despite the fact that Japan's population is growing faster than that of any other developed country, and despite the high level of density of population (second only to Holland amongst major industrialised nations) awareness of some twenty years of below replacement fertility has led many people to question the desirability of the small family pattern. A public opinion poll taken in 1969 showed that 35 per cent of respondents believed that population limitation was detrimental to the nation—a view shared by leading industrialists concerned about future labour shortages. Subsequently, a government report underlined the implications of existing fertility levels in the long term and made suggestions for the strengthening of social development programmes, including special child allowances for parents with three or more children. Whatever steps may be taken, it seems likely that future fertility levels will continue to be determined by individual couples, rather than government policy, and that most of these will continue to prefer smaller families, achieved by whatever means are available to them.

DEVELOPING WORLD

No country in the developing world has an achieved family size comparable to that of the unregulated fertility of the Hutterites. As in pre-industrial Europe, there is some control of fertility; although in some countries, such as Pakistan and Bangladesh, the degree of regulation is not as high as it was in sixteenth or seventeenth century Europe.

Patterns of family planning practice in the developing world often differ, in the profile of methods selected, from those in developed countries. The groups within a society who first adopt more modern methods of family planning are not necessarily the same as they were in the West. The balance of motivation between a desire to space pregnancies and a need to end fertility differs between countries. These variations need to be understood in order to attempt to make predictions about future changes in fertility within the developing world and to assist in the planning of those family planning services which will be most useful and acceptable to the communities concerned.

AFRICA

Throughout Africa populations are growing rapidly, with birth rates of around fifty, and an annual rate of natural increase of between 2 and 3 per cent. Such growth rates have existed only since the early 1960s and reflect a substantial fall in death rates in recent years, although life expectancy remains low and infant mortality high by world standards. Africa is not "over-populated" in the sense that many Asian countries are: Nigeria, the most densely populated of the major nations, has only 68 people per square kilometre, compared with nearly 200 in India and about 600 in Bangladesh. However, the rate of population increase is proving a major problem. *Per capita* income and food production remain low and have declined in some countries.

Africa is the only major world area in which a majority of couples believe four or more children to be the ideal number for a family. Six or more children are usually preferred here and most couples with as many as this number say they would like more. One source of the high fertility of the continent is, therefore, the continuing pervasive belief that it is good to have a large family, and that many children mean wealth, prestige and the blessing of God and ancestors. For the individual couple, sterility or limited fertility is a humiliating misfortune; on the other hand children are an important visible sign of success and achievement, bringing prestige and influence within the community and offering security in old age. For the father, children bring social status, proof of virility and help on the land; for the mother, a justification of her very existence. At the same time, traditional patterns limit reproduction by encouraging the spacing of births. Uncontrolled fertility is seen as animal-like and a threat to the health of existing children.

The Yoruba of Nigeria Further insights into African fertility patterns are provided by a series of studies by Caldwell of Yoruba women from the Western and Lagos states of Nigeria.

Like most peoples of sub-Saharan Africa, the Yoruba traditionally farmed communal land. Decisions about land use were made by the extended family, who lived together in what were often huge compounds. Traditional society was agrarian, based largely on subsistence production. Children had great economic value, so that family limitation made little sense for most couples in the face of high mortality in infancy. Even so, sexual abstinence was common in marriage and was supported by widespread polygamy, the marriage relationship being considered relatively unimportant in the context of the extended family system.

In recent years, life for the Yoruba has changed a great deal. Increasing numbers live in urban areas and are exposed to the influence of Western ideas. Old patterns of communal tenure of land and community residence are breaking down. It seems inevitable that this will weaken the extended family system and that nuclear family values will spread in the decades ahead, as the level of urbanisation, education and literacy increases.

A desire for many children remains strong amongst the Yoruba today. Practically all couples want at least four children and only a third see the ideal number as less than six. A large number of children is seen as essential to ensure that some will survive and be willing to help their parents as they grow older. Most of the wants of Yoruban society are satisfied within the household by human activities rather than machines, so that children are useful from an early age and many will further be involved in market-orientated activities (such as food processing, weaving and dyeing). Consequently, few couples see the birth of an additional child as problematic and there is no evidence that large families are economically disadvantaged.

Nevertheless, the marital fertility of the Yoruba falls well below that found in the Hutterites, as a result of substantial periods of sexual abstinence between births and a high frequency of female terminal abstention. Most women abstain from sexual activity for two or three years after the birth of a child. Such spacing of births is not the result of any "taboo" on intercourse, but rather a response to concerns over the health of the previous child and of the mother herself. The spacing of pregnancies can thus be seen as a means of maximising the number of surviving children and as such is fully compatible with the high-fertility values outlined above. There is a widespread belief that a further pregnancy diminishes the milk supply jeopardising the health of the nursing infant and many Yoruba believe that the man's sperm can actually enter and poison the milk. As a consequence, the period of post partum abstinence is linked to the period of lactation, but it is often extended beyond this in the interests of the mother's health, and it is the length of abstinence, rather than of lactation amenorrhoea, which determines the gap between births.

The continued existence of long periods of post-natal abstinence is supported by the high proportion of polygynous marriages, while amongst monogamous males extra-marital intercourse is common at such times. It is also helped by the belief that sex is primarily about reproduction, with very few women reporting that they missed having intercourse. There are indications that this traditional pattern is slowly breaking down. As infant mortality falls, with improved health and nutrition, the need for spacing is seen as less acute. In addition the availability of contraception makes possible an earlier resumption of intercourse even if spacing is desired, and this latter practice is becoming increasingly common amongst women with secondary or further education.

The most common reasons given for terminal abstinence are that the woman is too old or wants no more children, but this is often closely associated with the stage at which she becomes a grandparent. In traditional Yoruba society, women are expected to form strong and close relationships with their grandchildren and these are seen as threatened if she has a child of her own of comparable age. A majority of women in Caldwell's study were strongly opposed to grandmothers continuing sexual relations and he found that amongst women aged forty to forty-four, abstinence was much more common if they had grandchildren.

Use of contraception in Nigeria is still comparatively rare. In 1973, only 5 per cent of a sample of women aged fifteen to forty-nine were using modern methods of contraception; this figure rises to 11 per cent for the urban population of Ibadan, and is substantially higher amongst women with secondary education. The increase in birth-control practice in the urban population over the past decade has been dramatic and Caldwell predicts that by the 1980s a majority of couples in Ibadan will be practising contraception at some stage of their lives. The pattern of contraception is, however, an unusual one and seems to be compatible with a continuation of high fertility. More than a third of current users first practised birth-control before their first child, reflecting a strong motivation to avoid pre-marital pregnancy, especially amongst those receiving further education. At a later stage, birth-control is mainly employed as a substitute for traditional post-natal sexual abstinence. More than three quarters of all birth-control practice is by women who wish to have more children fairly soon. A preference for a large family continues and even amongst women with secondary education only 55 per cent of those with five surviving children said they want to prevent all future births. This is a pattern similar to that found in Caldwell's earlier study of the urban elite in Ghana.

The main sources of motivation to use birth-control seem to be the need to avoid extra-marital pregnancy and a desire to space children within marriage by means other than abstinence. It is possible, therefore, that for some years to come the Yoruba in Ibadan will increasingly possess the means to limit family without the motivation to do so. Nevertheless, the growing demand for birth-control amongst younger couples will mean that as social and economic changes begin to influence the desired number of children, married couples will be much more likely to find themselves already familiar with the means of achieving fewer children than was the case in most Western nations.

CHINA

China is the most populous developing country (850–900 million), but it has made most progress in effective family planning. All methods, including abortion and sterilisation, have been made available through realistic channels, and the age of marriage has been raised. Women are now discouraged from marrying before the age of twenty-five in the cities and twenty-three in the countryside (*see also* p. 60).

Nationwide vital statistics have not been published and may not even be available to the Chinese themselves. However, good records come from some cities and many communes. For example, in Shanghai, the birth rate is thought to have fallen from 30 per 1,000 in 1962 to approximately 10 in 1976 and maybe as low as 6 in the main city. One hospital which had 7,000 births in 1962 had only 3,000 in 1977. No urban population outside China has seen so rapid a decline in birth rate.

Wan-Tou Commune is an area in Kiangsu Province and has a population of 25,600. It is fairly typical of the more densely inhabited parts of China. In 1976 there were 3,797 women of child-bearing age; of these 2,382 had I.U.D.s, 405 used the Pill, 41 used condoms and 437 had undergone sterilisation. There were only 462 births in a year, which gives a rate of 18.3 per 1,000 and a natural increase of approximately 1 per cent.

Abortions are available on request and play a key role in controlling fertility. Again, national records are not available but institutional data is kept. For example, at the Shanghai International Maternity Centre there were 3,000 births and 2,000 abortions in 1977.

In 1977 Liu Ching-Shan, the responsible member of the State Council's family planning group, said to a visiting team from the American Planned Parenthood Federation, "in future, we must make every effort (to achieve an annual population growth of 10 per 1,000)." As the death rate is now between 7 and 8 per 1,000 the inference made was that the current birth rate may perhaps be 20 per 1,000. Some commentators believe that the birth rate is even lower. Whatever the level, it is uniquely low for any large developing country.

Taiwan provides an interesting comparison to the Peoples' Republic of China. An island with 3 million people in 1905, the estimated population reached 8.2 million in 1946 and then grew to 14.3 million in 1969, as a result of natural increase and due to immigration as the Communists triumphed on the mainland. Family planning began ten years earlier than on the mainland, but it moved slowly. It started timidly in the maternal and child sector and from 1963 onwards attempted a "one-shot" solution using I.U.D.s. When Pills were first made available in the programme, it was only to women who had discontinued the loop; a "single insertion" was judged by the experts to be preferable to "something you have to take every day".

The programme represented a profound clash of cultures and achieved its aims in a tortuous way. The fact that progress was made at all is a testimony to the dedication of the Chinese and American experts who worked in the field and to the common sense of married couples in the country.

In a traditional society where men take many of the fertility decisions, female methods were offered predominantly. Family planning was bracketed with health, as had occurred in the U.S.A. Although Taiwan is a very health conscious society, the structure of health care differs from that in the U.S.A. Western trained doctors are expensive and often remote and people turn to pharmacies, selling a range of over-the-counter and traditional herbal remedies.

By 1969 the programme had inserted over 600,000 I.U.D.s, reaching 30 per cent of the 1.7 million women aged twenty to forty-four. However, less than half the women who adopted the method were using it at any one time (14 per cent). Pills became increasingly popular in the late 1960s, but apart from the women who made the journey to a doctor and underwent the ordeal of examination, approximately 50,000 purchased them directly from pharmacies, even though they cost approximately five times as much as those sold by the official family planning programme.

The tangential nature of the programme is symbolised most vividly by what for some is its proudest achievement—its army of field workers. Field workers, one of the oddest aberrations of family planning, were supposed to motivate women to go to doctors' clinics, but never carried contraceptives themselves. They became even more irrelevant when the government began to take up the programme which the Population Council had started and raised the minimum educational standards for those who would become field workers. Not surprisingly, by the late 1960s, 40 per cent of the annual budget went on staff salaries and professional fees and 24 per cent on supervision and travel.

By 1977, the birth rate in Taiwan was 23 per 1,000, which may have been no lower than in the Peoples' Republic of China, although the *per capita* income of Taiwan is twice as high.

BRAZIL

Brazil is a country of extremes. It has above average natural resources, but is unlucky in not having any oil fields. It has great wealth and by the end of the 1960s 1 per cent of the population had an income of $15,000 and over. But 8 per cent of the population earned less than $226 a year and 20 per cent had a disposable income of only $100. It is an urbanising country, yet one which still has a high population growth rate. In the 1960s the population expanded by over 3 per cent per annum and even in 1975 the rate was as high as 2.8 per cent. Tens of millions of people were migrating from the countryside to the cities and 60 per cent of all the urban population are recent migrants. The cities grow by over 5 per cent per annum and the countryside population by less than 1 per cent, because of the outward migration. Unemployment is not honestly measured in the country, but is at a high level.

In 1870, there were 10 million people in Brazil, mostly settlers from Europe, themselves the diaspora of the European population explosion. By 1900, there were 19 million and by 1940, 43.5 million: this growth came both from immigration and natural increase. In 1960, there were 73.5 million and in the following decade over 20 million were added. Today, the population is approximately 100 million and has multiplied ten times in a century. By the year 2000 it is estimated that it will double again.

As in many countries, the population is concentrated in relatively few areas. This has created an illusion of unexploited space which has lulled many Brazilians into a false belief that rates of population growth are irrelevant to economic progress. In practice, the early settlers exploited the coastal forest belts and over a period of 400 years they destroyed 1.5 milllion square kilometres of forest and burnt or cut down approximately 15,000 million trees. The soil they tilled became denuded and now the agricultural population is migrating to the towns. This migration has been vividly described as involving people "displaced in an ecological war to live in urban concentration camps". It is expected that the megalopolis of Rio–Sao Paulo will contain 60 million people by the year 2000.

In the years 1960–72 the economy of Brazil exploded, growing by 156 per cent, yet the *per capita* income only rose by a mere fourteen dollars per person per year. Although a few brave intellectuals like Van de Costa have tried to draw the attention of Brazilians to their population problems, the government has persistently looked the other way. In the mid 1970s, the first timid efforts at family planning at a national level seemed to be emerging with cautious programmes directed towards women of very high partity. Non-governmental agencies, and in particular the I.P.P.F. affiliate BEMFAM (Sociedade Civil de Bem Estar Familiar no Brasil), have tried to meet the needs of people in local areas. In the north east of Brazil which has the poorest states, successful community-based family planning schemes have been run since the late 1960s. Whereas prior to the setting up of these schemes a handful of clinics were attempting to serve a million people, now many hundreds of schoolteachers were recruited as volunteers to distribute contraceptives and they have done this with considerable success.

Abortion is a major variable in fertility control and the estimated rate in Rio is 21 per 1,000 women per year. The average family size in Rio of 2.3 children suggests that there is quite a rigorous control of fertility. In Sao Paulo there are two abortion deaths per 100,000 women aged fifteen to forty-four per year, which is approximately ten times the rate observed in countries with high abortion ratios but legal operations, such as Poland or Japan.

To conclude, Brazil is a country in desperate need of fertility control; a country where the wealthy already have a small family size, but where the non-availability of family planning and of the surgical means of fertility regulation for the bulk of the population both keep fertility high, at a time when it could and should be declining.

CONCLUSION

The Hutterites of North America are of interest because this small group of people is extremely rare in that they have approached the maximum biological potential for human reproduction and have maintained this despite low levels of mortality. Even here a ceiling is imposed on total fertility by delayed marriage. The rest of mankind, from primitive groups through historical times to the contemporary world, have placed varying degrees of restriction on their final family size. The extent and nature of such restrictions differ considerably from society to society and we have tried in this chapter to show the diversity of means by which different communities have controlled their fertility, and also to consider some of their reasons for so doing.

One theme to emerge is that fertility behaviour reflects the values of a society. For the Hutterites many children are seen as a blessing and there are no social costs in frequent child-bearing. Rapid population increase has ensured expansion of membership of the Church, and for many years has posed no threat to a continuation of their traditional way of life. In contrast, fertility regulation has been seen to reflect the importance attached to preserving a valued way of life threatened by excessive reproduction, whether this is manifested in the Tikopia's concern over their food supplies, the !Kung's need for women to be mobile and unencumbered by too many infants, or the Victorian middle class determination to maintain living standards for themselves and their children. Linked to this is the importance of a new threat to such a way of life as a factor in demographic change, examples being the Great Depression in Britain, adverse economic conditions in pre-industrial Europe, or the aftermath of the Second World War in Japan. In many cases the pattern seems to fit in with Douglas's suggestion that oysters and champagne are more relevant to fertility than bread and butter. This highlights the problems encountered concerning motivation to fertility control amongst the most deprived people of the world.

We have also seen that there can be a concern for controlling fertility even in a country such as Africa, where the number of children desired is high as couples still wish to avoid extra-marital pregnancies and to space their children. Interest in being able to defer and ultimately terminate child-bearing can, therefore, be seen as almost universal, so that access to acceptable means of doing so becomes an important secondary determinant of achieved fertility levels.

We have looked at the process of demographic change in outlining the experience of the United Kingdom and Japan over the past century. In the next chapter we shall pursue this further by examining the nature of the "demographic transition" in developed nations and looking at the relevance of such a model to the developing nations of the world. In doing so, we shall explore the importance of economic development as a precursor of fertility decline, and the role of family planning provision in initiating or accelerating such a decline. It seems probable that the rate of population growth at a global level reached its peak in the early 1970s and has now begun to decline, after climbing steadily in the quarter of a century following the Second World War. Age at marriage is rising in many countries and child-bearing in the later years of fertile life is increasingly coming under voluntary control. Yet while the percentage growth rate may be falling, the absolute numbers added continue to grow. Such is the momentum of demographic change. Interest rates, as it were, have fallen, but the debt continues to increase.

We shall argue that both socio-economic development and family planning programmes are relevant to the continuation of this decline in fertility and that an unnecessary and artificial polarisation has emerged in the debate over the mechanisms of demographic change. Economic progress may indeed be a sufficient condition for fertility reduction in the long term, but recent experiences of developing countries suggest that it is not a necessary condition, and that modern methods of family planning can be adopted—and be associated with demonstrable demographic effects—in advance of major improvements in *per capita* income or education. The World Fertility Survey conducted in 1974 shows a higher prevalence of contraceptive use in countries with effective family planning programmes than was previously suspected. For example, in Thailand a third of couples now take contraceptive precautions and the T.F.R. has fallen from 6.6 in 1965 to 4.9 in 1974.

The fifth of the world's population that lives in China is the most vivid example of a community where fertility is declining rapidly in the absence of some of the economic changes which were associated with similar declines in the West. China is still a predominantly rural society where *per capita* income remains very low, but in recent years the birth rate has fallen to a level comparable to many more prosperous Asian communities and well below that of the other Asian giants such as India, Pakistan and Bangladesh. China is unique amongst the poorer nations of the developing world in providing easy access to all methods of fertility regulation, including abortion and sterilisation, for a substantial proportion of its people. At the same time it has created strong social pressures towards late marriage and small families. These pressures are linked to important social changes (which are taking place, despite limited economic growth) which have affected the role of women and lessened dependence on the family for individual prosperity and security in old age. We shall see that there are significant populations in other parts of the developing world where fertility has also declined, either in the absence of significant economic development, or more rapidly than the change of other variables in the community.

SELECTED REFERENCES AND BIBLIOGRAPHY

Banks, J. A. *Prosperity and Parenthood.* Routledge & Kegan Paul, London 1954

Birdsell, J. B. "Some Predictions for the Pleistocene Based on Equilibrium Systems Amongst Recent Hunter-gatherers." In Lee, R. B. and De Vore, I. *Man the Hunter*. Aldine, Chicago 1968

Borrie, W. D. *The Growth and Control of World Population*. Weidenfeld & Nicolson, London 1970

Caldwell, J. "The Economic Rationality of High Fertility; An Investigation Illustrated with Nigerian Survey Data." *Population Studies*. 31, 5 1977

Caldwell, J. and P. "The Role of Marital Sexual Abstinence in Determining Fertility: A Study of the Yoruba in Nigeria." *Population Studies*. 31, 193 1977

Caldwell, J. and Ware, H. "The Evolution of Family Planning in an African City; Ibadan, Nigeria." *Population Studies*. 31, 487 1977

Carr-Saunders, A. *The Population Problem*. Clarendon Press, Oxford 1922

Cartwright, A. *Parents and Family Planning Services*. Routledge & Kegan Paul, London 1970

Cartwright, A. *How Many Children?* Routledge & Kegan Paul, London 1976

Chang, M. C. and Chow, L. P. "Study by Matching of the Demographic Impact of an I.U.D. Program." *Millbank Memorial Fund Quarterly*. 1977

Chow, L. P. "Family Planning in Taiwan, Republic of China: Progress and Prospects." *Population Studies*. 24, 339 1970

Davis, K. "The Theory of Change and Response in Modern Demographic History." *Population Index*. 29, 345 1963

Devereux, G. "A Typological Study of Abortion in 350 Primitive, Ancient and Pre-industrial Societies." In Rosen, H. (ed) *Abortion in America*. Beacon Press, Boston 1967

Douglas, M. "Population Control in Primitive Groups." *British Journal of Sociology*. 7, 263 1966

Drake, M. *Population in Industrialisation*. Methuen, London 1969

Dumond, D. "The Limitation of Human Population: A Natural History." *Science*. 187, 713 1975

Eaton, J. W. and Mayer, A. J. "The Social Biology of Very High Fertility Among the Hutterites; The Demography of a Unique Population." *Human Biology*. 25, 206 1953

Firth, R. *We, the Tikopia: A Sociological Study of Kinship in Primitive Polynesia*. Allen & Unwin, London 1936

Firth, R. *Social Change in Tikopia*. Allen & Unwin, London 1965

Ganiage, J. *Trois Villages de L'Ile de France au XVIIe Siècle*. I.N.E.D. Cahier no. 40 Paris 1963

Glass, D. V. and Eversley, D. E. C. *Population in History*. Edward Arnold, London 1965

Gautier, E. and Henry, L. *La Population de Crulai*. Presses Universitaires de France, Paris 1958

Henry, L. "The Population of France in the Eighteenth Century." in Glass and Eversley (op. cit.) 1965

Hollingsworth, T. H. "A Demographic Study of the British Ducal Families." *Population Studies*. 11, 4 1957

Howitt, A. W. *The Native Tribes of South East Australia*. Macmillan, London 1904

Kolata, G. "!Kung Hunter Gatherers: Feminism, Diet and Birth-control." *Science*. 185, 932 1974

Leach, E. R. "Virgin Birth." *Proceedings of the Royal Anthropological Institute*. 39 1966

Lee, R. B. and Devore, I. *Man the Hunter*. Aldine, Chicago 1968

Meuvret, J. "Demographic Crisis in France from the Sixteenth to the Eighteenth Century." in Glass and Eversley (op. cit.) 1965

Mitchison, R. *British Population Change since 1860*. Macmillan, London 1977

Molnos, A. *Cultural Source Materials for Population Planning in East Africa*. Institute of African Studies, Nairobi 1972

Muramatsu, M. *Japan*. Country Profile, Population Council, New York 1972

Peel, J. and Carr, G. *Contraception and Family Design*. Churchill Livingstone, Edinburgh 1975

Rasmussen, K. *Across Arctic America: Narrative of the Fifth Thule Expedition*. G. P. Putnam & Son, New York 1927

Smith, T. E. "The Cocos-Keeling Islands: a Demographic Laboratory." *Population Studies*. 24, 94 1960

Sweeney, C. "The Last Raj Sells Out." *The Guardian*. 7th July 1978

Taeuber, I. B. *The Population of Japan*. Princeton University Press, Princeton 1958

Wilkinson, R. *Poverty and Progress*. Methuen, London 1973

Wrigley, E. A. "Family Limitation in Pre-industrial England." *Economic History Review*. 2nd series. 19, 82 1966

Wrigley, E. A. *Population and History*. Weidenfeld & Nicolson, London 1969

Wynne-Edwards, V. C. *Animal Dispersion in Relation to Social Behaviour*. Oliver & Boyd, London 1962

Chapter 8

Demographic Change

The very rapid rates of population growth which have characterised world population since the end of the Second World War represent what must be a temporary deviation from the annual growth rates that have prevailed during most of man's history and must prevail again in the future. The so-called "population explosion", which manifested itself in a population increase of over 2 per cent per annum in less developed countries, followed a period of relatively rapid population growth in what are now called the developed nations of the world. This growth began as early as the eighteenth century. It is easily visible and has been partly analysed. Current demographic changes are not yet complete at a global level, but clearly relate to the major technological changes of the period; nor are they unique within man's history.

There are at least two previous periods during which there occurred breaks in the prevailing population equilibrium, with rapid population growth, technological change and family adjustments to new demographic circumstances. Towards the end of the upper palaeolithic period (about 30,000 years B.C.) the small populations of hunters and gatherers improved their capacity to take food from an environment rich in large game mammals that roamed the grasslands characteristic of much of their environment after the last ice-age. Skeletal remains from the period suggest that adults lived on average to their mid-thirties and their stature suggests good nutrition. After many hundreds of thousands of years, during which population growth was minimal, man's numbers began to increase significantly, as they enjoyed the benefits of this new food supply.

In addition to the exploitation of the food resources of the large game animals, it was at this time that man learned how to keep warm by putting fire to domestic use and clothing himself in the skins of other animals. This enabled him to move into new areas of the globe and between 40,000 B.C. and 10,000 B.C. human hunting groups spread to occupy all the main land masses of the earth, with the exception of the Antarctic. According to McNeill, this had the additional advantage of enabling many to escape the parasites and disease organisms of their tropical environment, so that health and longevity improved.

However, mankind slowly overexploited this first Eden, exterminating some of his main sources of food, such as the mammoth in Asia and the giant sloth in the U.S.A. This gradual extinction of the large-bodied game animal must have brought an end to population growth locally, while the spread of hunting groups to new areas eventually came up against the limitation of available land space. Anthropologists and historians have suggested that before the introduction of agriculture, the world could have supported a hunting and gathering population of only 5 to 10 million. By mesolithic and early neolithic times, the evidence of skeletal remains suggests diminished stature and poorer nutritional standards.

With the loss of the big game mammals, man was forced to turn to new sources of food; initially these were probably fish, molluscs and vegetables. Only with the development of agriculture and the domestication of animals did a new era of expansion become possible. The so-called Agricultural Revolution, which is variously dated between 10,000 and 5,000 B.C., may have begun on a world population base of 8 to 10 million. By A.D. 1 the population had increased to about 300 million, representing an annual growth rate of 0.36 per 1,000 people.

The shift to agriculture brought new forms of over-exploitation of the environment, deforestation and soil erosion, which was in turn partially offset by the development of new techniques of irrigation and manuring. Nevertheless, there is much to suggest that the population of the period did not regain the levels of health achieved at the peak of the hunter's era. The growth of cities and slave economies which partly supported them eventually proved unstable and self-destructive; by the early centuries after Christ, the carrying capacity of the land had fallen and skeletal remains suggest a fall in life expectancy. For this reason, it has been suggested that the increased growth of the agricultural period may reflect higher birth and death rates; the increase in the former relates to the social changes involved in the shift from a nomadic hunting and gathering way of life to a more settled agriculture (*see also* Chapter 7).

The size and pace of mankind's previous spurts of population growth differ greatly from today, when the annual increase in India's population exceeds the total world population at the time of the agricultural revolution. Our palaeolithic ancestors in their hunting bands had densities of population as low as one person per ten square kilometres—just as today the Caribou Eskimos require land with a radius of up to forty-five kilometres for a band of twenty-five. In

Mexico City, in contrast, there would be over 10 million people in the same area.

What has not changed is man's capacity to over-exploit his environment. Falling fish yields and the extermination of the whale should remind us of our ancestors' experience with the mammoth and the sloth.

THE DEMOGRAPHIC TRANSITION

The "theory" of the demographic transition was first elaborated some forty years ago, as an attempt to explain the shift from high to low birth and death rates in the course of industrialisation in Western nations (*see* Fig. 34). Since then, various attempts have been made to apply the theory to the process of modernisation in developing countries.

THE THEORY OUTLINED

In its classical form the "theory" is essentially a description of an historical process that is supposedly the common experience of industrialised nations in the West. The population growth in Western nations is seen as due to a decline in mortality ahead of fertility, so that for a period births are far in excess of deaths. After a time-lag, fertility is reduced and a new equilibrium achieved, thus completing the "transition" from high birth and death rates to low levels of both mortality and fertility, and so from one form of stable population to another. The process of population change can be divided into four stages (*see* Fig. 36) representing the two periods of equilibrium, and two intervening stages of disequilibrium and transition. The whole process is seen as closely related to stages in economic development in a country.

Stage one represents the pre-transition period, prior to industrialisation, during which agrarian peasant economies experience slow population growth as a result of high average birth and death rates. Birth rates are seen as stable and subject to little restraint apart from traditional patterns of marriage; death rates are more liable to fluctuate as a result of variations in crop production and the incidence of disease, but are generally high as a result of poor diet, primitive sanitation and the absence of any effective medical practice. Any excess of births over deaths in years of low mortality is countered by loss of population in years of war, famine or epidemic. High birth rates are essential to the survival of society and so tend to be supported by social beliefs and customs which develop in response to the threat of high mortality.

Stage two commences with the advent of sustained economic

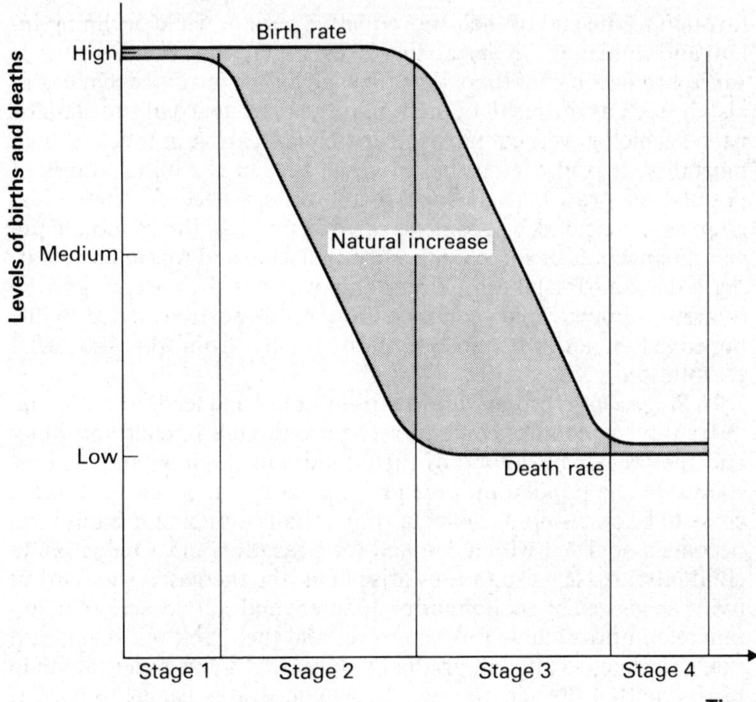

Fig. 36. *The demographic transition.*

growth and the evolution from a predominantly agrarian peasant economy to an economy with a greater division of labour, changing technology and all the other factors associated with industrialisation. These changes remove the ceiling of resources imposed on pre-industrial societies and encourage a fall in mortality for various reasons. Food supplies become more regular, aided by better communication and improvements in agricultural technology, so that diet improves and death from starvation or lack of resistance to infectious diseases becomes less frequent. Other contributory factors are seen as indirect consequences of economic change—improved sanitation, better personal hygiene, hospital building and other medical advances.

The birth rate remains high and consequently there is a period of rapid population growth, often lasting several decades; this occurs despite growing population pressure and increased survival of children in a family, which might be expected to lead to early fertility reductions. In part, the reasons for this are demographic—fewer women are widowed in their child-bearing years and more live through to the end of their reproductive period, while declining infant and child mortality mean that an ever increasing number of girls survive to become mothers. The time lag before fertility declines can also be seen as the result of inertia, or the persistence of pro-natalist values which governed marriage and child-bearing in times of high mortality. It is also plausible to argue that in the initial stages of population growth in Europe there was no need for individual couples to respond by reducing their fertility, as the economic development could absorb additional population and was in fact creating a demand for labour. Where this was not the case, migration to areas of more rapid economic growth was possible, aided by the improved means of transportation arising from the Industrial Revolution.

In *Stage Three*, economic growth continues and leads to reduction in fertility, as couples come to recognise the fall in child mortality and the greater likelihood of their children surviving, and as a response to the population pressure created by *Stage Two*. Children cease to be an economic asset, as industrialisation and urbanisation become associated with a demand for education and a reduction in child labour. New aspirations arise from the increased standard of living generated by economic development and couples seek to maintain and improve these for themselves and their children. The death rate continues to fall, but gradually does so at a less rapid rate than births, so that the gap between births and deaths begins to narrow and the rate of population growth slackens.

Finally, in *Stage Four*, both birth and death rates level off, producing a new equilibrium, in which population grows only slowly and may eventually stabilise or begin to decline.

THE DEMOGRAPHIC TRANSITION IN THE WEST

In recent years, the theory has come under increasing attack from anthropologists and historians, who challenge its accuracy even as a description of historical processes in the West. Although clearly population growth on average must have been very slow before the seventeenth century, it is probably wrong to believe that there were no periods of sustained growth before this (we have already mentioned the aftermath of the agricultural revolution some ten thousand years ago).

In the previous chapter, we cited evidence from primitive societies of population being kept stable by a control over fertility, rather than by high mortality alone. Most contemporary hunters and gatherers do not seem to live in misery, faced with the threat of extinction from famine and disease. On the contrary, they seem to be well-nourished and free from most infectious diseases. Evidence from such societies of widespread use of infanticide, abortion and abstinence to keep down the level of reproduction suggest that similar mechanisms may have existed in our ancestors living before the Agricultural Revolution, when any rapid population growth (given the limited carrying capacity of the earth for a society based on hunting and foraging) would have been potentially disastrous.

We have also seen that in pre-industrial Europe there were periods of population growth and stagnation which cannot be simply attributed to prevailing mortality and that marriage was delayed and family size limited in response to adverse economic conditions. To characterise pre-industrial populations as having universally high and virtually uncontrolled fertility, as a response to very high mortality, is clearly an over-simplification.

Doubts have also been raised about the picture presented of *Stage Two* of the transition; these are particularly concerned with the insistence that mortality decline caused the population growth and that this was in turn the result of economic developments. Many of the highest rates of growth occurred far from the centres of industrialisation. Consequently anyone who attempts to explain the fall in mortality that occurred throughout Europe at this time has to consider the possible relevance of a number of factors which are not directly linkable to industrialisation (such as the introduction of potato cultivation and the disappearance of plague). It has also been argued that an increase in fertility may have been at least partially responsible for the acceleration in population growth through the demand for child labour, or an increase in money wages which enabled men to marry earlier.

The decline of fertility in *Stage Three* of the transition has been subjected to detailed study by Ansley Coale and his colleagues, who have attempted to clarify the mechanisms of fertility decline in Europe and to identify thresholds of economic development at which birth rates begin to fall. He notes the importance of late age at marriage, attributed to the societal expectation that a couple would not marry until they had acquired economic independence, in keeping birth rates relatively low even before the transition, and points to the early fertility reductions in late eighteenth century France, where *Stage Two* and *Stage Three* overlap considerably.

Various factors have been considered important in the decline in births:

(*a*) the process of urbanisation;
(*b*) reduced infant mortality;
(*c*) rising costs and diminished economic advantages of children;
(*d*) the growth of literacy;

(*e*) the higher status of women;

(*f*) religious changes;

(*g*) the development of secular, rational attitudes.

All seem to be relevant in at least some European societies but there are many exceptions. France reduced its fertility prior to any major industrialisation and urbanisation. The birth rate fell in Spain and Bulgaria while mortality was still high. In several countries, rural and urban fertility fell simultaneously, and in Northern Italy Catholicism proved no barrier to a reduction in family size. Only a growth in literacy seemed to be common to all countries as their birth rates fell, but no correlation could be found between the onset of fertility decline and any particular level of literacy. There seems, therefore, to be no specific threshold of socio-economic development which triggers off a decline in births. The explanatory value of the classical demographic transition theory is weak.

At a very general level, however, the theory clearly does provide a description of the process of demographic change in Europe. Basically, in order for fertility to decline it seems that couples must be able to consider family size a suitable matter for rational choice, must be able to see advantages to themselves in controlling fertility and, all other considerations apart, must have access to an effective means, or combinations of methods, of fertility control.

The European experience shows that a high level of development is sufficient to ensure the emergence of all three factors, but provides no evidence that any threshold of development is necessary. In France and Hungary they seem to have been acquired prior to any major socio-economic change.

Finally, it is worth mentioning that *Stage Four* needs to be reconsidered in the light of rising birth rates in many developed countries after the Second World War. Some have seen this as a reaction to "overshooting" in the 1930s. Roberta Hall, however, suggests that we should rather characterise the immediate post-transition stage as one in which death rates are at a low stable level and birth rates comparatively low (but tending to fluctuate with economic conditions, at times being high enough to produce a mini-population explosion). This stage is only reached with full industrialisation. Hall goes on to propose a hypothetical *Stage Five* in which population finally tends towards stability, with a very low average birth rate, but increased variation over time; this stage is associated with developing automation, equal social and employment status for women, and an increase in voluntary childlessness.

PROSPECTS FOR THE DEVELOPING WORLD

The crucial question in relation to the application of demographic transition theory to the developing countries of the Third Wor in the area of the move from *Stage Two* to *Stage Three*. Death ra have fallen in most areas, so that slow rates of growth have give way to rapid population increase. As birth rates in the pre-transitional stage were higher than in Europe and death rates have fallen more rapidly, growth rates have accelerated sharply to a level substantially above that experienced in Europe resulting in a youthful age-structure which will perpetuate growth for decades to come.

Initially, debate about the relevance of the theory centred on the possibility of matching this rapid growth in *Stage Two* (which was seen as largely the result of an "artificial" lowering of mortality through public health measures imported from the West) by ensuring an equally rapid decline in fertility through introducing family planning programmes using modern technology. Today such programmes are being re-evaluated and some writers have argued that the move to *Stage Three* is only possible through socio-economic development. They point out that in the West fertility decline was achieved without family planning programmes, and argue that the developing countries should be allowed to follow the same path, with outside aid put into promoting economic development rather than population control. "Look after the people and the population will look after itself." This is an issue to which we will return several times.

In many respects, the developing world today seems to face a very different situation from that of the European countries on which the model of the demographic transition was based, and it has been suggested that the transition is likely to follow a substantially different course. A review of the differing circumstances points to some factors which, it appears, present greater obstacles to a natural transition to stable population without any increase in mortality, and to others which offer the prospect of a more rapid natural transition than was experienced in the West.

Obstacles to a timely reduction in growth rates include the rapidity of mortality decline and the higher initial levels of fertility, which have resulted in growth rates which are often double those typically found in Europe. Death rates have fallen mainly as a result of imported technologies, rather than socio-economic change, which in Europe was seen as containing the seeds of later fertility decline. The current rates of growth can be seen as impeding the continued economic development necessary to trigger *Stage Three* of the transition. The growth rates also have a greater momentum because of the higher proportion of young people in these countries, so that, even if replacement fertility is achieved, populations will continue to expand for at least half a century. The increase in literacy which cial is inhibited by the growth in numbers requir- ally, the safety valve of migration, available to y European countries in the nineteenth century, ıost developing nations today.

are several factors likely to favour more rapid ome countries, particularly in Latin America, d economic development has been more rapid ntury Europe. Current low ages of marriages beginning to rise and offer a potential for reducing birth rates which did not exist in the West. Acceptance of a small family norm may also proceed more rapidly amongst young people in the Third World, especially those who have travelled or been exposed through education to the fertility patterns of the developed world.

The fall in marital fertility in Britain and other European countries occurred as a result of widespread use of traditional methods of fertility control, such as abortion and coitus interruptus, which were either dangerous or of limited effectiveness; whereas in an increasing number of developing nations, there is access to more reliable contraception, sterilisation and safer abortion. Finally, it must be remembered that (in sharp distinction to the official opposition to any form of birth-control found in nineteenth century Europe) a majority of governments in the developing world do now recognise population growth as a matter of public concern. Therefore they devote money from their budgets to providing family planning services, while also being able to call on international assistance in tackling the problem.

ROLE OF ABORTION IN FERTILITY DECLINE

We have pointed out how abortion is an essential element in fertility regulation (*see* p. 140). It is used by individuals whether legal or illegal. Indeed, the law seems an unimportant determinant of total numbers taking place, although it does decide the potential health and economic costs to the woman.

Abortion is known in all societies and, although not frequent in the traditional village society of the developing world, is recognised, available and openly used. In the Indian subcontinent the woman seeking a traditional method of abortion is sometimes asked to squat over a stick held upright between a number of stones. An attempt is made to align it with the cervix and then the woman's friends suddenly push on her shoulders. The hope is that the stick may enter the womb, although it may pass into the *posterior fornix* of the vagina and perforate the abdominal cavity or rectum.

In the Orient, the traditional village midwife will perform a "massage" abortion. The woman lies on the floor, or on a firm split-bamboo bed, and the midwife begins to massage the abdomen with her fingers and thumbs trying to reach as far as possible below the pubic bone. The rate-limiting factors are the midwife's strength and the woman's ability to withstand pain. The intention is to produce vaginal bleeding. If the initial procedure doesn't work, the midwife may change to using her bare heel or the point of her elbow, or even the pestle used for pounding rice, as a mechanism for attempting to crush the embryo within the womb. The procedure may go on for up to an hour and may be repeated on successive days. If bleeding is produced, the midwife will receive a small gift, such as a chicken. Gynaecologists describe complications such as bleeding from the rectum, damage to the bladder and a clinical syndrome rather like acute appendicitis with fever and rigidity of the abdominal wall.

The Western world entered the Industrial Revolution with a similar knowledge of abortion techniques. Some, such as insertion of foreign bodies into the uterus, worked, whereas others, such as the tradition of pulling a tooth to produce a "shock", did not. In the U.S.A. abortion has always been near the surface of public awareness and before the second half of the nineteenth century abortion services were widely advertised. This, combined with an aggressive press and the publicity associated with courts of law, made the subject one of extreme public reaction. At the beginning of the nineteenth century no state had made abortion illegal; by 1900 the operation was outlawed throughout the country.

Mohr has shown that the evolution of public and legal attitudes was not initially related to moral judgments. Abortion became a symbol of the early nineteenth century battle between qualified doctors and quacks: the initial publicity and attempts to restrict abortion were, in a sense, restrictive practices by the medical trade union. The debate heated up after the founding of the American Medical Association in 1847 and the well orchestrated campaign by Horatio Robinson Storer. (A man who resisted the entrance of women into medicine and who wrote, "in loosing, as I hope to do, some of women's chains, it is solely for professional purposes, to increase her health, prolong her life, extend the benefits she confers upon society—in a word, selfishly to enhance her value to ourselves.")

The first restrictive abortion law was passed in New York (1828) and those who supported it initially intended to punish anyone who performed "a surgical operation, by which human life should be destroyed or endangered, such as amputation of a limb, or of the breast, trepanning, cutting for stone or for hernia ...".

In 1800 the average American woman had 7 children, but in 1900 she had only 3.5. Mohr accepts estimates of induced abortion rates as high as one in five of all pregnancies, for the second half of the nineteenth century. Prices varied from $10 to $50 (a great deal in those days) and certainly some abortionists were very wealthy and apparently were able to jump bonds (bail) of up to $5,000 at the time of trial with apparent ease. Madame Restell is said to have been worth $1,000,000 at the time of her suicide (in 1878) when she was finally brought to trial by Comstock, the American fanatic who did so much to introduce anti-contraceptive legislation.

The picture in Britain was similar. In 1868 the *British Medical Journal* quoted one of innumerable such advertisements:

> Consulting Accoucheur No... after many years devoted to the practice of midwifery in its most intricate forms, is enabled to afford immediate relief in all cases of female irregularity however difficult. Immediate applications preferred. 20% allowed for recommendations.

The mid-nineteenth century advertisement is more open than that allowed for legal abortion today. The London Underground has been particularly coy about permitting the Pregnancy Advisory Service to mention abortion by anything but inference.

The *British Medical Journal* investigated nineteenth century abortion practices in some detail. They were often linked to baby-farming. The alternative to abortion was to disappear from society for six or more months and have the baby secretly, pretending a pregnancy had never taken place. One illegal abortionist, who had been working since the early days of Queen Victoria's reign, told a *British Medical Journal* reporter that she had clients who "came back six or seven times". This particular abortionist had a happy, hearty attitude: "I am a jokeler (jocular) person, I am; and I says funny things and cheers 'em up. She needn't mind and musn't fret and I will see her alright. I am the old original I am and I have had hundreds."

Fee-splitting, inflated prices and all the practices associated with illegal abortion are documented from the nineteenth century onwards. When two brothers called Chrime were convicted and sentenced as abortionists in 1898, the police found that £800 had changed hands within three or four days of their practice. The prosecution claimed that 12,000 women had approached them for abortifacients.

By 1868, one French observer claimed that abortion had grown "into a veritable industry". Hospital admission records for incomplete abortion in the late nineteenth and early twentieth century show rising trends in nearly all cities which are very similar to those indicated by hospital records for contemporary Latin America.

The desire to control fertility and the acceptability of abortion are both vividly illustrated in North America and Europe during the nineteenth and early twentieth century by the massive trade in abortifacients. In 1871, Ely van der Warker described abortion practices in Syracuse, New York State. He believed "injection of water into the cavity of the womb is the means generally relied on by the abortionist", and he complained that "the luxury of an abortion is now within the reach of a serving girl. An old man in the city performs this service for $10 and takes his pay in instalments." When he reviewed twenty-one deaths due to abortion, he claimed that ten followed the use of abortifacient drugs and he attempted to collect abortifacients from shops in the town. Interestingly, he took a number himself and gave the remainder to his dog.

One of the most ancient abortifacients is savin. It was described by Culpepper (1616–56) in his book *The Complete Herbal* as a plant being found "in almost every garden" which "cannot be taken without manifest danger, particularly to pregnant women and those subject to flooding". When van der Warker took a preparation of savin he had purchased in Syracuse he suffered from "a violent pain in the abdomen, vomiting and powerful cathartic action with tenesmus (pain in the anus), strangury, heat and burning in the stomach, bowels and anal regions". Beechams Pills, which had a remarkably successful sale from the late nineteenth century onwards, often included savin or other derivatives of juniper. In the popular culture they were associated with bringing on late periods and the nineteenth century advertisement for Beechams Pills often suggested the hopeful abortifacient action of the drug.

As late as 1937, the Midwives Institute in evidence to the Government Interdepartmental Committee on Abortion quoted a widespread trade in abortifacients. One midwife thought the reason women so frequently asked if the baby was "all right" was because they had so often taken remedies in attempts to end the pregnancy.

It appears that when a community first begins to regulate its fertility, both the use of contraception and the resort to abortion rise together. This seems to have been true of nineteenth century Britain. Contemporary Korea, Latin America and Egypt appear to be in the same stage of evolution of family planning practices as England was a 100 years ago. The incidence of illegal abortion in Korea doubled between 1964 and 1968 when during the same years contraceptive practice also increased.

With the passage of time it seems that the number of abortions increases dramatically and then begins to decline, although the resort to abortion is never eliminated (*see* Fig. 37). The fact that abortion has been legal in Japan since the end of the Second World War is well known. The number of abortions done in the country is very high, but it may be no higher than the number taking place in

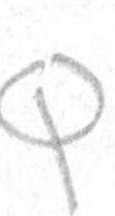

England during the years of the Depression, when the birth rate was as low as it is today and the family planning services much less developed. The important thing about Japan is that there has been a

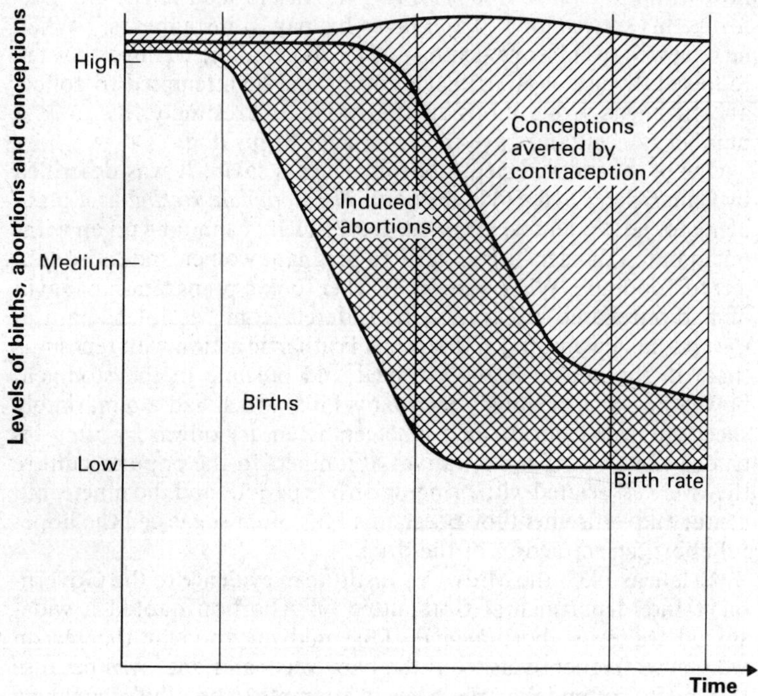

Fig. 37. *Abortion in the demographic transition.*

measurable improvement in contraceptive usage throughout the 1960s and a slow but significant fall in the total number of abortions taking place. A similar change has taken place in Hungary and may be beginning in Tunisia.

In Romania in 1966 a previously liberal abortion law was reversed for political reasons (*see* Fig. 38). Nine months later the birth rate doubled, but illegal abortion networks were slowly re-established. Today the birth rate has almost returned to the low level achieved before the legal restrictions, but several hundred women now die each year from illegal operations. Abortion is an inescapable part of fertility control.

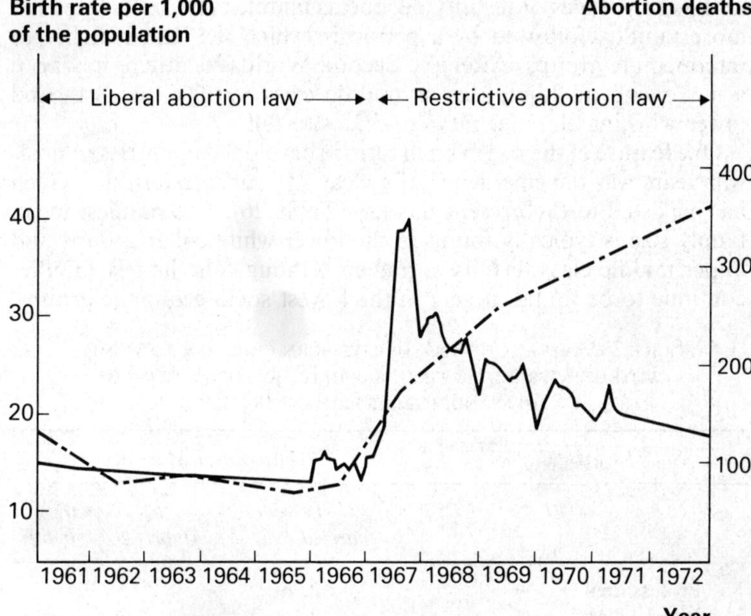

(*Source:* Potts, M., Diggory, P. and Peel, J. *Abortion.* Cambridge University Press 1977)

Fig. 38. *Romanian birth rate per 1,000 of the population* (——) *and deaths attributed to abortion* (- - -) *1961–72.* NOTE: the birth rate is plotted monthly for the years 1966–71.

DIFFERENTIAL FERTILITY

The decline in family size in Britain (*see* Chapter 7) did not proceed uniformly in all social groups. Doctors and clergy seem to have been among the first to recognise the advantages of having fewer children, despite the antagonism of their respective professions to the practice of birth-control by less worthy members of society. By the 1870s, fertility control was practised widely within the upper middle class and gradually the practice spread to the lower middle classes and skilled artisans. There remains much uncertainty about the nature of this process, especially concerning the relative importance of the diffusion of knowledge of (and access to) birth-control, as opposed to changing motivation to control fertility.

The trends in class differentials in fertility in the West are well described by Dennis Wrong. He points to a widening in differentials in the early stages of fertility decline as middle class birth rates fall more rapidly, followed by a period in which the lead switches to intermediate groups. After the Second World War there has been a narrowing of differences as middle class fertility increases and lower working class fertility continues to fall.

One feature of the rise in birth rates in developed countries in post-war years was the emergence of a clear "J" curve in fertility, which has persisted to the present day (*see* Table 26). The smallest mean family size is typically found in the lower white collar groups and upper middle class fertility is higher, although the largest families continue to be found largely in the lowest socio-economic groups.

TABLE 26: AVERAGE NUMBER OF LIVE-BORN CHILDREN TO WOMEN WITH UNINTERRUPTED FIRST MARRIAGE, BY SOCIAL CLASS OF HUSBAND, (GREAT BRITAIN, 1971)

	Social Class	*Duration of Marriage*	
		15–19 years (married 1951–5)	*10–14 years (married 1956–60)*
1	Professional	2.26	2.23
2	Intermediate*	2.18	2.13
3N	Skilled non-manual	2.02	2.00
3M	Skilled manual	2.37	2.31
4	Semi-skilled manual	2.40	2.32
5	Unskilled manual	2.74	2.62
	All	2.33	2.26

(*Source:* 1971 Census, 10 per cent sample data)

NOTE: * includes most managerial and senior administrative occupations.

The emergence of a curvilinear relationship led commentators to argue that we were witnessing a gradual shift to a situation in which fertility would be positively related to social class and especially to income, thus reversing the traditional relationship. Economist Gary Becker has argued that children in developed societies are essentially "consumption goods" and that those who are better-off are able to afford more; so that fertility would be positively related to income, if it were not for the less effective use of birth-control by the poor. This view of children as "consumer durables" has been challenged by Judith Blake, who points out many ways in which the two differ and suggests that there are good reasons for thinking that the poor may want more children and little evidence that they will behave with economic rationality and have few or none. Later developments in the Economic Theory of Fertility have made it into a more sophisticated model, stressing the inter-relationship between income, tastes and costs, and looking at the latter in broad terms. These include the opportunity-costs to parents in relation to the value of their time, and the human capital represented by the mother's investment in education.

INCOME

The relationship between income and fertility in developed societies is particularly problematic. The long-term fall in birth rates has clearly been associated with rising incomes, but in the post-war fluctuations of fertility, rising birth rates and falling age at marriage have been associated with periods of prosperity. David Heer has argued that in the process of economic development rising *per capita* income would have exerted an upward pressure on fertility, but that this is countered by other factors associated with development such as increased education, the rising costs of children and the declining levels of infant mortality.

Similarly in cross-sectional studies an over-all association between higher income and low fertility may conceal a direct relationship between income and family size within occupational or other groupings. Such a relationship has indeed been found within each broad socio-economic group in West Germany and within educational strata in Canada and the U.S.S.R., although in both of the latter countries there is an over-all inverse relationship arising from the close links between education and income level. In America, Deborah Freedman found that income above the mean for the husband's age, occupation and educational status was associated with above average fertility (while an income below the mean for his status was associated with fewer children). It has also been pointed out by Mincer that, while a husband's income may have a positive effect on fertility, wife's income can be expected to show a negative association with family size, as it reflects the opportunity costs to the couple of an additional birth. There are, therefore, considerable problems in determining the influence of income on fertility and these are exacerbated by the difficulty in conceptualising and measuring "income", which is all too often simply taken as "current" income at one point in time, when past, potential or anticipated income may be much more relevant measures.

Sweden is often cited as an example of a country where birth-control is widely available and used and where an emerging, positive relationship between economic status and family size might be first seen. In a recent study, Bernhardt showed that the relationship was still negative, except at the top end of the scale, so that there is a "J" curve comparable to that described for Britain (*see* Table 26). At higher incomes, above-average fertility results from a large proportion of parents having at least two children; while in the poorer groups the key factor seems to have been the continued occurrence of many births to women with three or more previous live-born children. She concludes that the higher the economic status the more likely it is that couples will fulfil the social norm of having at least two children; while the proportion of marriages with four or more children is high amongst the poor and derives from a lesser ability to control unwanted fertility after the third child.

The continued existence of large unplanned families in the poorer sections of many developed societies, reflecting as it were a microcosm of the world population situation, has led to many studies of the relationship between fertility and poverty. There has been dispute about the extent to which the poor have more children because they want more. Some writers such as Judith Blake argue that this is a major factor, while others have seen the differences as largely due to unwanted births and a lack of realistic opportunities to plan their families. This can be seen partly as being a reflection of the failure of family planning provision and difficulties over access to effective means of birth-control (*see* p. 92). Effective use of birth-control also requires an orientation to the future and a belief in the possibility of controlling future events, together with the existence of tangible benefits from limiting family size, which can offset the costs of practising consistent birth-control. Such conditions are less likely to exist amongst the disadvantaged found in the lower socio-economic groups in a highly stratified society, and are reinforced by the inadequacy of birth-control provision.

EDUCATION

The importance of education and especially that of women has often been stressed as contributing to a decline in family size. Heer sees it as a crucial factor in the link between economic development and fertility decline, and an inverse relationship between education level and family size has been established in many countries.

In post-war Japan a clear inverse relationship between fertility and education was found at all ages and at most marriage durations in the 1950 and 1960 censuses. An official survey carried out in 1965 showed a mean family size for women aged thirty-five to thirty-nine, which ranged from 1.69 for those with a university education to 4.07 for those with only elementary schooling. A comparable study in the U.S.A. in 1965 found a similar inverse relationship, but less striking differences, with the average number of children ever born rising from 1.63, for women aged forty-five to forty-nine with four years of college education, to 2.9 for those with less than eight years elementary schooling. The Japanese figures reflect the widening differentials often associated with a period of initial fertility decline. Similar patterns have been found in the U.S.S.R., Hungary, Canada and several European countries. In the latter, however, there have been signs of a curvilinear relationship similar to that noted for occupation, with university graduates having especially high numbers of children. In the 1961 British Census the highest mean family size was found where both partners left school before the age of fifteen, and in marriages where the husband continued in full-time education to the age of twenty and over, and the wife to seventeen or over.

There are many reasons why a higher education level in women might be expected to lead to lower fertility. The more educated are likely to have a greater knowledge of, and easier access to, effective means of birth-control. They will tend to marry later and will face higher "opportunity" costs in having children. They have a wider choice of extra-familial roles which will conflict with child-bearing and a greater ability to plan ahead in a rational way. In the context of rapid social change and a declining birth rate, the more educated may be expected to be exposed to and perceive such changes earlier and to adapt their child-bearing more rapidly if it seems appropriate.

The higher fertility of the most educated in some European countries may reflect essentially higher family size preferences and be associated particularly with those highly educated women who choose not to work. Alternatively, it may arise from a conviction that at least two children are necessary, and an ability to afford these, as Bernhardt suggested for the higher income groups in Sweden. Population concerns and improved opportunities in careers in more recent times may be changing this pattern yet again. Certainly, many recent studies have indicated the importance of female employment as a factor in determining family size and spacing.

FERTILITY DIFFERENTIALS IN DEVELOPING NATIONS

The widening of class differentials in the West at the beginning of fertility decline has led to a great interest in the existence of possible parallels in developing countries, and even to a belief that the emergence of such differentials is an indication of the commencement of the later stages of the demographic transition.

There is little doubt that there are wide variations in fertility according to socio-economic levels in many developing countries which have recently experienced falling birth rates. One example is Colombia; this Latin American country has experienced major reductions in fertility in recent years. A recent study in Bogota indicated a wide range of fertility-rates in different social strata in the

TABLE 27: GENERAL FERTILITY RATES BY SOCIO-ECONOMIC STATUS (BOGOTA, COLOMBIA, 1973)

Economic status of neighbourhood	*Births per 1,000 women aged 15–44*
Upper	35
Upper-middle	50
Middle	56
Lower-middle	117
Lower	129
Lower-lower	158
Total	97

(*Source:* Bailey, J. "Fertility and Contraceptive Practice, Bogota, 1964–74." *Studies in Family Planning*. 7 (9) 1976)

society (*see* Table 27). In contrast fertility in rural areas of developing countries is often found to be positively related to socio-economic status, as in Ajami's study of six Iranian villages (*see* Table 28).

In many countries, from Iran and Egypt to India and Bangladesh, the fertility patterns of the educated urban elite are being increasingly Westernised, although over-all birth rates remain high. The more privileged classes are increasingly exposed to an awareness of Western pattern of reproduction, through a variety of contacts from mass media to travel, while the economic and personal advantages of reduced fertility are evident, especially if the wife has also been exposed to a long education. For the poor peasants of such countries, who make up the bulk of the population, fertility remains high, reflecting both a lack of access to the means of birth-control and also a social situation in which the achievement of a small family is unlikely to have a high priority.

TABLE 28: MEAN NUMBER OF CHILDREN DESIRED, EVER BORN AND CURRENTLY LIVING, BY SOCIO-ECONOMIC STATUS (IRAN 1974)

	Mean number of children		
Socio-economic status	*Desired*	*Ever Born*	*Currently Living*
High	6.1	5.4	4.4
Medium	5.9	4.9	3.7
Low	5.7	3.8	2.9
Total	5.9	4.7	3.6

(*Source:* Ajami, I. "Differential Fertility in Peasant Communities." *Population Studies*. 30, 453 1976)

The emergence of fertility differentials in a high fertility developing country can be seen clearly in recent data from Jordan, which shows that women with no education have a greater number of live births, a larger number of living children and also want more additional children, especially sons (*see* Table 29).

Such differentials are often perceived as a threat by the more prosperous and educated, who are not convinced that fertility control will diffuse through the society and who may advocate coercive measures to restrict the families of the less privileged, as happened in India during 1976 and 1977. The challenge to certain groups is most marked when fertility differentials coincide with language, ethnic or religious groupings, as occurred in Singapore, where fertility declines amongst the Chinese preceded those among the Indian and Malay populations. However, in this case, all three groups eventually achieved comparable levels of fertility control.

TABLE 29: MEAN NUMBER OF CHILDREN BORN, LIVING AND WANTED (JORDAN 1972)

Educational level	*Live births*	*Living children*	*Additional children wanted*	
			Male	*Female*
University	3.6	1.3	1.5	0.8
Higher institutions	4.0	2.0	1.3	0.8
Secondary	4.0	1.6	1.6	0.8
Preparatory	4.8	1.6	2.4	0.7
Primary	6.0	2.5	2.8	0.7
Illiterate	8.3	3.8	3.9	0.7
Total	7.1	3.1	3.3	0.7

(*Source:* Rizk, H., "Trends in Fertility and Family Planning in Jordan." *Studies in Family Planning*. 8 (4) 1977)

RELIGION

Fertility differentials within societies are not confined to socio-economic variations. Religious differentials have been noted. Most striking is the higher fertility of some Catholic couples. In the U.S.A., family size is somewhat higher in Catholics than in Protestants. These differentials can be important, although it also needs to be emphasised that they are relative. The lowest fertility level occurs among Jews, and this pattern persists within all socio-economic groupings. Indeed, it has been suggested that religion is now a greater influence on fertility than socio-economic status. This certainly seems to be true in Holland where over-all Catholic fertility at a marriage duration of twenty-one to twenty-five years is higher than that for any occupational group, while the fertility of those claiming no religion is lower than any socio-economic grouping. In each occupational group, fertility is highest among Catholics and the cross-classification of religion and occupation gives a range of family size from 2.00 for lower middle-class couples with no religion, to 6.21 for Catholic farmers.

The most striking example of a country where religion is dominant as an influence on fertility is Ireland (*see* Table 30). In both Eire and Northern Ireland, religion is clearly a much more important factor in differential fertility than occupational grouping. After twenty years of marriage, the difference in numbers of children between

TABLE 30: MARITAL FERTILITY AFTER 20–24 YEARS OF MARRIAGE, BY RELIGION AND SELECTED SOCIO-ECONOMIC GROUPING (IRELAND 1961)

Occupational Group	*Eire, 1961* *Religion*		*Northern Ireland, 1961* *Religion*	
	Catholic	*Others*	*Catholic*	*Others*
Farmers/managers	4.26	3.13	4.37	2.94
Higher professional	3.63	2.15	3.80	1.98
Intermediate non-manual	3.66	1.94	3.54	2.06
Skilled manual	4.45	2.59	4.45	2.34
Unskilled manual	4.96	3.57	4.54	2.59

(*Source:* Eire, Census of Population, 1961, Vol. 8; Northern Ireland, 1961 Census, Fertility Tables)

Catholics and others in each social grouping is at least one and often as many as two. There is more variation by socio-economic status within the non-Catholic groups, but in both countries the lowest Catholic fertility level is above the highest level of the non-Catholics. Thus, in Northern Ireland, lower middle class Catholics have a significantly higher number of live births than non-Catholic farmers or manual workers. There have recently been signs of a more relaxed attitude towards contraception on the part of the Roman Catholic hierarchy in Ireland, which may in time lead to a narrowing of differentials.

In contrast to social class differences, there is little doubt that variations in fertility amongst religious groups reflect differing values about family size, as well as birth-control. Studies in Britain and the U.S.A. have consistently shown that Catholics see a larger number of children as ideal, and are less likely to approve of birth-control, although a large majority do practise contraception for much of their married lives. The main difference lies in the methods of contraception chosen; in Britain, Catholics are more likely to rely on the safe period and withdrawal and less likely to use appliance methods, but show no significant difference from other groups in use of the Pill or sterilisation. Nor is there any evidence that Catholics seek abortion less frequently. Indeed in some areas of Switzerland, Catholics have more abortions, possibly in an effort to make up for less effective contraception.

Despite the strong and continuing opposition of the Catholic Church to abortion and most modern methods of contraception, individual members of the Church seem to make up their own minds about what to do. In Latin America and the Philippines Catholicism has not been a barrier to the adoption of family planning by the poor, and it is worth remembering that Roman Catholics in Northern Italy have one of the lowest fertility levels in the world.

ECONOMIC DEVELOPMENT AND FERTILITY DECLINE

If socio-economic development is the key to a decline in birth rates, we might expect to observe a fall in the fertility of those developing countries which are approaching Western levels of prosperity. Most developed nations now have birth rates near to or below 20 per 1,000 people. This level has so far been achieved among developing countries only by the two "city-states" of Singapore and Hong Kong, where living standards, mortality levels and *per capita* Gross National Product are comparable with those of many Western nations. When we look at other developing countries where birth rates have fallen, we find a wide range of levels of prosperity, as measured by *per capita* G.N.P. Table 31 lists selected developing nations according to recent figures provided by the World Bank on *per capita* G.N.P., contrasting in each income band countries with high and low birth rates, measured arbitrarily as above 35 per 1,000 and below 30. It is clear that high fertility can persist despite high levels of G.N.P. and that lower rates have been achieved in some very poor nations, although it remains true that a large majority of those countries with a *per capita* G.N.P. below $500 have birth rates well above 35.

Most of the countries listed as having low birth rates have had vigorous family planning programmes over the last ten years or so, while these have been noticeably absent from the "high fertility" countries. Noting this, Ravenholt has argued that fertility reduction is not dependent on the existence of major socio-economic development. He points out that Brazil, Mexico and Kuwait all experienced very high rates of economic growth during the 1960s, but that in the absence of family planning programmes and ready access to improved means of fertility control, these socio-economic gains were not translated into lower birth rates. He demonstrates his point by the use of fertility silhouettes (*see* Chapter 3), which show the changes over time in age-specific fertility rates. Figure 39 shows the contrasting patterns of change in a selection of countries from Table 31, indicating the nature of fertility decline in countries with and without vigorous family planning programmes.

TABLE 31: HIGH AND LOW FERTILITY IN COUNTRIES WITH SIMILAR LEVELS OF G.N.P. 1974
(BRACKETED FIGURES REFER TO CRUDE BIRTH RATE IN 1974)

Per Capita G.N.P. (U.S. $)	*Low Fertility*		*High Fertility*	
$2,000+	Puerto Rico	(23.1)	Kuwait	(45)
	Singapore	(17.8)	Saudi Arabia	(50)
$1,000–2,000	Trinidad and Tobago	(24)	Venezuela	(36)
			Iran	(42–43)
	Hong Kong	(18.3)	Mexico	(40)
	Barbados	(21)		
$700–1,000	Costa Rica	(29.5)	Brazil	(38–40)
	Taiwan	(23)	Peru	(42.9)
	Cuba	(22)	Algeria	(48–50)
$400–700	Mauritius	(25.1)	Syria	(45–50)
	Martinique	(22)	Ecuador	(42)
	Colombia	(30–33)	Ivory Coast	(46)
$100–400	S. Korea	(24–28)	Bolivia	(47)
	China	(26)	Bangladesh	(46–50)
	Sri Lanka	(27.3)	Ethiopia	(46–50)

(*Source:* World Bank Atlas, 1976; *Population and Family Planning Programes; A Factbook.* Population Council, New York 1976)

A contrasting analysis of the reasons for the differences is provided by William Rich, who has argued that a key factor is the distribution of income within a country. In other words, a particular level of average income is meaningless unless we know whether the bulk of the population has shared in the benefits of economic progress. In his monograph, "Smaller Families through Social and Economic Progress", he states his belief that "policies combining economic growth, more equitable distribution of the economic and social benefits of progress and easy access to family planning services can bring about a much greater reduction in fertility than can any one of these factors alone."

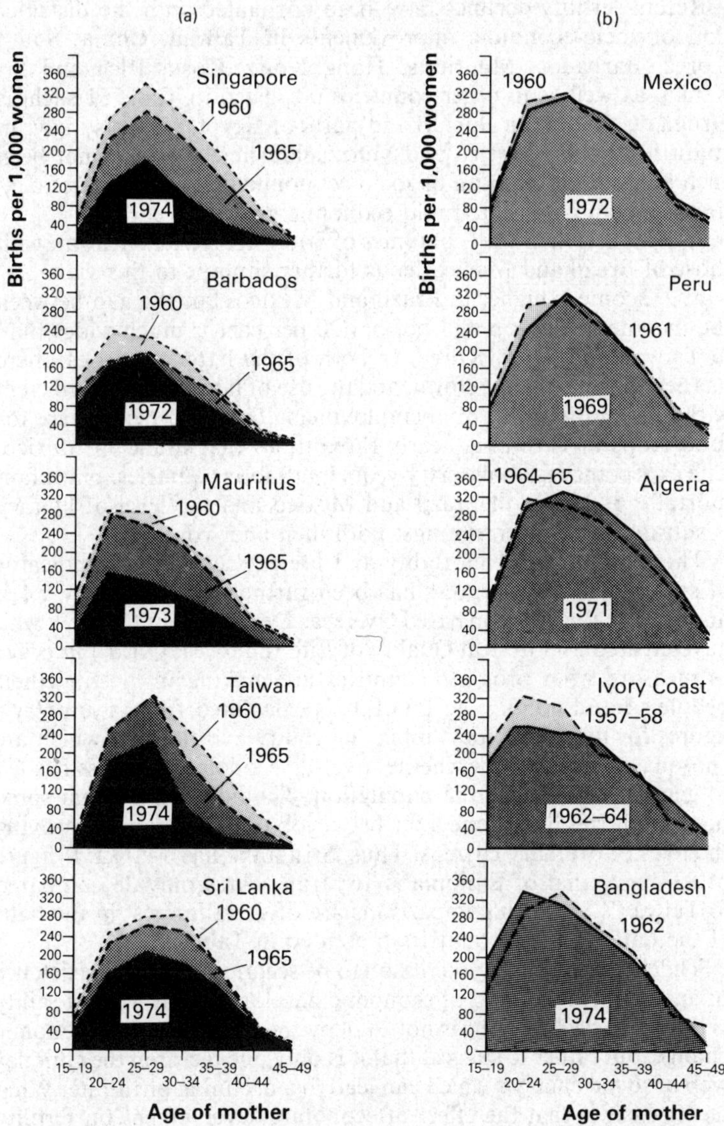

(*Source:* Ravenholt, R. T. and Chao, J. *World Fertility Trends 1976*. George Washington University Medical Center 1976)

Fig. 39. *Age-specific fertility rates for countries* (*a*) *with and* (*b*) *without vigorous family planning programmes.*

Recent fertility declines have been correlated with the distribution of socio-economic improvements in Taiwan, China, South Korea, Barbados, Mauritius, Hong Kong, Costa Rica and Sri Lanka, as well as in other countries not listed in Table 31 such as Uruguay, the Indian Punjab and parts of Egypt. Contrastingly, in countries such as Mexico and Venezuela where there has not been such a broad distribution of socio-economic gains, birth rates continue to be high despite rapid economic growth.

A comparison of the economies of South Korea and Taiwan with those of Brazil and Mexico lends further support to this view. *Per capita* income is higher in Brazil and Mexico, but the gap between the income of the top and bottom 20 per cent is much wider than in Taiwan and South Korea. In both of the latter countries, there has been effective land reform, and the use of labour is more efficient with much lower rates of unemployment. The yield per hectare for food crops in Taiwan is nearly three times that found in Mexico. Life expectancy is above sixty years in all four countries, but infant mortality is higher in Brazil and Mexico and the level of literacy is substantially lower amongst both men and women.

The importance of mortality and literacy levels as an indicator of socio-economic progress has been further highlighted by work done by the Washington based Overseas Development Council, who have created a "Physical Quality of Life Index" (P.Q.L.I.) in order to measure what progress countries are making in meeting their people's basic needs. The P.Q.L.I. is calculated from a country's figures for life expectancy, infant mortality and literacy, which are chosen as likely to show whether over-all economic progress has led to general benefits for the population. The index shows that some poor countries have done a far better job than others in improving the lives of ordinary citizens. Thus, Sri Lanka has a P.Q.L.I. figure of 83, while that of Ethiopia is 16; Iran scores only 38 compared to Taiwan's 88. Such comparisons are of great interest in the light of the data on these countries presented in Table 31.

There is, therefore, good reason to be sceptical about the existence of any simple threshold of economic development at which fertility is bound to decline. This is not to deny the importance of economic change, but rather to suggest that it is only one factor in the complex web of social changes which can lead to a declining birth rate. What seems clear is that the effect of economic development on fertility is probably greatest where the benefits—no matter what their level—are shared by a majority of the people and are translated into tangible gains in improved literacy and reduced mortality, and where any increased motivation to reduce family size is supported by the availability of family planning services and up to date contraceptive methods.

CONCLUSION

In demographic as well as human terms, the story of the changes in the past 150 years in the West was a sad one. It took approximately one century for births and deaths to come into kind of balance and not only did populations grow four or five times in many countries, but a significant proportion of the population growth was exported as immigrants—a process which the contemporary developing world cannot repeat.

In exploring the role of birth-control in the fertility transition of Europe in the nineteenth century and of developing countries today, the central question is whether the transition should be viewed as a simple adjustment to new socio-economic circumstances based on previously established behavioural mechanisms. Will birth rates in contemporary Asia fall only when people wish to adjust their fertility to a new set of structural and motivational forces? Or is there already an unmet need for family planning?

One group asserts that family planning programmes will achieve little until socio-economic circumstances alter—hence the current vogue for stressing the importance of economic development as the only way to achieve low fertility levels in developing countries. It is argued that development programmes should pay special attention to those features of socio-economic advance which are most likely to affect motivation to use family planning, such as literacy, lowering infant mortality, more equitable income distribution and raising the status of women.

Others see the decline of fertility as an example of the diffusion of an innovation. Birth rates fall as an increasing proportion of the population acquire knowledge of the techniques of birth-control and as the idea of limiting family size and delaying the occurrence of birth becomes widely accepted. This model assumes a prior motivation to have fewer children, reflected in the occurrence of unwanted pregnancy and the use of post partum abstinence, induced abortion and infanticide.

The strength of the "adjustment" model lies in its explanation of the "failure" of birth-control programmes in India and other underdeveloped countries, and the dramatic decline of fertility in countries such as Japan. It also offers a plausible explanation for socio-economic differentials in fertility decline and for the persistence of pockets of high fertility in some social groups in developed countries long after knowledge of methods of birth-control have spread throughout such societies.

In contrast to this position, those seeing the deliberate prevention of births as innovatory behaviour for the vast majority of a population, in the course of the fertility transition, cite the fact that in Europe non-marital fertility declined at the same time as marital fertility. They argue that the reduction in both illegitimate and legitimate births is due to the diffusion of knowledge and skills which enable people effectively to avoid unwanted births. It is pointed out that the pattern of social class differentials in fertility suggest a process of diffusion, as do initial declines in urban rather than rural areas, and that the pattern of growing use of birth-control and reductions in family size is a continuous one which suggests a steady spread of contraception practice. Later fluctuations in the birth rate are seen as explicable by changes in the number of children desired, and the spacing of these, and it is pointed out that these changes often accompany an increase in the actual use of birth-control, especially the more reliable methods, so that the long term secular decline is maintained.

In respect of the application of such ideas to the Third World, it is pointed out that evidence of deliberate family limitation in pre-industrial Europe does not necessarily mean that all developing countries have the same pattern and there is evidence which suggests that this is not the case. Age at marriage is typically much younger, and those mechanisms which reduce fertility below its biological potential are usually related to patterns of lactation and sexual abstinence which are not practised for demographic reasons.

Caldwell has recently suggested that a distinction should be drawn between "demographic" innovation—the growth and diffusion of beliefs about the desirability of a smaller family size—and "contraceptive" innovation—the development and spreading of knowledge about effective methods of fertility control. He argues that in Africa, in contrast to the West, the former may not be the crucial factor, and that countries may show interest in modern forms of contraception (even though most married couples still want many children) because it provides a means of avoiding extra-marital pregnancy and the need for prolonged sexual abstinence to ensure adequate spacing of births.

Coale suggests that there are three general prerequisites of major declines in marital fertility:

(*a*) fertility must be considered as a matter for rational choice;

(*b*) reduced fertility must be seen as advantageous in the context of perceived social and economic circumstances;

(*c*) effective techniques of birth-control must be known and accessible.

If we consider the above arguments in the light of this suggestion, we can see that the "adjustment" model sees (*b*) as the key factor, assuming that (*c*) already exists and that (*a*) is either already present or arises from socio-economic changes. The "innovation" model stresses the importance of (*c*) and to a certain extent (*a*).

If all three are considered to be important, there is clearly a need for an approach which stresses both innovation and adjustment, with one or other process being of possibly greater relevance in any particular instance. This would indicate that there is relevance in the development of family planning provision in all countries (quite apart from the arguments for these on personal and health grounds) but that their impact will be dependent on the social and economic conditions in which potential users live. Consequently birth rates may remain high, if individual views on family size are that many children are needed. However, the adoption of birth-control (alongside high family size preferences) and the availability of effective means of birth-control may influence fertility attitudes. The result would be not only a reduction in the number of unwanted pregnancies and the postponement and spacing of wanted births, but also the reduction of the number of children seen as necessary.

The truth lies in neither extreme. It is reasonable to argue that family planning programmes in the Third World may have been too optimistic in assuming that they alone can rapidly bring fertility down to replacement level, but there is no warrant for asserting that they are irrelevant to such a goal. As has been pointed out earlier, failure should be examined both in relation to demand and supply and the possibility that programmes may have identified wrong targets, ignored questions of cultural appropriateness and overemphasised medical approaches. The widespread availability and legitimisation of all methods of fertility control is essential, alongside encouragement of economic development and attempts to ensure that its benefits are shared equally by all members of society. The tragedy is that for many countries in the Third World, neither approach is being fully sustained.

There are still commentators who maintain that if you put electricity in a traditional village the birth rate will come down. On a lesser level, there is a considerable body of thinkers who press for socio-economic development as not only the prerequisite for fertility decline, but as the only policy to be preferred. Conversely, there seems to be a group of policy makers who consider that family planning can be promoted as not only a major but even the sole solution to the imbalances and inequalities visible in the contemporary world. Perhaps it is blindness to the past which creates these extremes of opinion. A more sober and common-sense review of the situation is to realise that there is every advantage in the community attempting to assist individuals to control their fertility, whatever their socio-economic background. Observation suggests that, left to their own devices, people's achievements tend to lag behind their goals and that, all other considerations apart, the control of fertility through the less effective methods of contraception combined with illegal abortion is a costly and unpleasant set of choices, which it is humane and in the interests of public health to replace. Certainly, during the beginning of the demographic transition in the West, society did not have the maturity to assist people in the difficult process of controlling their own fertility. Birth rates fell in the West despite public and professional opposition to any type of assistance in family planning: perhaps this is a mistake from which the contemporary developing world can learn.

SELECTED REFERENCES AND BIBLIOGRAPHY

Ajami, I. "Differential Fertility in Peasant Communities. A Study of Six Iranian Villages." *Population Studies*. 30, 453 1976

Becker, G. "An Economic Analysis of Fertility." In Universities National Bureau Committee for Economic Research, *Demographic and Economic Change in Developed Countries*. Princeton University Press, Princeton 1960

Bernhardt, E. N. "Fertility and Economic Status: Some Recent Findings on Differentials in Sweden." *Population Studies*. 26, 175 1972

Blake, J. "Are Babies Consumer Durables?" *Population Studies*. 22, 5 1968

Callahan, D. *Abortion: Law, Choice and Morality*. Macmillan, London 1970

Carlsson, G. "The Decline of Fertility: Innovation or Adjustment Process?" *Population Studies*. 20, 149 1966

Coale, A. J. "The Decline of Fertility in Europe from the French Revolution to World War II." In Behrman, S. J., Corsa, L. and Freedman, R. *Fertility and Family Planning: A World View*. University of Michigan Press, Ann Arbor 1969

Coale, A. J. "The History of the Human Population." *Scientific American*. 231 (3), 41 1974

Davis, G. *Interception of Pregnancy*. Angus & Robertson, Sydney 1974

Freedman, D. "The Relation of Economic Status to Fertility." *American Economic Review*. 53, 414 1963

Gille, H. "Summary Review of Fertility Differentials in Developed Countries." *International Population Conference, London 1969*. Vol. 3. I.U.S.S.P., Liege 1971

Glass, D. V. "Fertility Trends in Europe Since the Second World War." In Behrman, S. J., Corsa, L. & Freedman, R. *Fertility and*

Family Planning; A World View. University of Michigan Press, Ann Arbor 1969

Hall, R. "The Demographic Transition; Stage Four." *Current Anthropology*. 13, 212 1972

Heer, D. M. "Economic Development and Fertility." *Demography*. 3, 423 1966

Kocher, J. E. *Rural Development, Income Distribution and Fertility Decline*. Population Council, New York 1973

Loraine, J. A. *Syndromes of the Seventies*. Peter Owen, London 1977

McNeill, W. *Plagues and Peoples*. Basil Blackwell, Oxford 1977

Mincer, J. "Market Prices, Opportunity Costs and Income Effects." In Christ, C. F. (ed.) *Measurement in Economics*. Stanford University Press, Stanford 1963

Mohr, J. C. *Abortion in America*. Oxford University Press, Oxford 1978

Polgar, S. (ed.) *Culture and Population*. Schenkman, Cambridge, Mass. 1971

Polgar, S. *Population, Ecology and Social Evolution*. Mouton, The Hague 1975

Ravenholt, R. T. and Chao, J. "World Fertility Trends, 1976." *Population Report*. Series J–12, George Washington University Medical Centre 1976

Rich, W. *Smaller Families through Social and Economic Progress*. Overseas Development Council, Washington 1973

Teitelbaum, M. J. "The Relevance of Demographic Transition Theory for Developing Countries." *Science*. 188, 420 1975

Van der Tak. *Abortion, Fertility and Changing Legislation; An International Review*. Lexington, New York 1974

Wrong, D. H. "Trends in Class Fertility in Western Nations." *Canadian Journal of Economic and Political Science*. 24, 216 1958

Chapter 9

The Individual and the Family

We stressed at the start of this book our belief that fertility is a matter of profound significance in the lives of individual members of society, affecting the life styles and life chances both of parents and of the children born. Our aim in this chapter is to pursue further some of the consequences of fertility patterns for individuals and families, concentrating on the effects on health, the implications of a reduction in family size for both parents and children, and the consequences of unwanted births. Illegitimacy and childlessness are considered in some detail and lead into an exploration of adoption in human society.

HEALTH

The age of the mother, her parity and social class are all important and interlocking variables affecting human reproduction.

The risks of pregnancy to the mother are higher than average immediately after puberty, reach their lowest level during the late teens and twenties, rise slowly in the early thirties and more steeply in the later thirties and forties. The pattern is a persistent one and applies whatever the basal level of maternal mortality in a country. The risks of death to the baby during delivery and in infancy follow a similar curve.

The risks to the mother and baby are lowest for the second and third children, somewhat higher for the first and considerably higher for the fourth and subsequent pregnancies (*see* Fig. 40). This variation is independent of age, although naturally women with large numbers of children are usually in the older age bracket (which compounds the problems facing them).

The interval between births is another factor affecting the health of mother and child (*see* Fig. 41). A second conception within twelve months of a delivery is particularly at risk. Very long intervals, of more than five to seven years, are also associated with some rise in risk to mother and baby.

In all countries, but particularly developing countries, the children of large families receive less care than those of small. This is partly

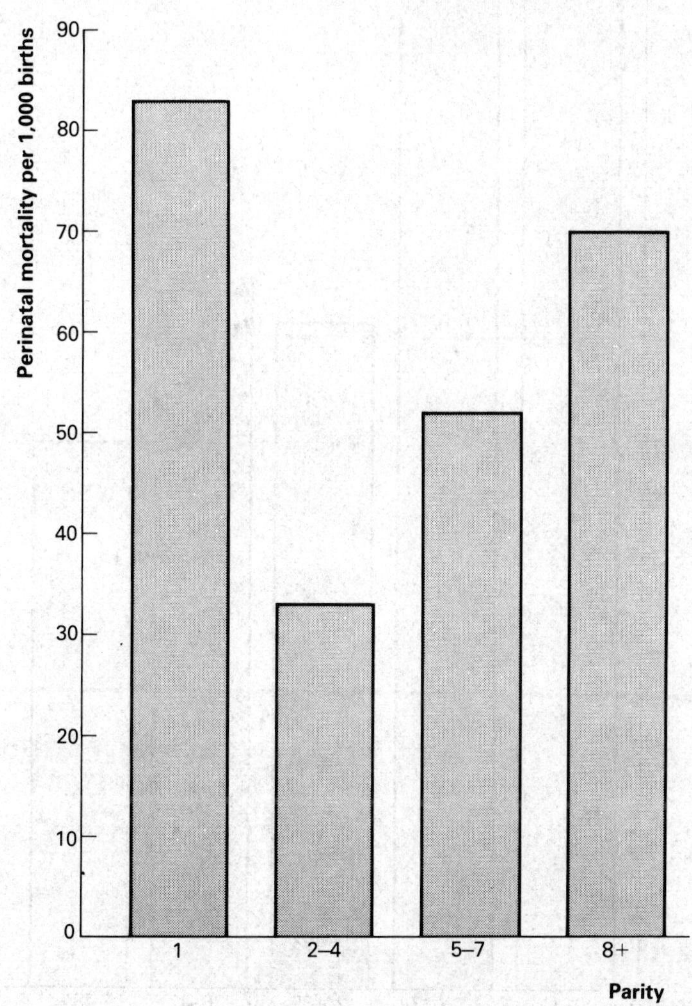

(*Source:* Omran, A. R. *The Health Theme in Family Planning*. Carolina Population Center 1971)

Fig. 40. *Perinatal deaths* (*stillbirths and deaths in first week of life*) *and parity* (*India 1957*).

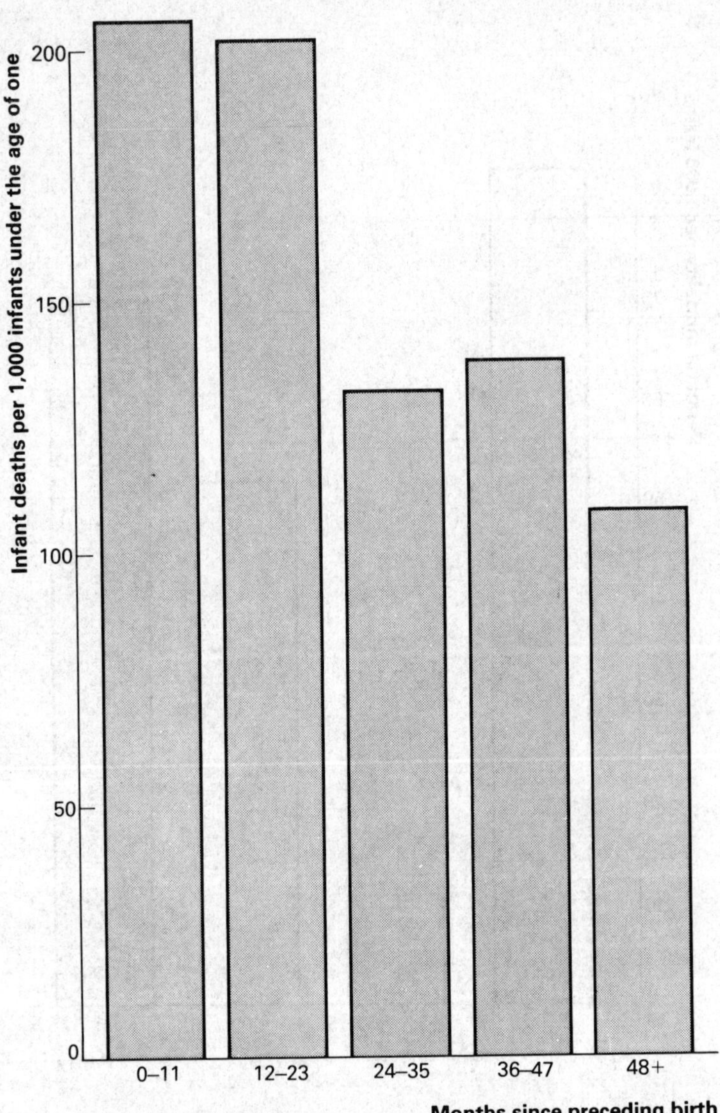

(*Source:* Omran (op. cit.))

Fig. 41. *Infant deaths by birth interval* (*India 1955–58*).

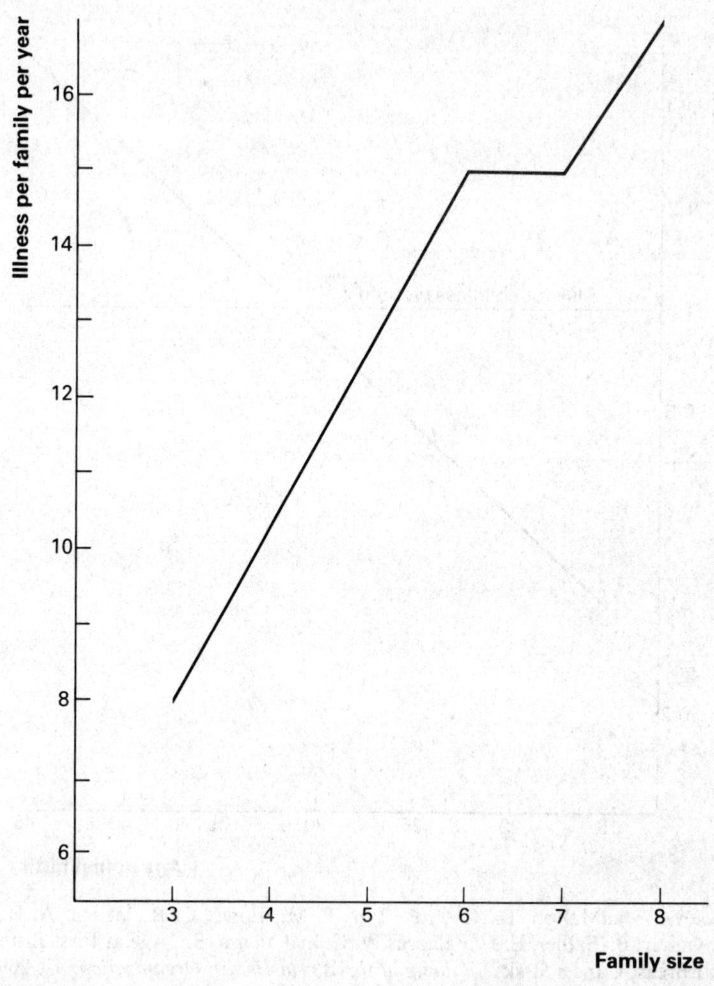

(*Source:* Omran (op. cit.))

Fig. 42. *Cases of gastro-enteritis per family per year (U.S.A. 1960s).*

a matter of how the disposable income is divided and partly of how much time a mother has to devote to each child. Children of large families are more at risk for infectious diseases (*see* Fig. 42).

Not only are older women at greater risk for delivery, but the incidence of a number of congenital abnormalities rises with maternal age. There may be a biological factor due to ageing of the ova, which have been set aside unchanged since the birth of the mother,

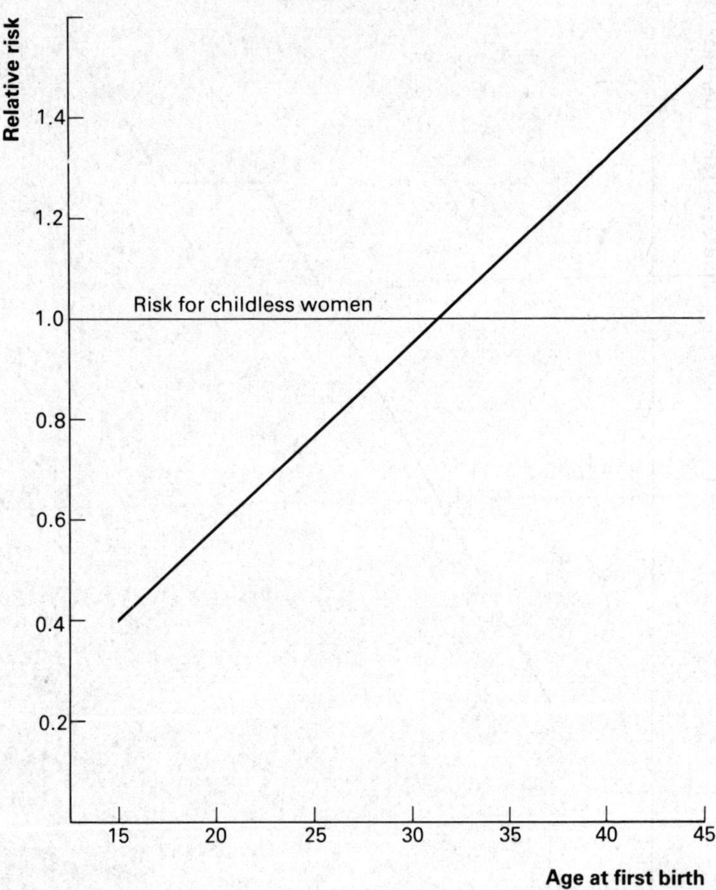

(*Source:* MacMahon, B., Cole, P., Lin, T. M., Lowe, C. R., Mirra, A. P., Ravuihar, B., Salber, E. J., Valaoras, V. G. and Yuasa, S. "Age at First Birth and Breast Cancer Risk." *Bulletin of the World Health Organisation*. 43, 209 1970)

Fig. 43. *Relative risk of cancer by age at first birth.*

although other biological explanations are also possible. The effect is particularly striking in the case of mongolism (*see* Table 32).

Family planning, by restricting births among older women, has a direct effect on maternal and infant mortality. In developing countries, one of the most straightforward ways of improving maternal and child care is to extend family planning services as rapidly as possible. If births could be concentrated in the age group twenty to thirty-four, the mortality in Thailand would be reduced by 20 per cent, while in Bangladesh a family planning campaign aimed at mothers with four or more children could reduce maternal mortality by 30 per cent.

At the same time, it is also honest to recognise that the postponement of the first pregnancy, which is common as societies develop, also carries with it some penalties. The human animal was evolved to begin bearing children within a few years of puberty and the risk of the first birth, when postponed to the later twenties or earlier thirties, is greater than if the woman had borne that child when she was nineteen. Postponement of the first pregnancy has one spectacular pathological effect which is rarely remarked upon, but outweighs all others in its significance. Cancer of the breast is the

TABLE 32: INCIDENCE OF DOWN'S SYNDROME (MONGOLISM) BY MATERNAL AGE

Age	Incide[illegible]
Under 15	[illegible]
15–19	[illegible]
20–24	[illegible]
25–29	[illegible]
30–34	[illegible]
35–39	[illegible]
40–44	[illegible]
Over 45	[illegible]

(*Source:* Omran, A. R. *The Hea*[illegible] *Family Planning*. Carolina Popula[illegible]re 1971)

commonest lethal malignancy in the Western world, killing one in twenty in the United Kingdom and approximately one in eighteen in the U.S.A. It is still relatively rare in the developing world, only reaching one seventh of the incidence in Taiwan that it does in Boston. Like cancer of the lung, cancer of the breast is an environmental disease of some type. Among the Japanese it is still a comparatively unusual disease, but if a Japanese woman migrates to the U.S.A., her chance of getting the disease rises and those of her children are the same as for the Caucasian inhabitants of the U.S.A. If we are to look for an explanation of this disease, it is likely to be found in the way in which we use our reproductive systems. There is a direct relationship between the age at which a woman has her first child and the chance of developing cancer of the breast later in life: the earlier she has her first child, the less the risk (*see* Fig. 43). In the long term, medical science must not only look for methods of controlling human fertility but also select those which are likely to leave a healthy woman at the menopause. Those who say oral contraceptives are "unnatural" overlook the fact that the control of reproduction and the postponement of the first pregnancy is also "unnatural" and has a proven mortality. As has been pointed out earlier, women who take the Pill have a lower chance of developing lumps in the breast than those that do not. While it would be superficial to suggest that oral contraceptives as they currently exist will necessarily protect against cancer in later life, it is realistic to point out that interest in hormonal methods of controlling fertility in women is likely to continue for as far as can be seen into the future. Ultimately, we may expect to develop some type of oral, hormonal contraceptive which controls fertility and protects the breast (and to a lesser extent the uterus) against diseases which are associated with the long intervals of non-pregnancy which are a necessary part of modern living.

EFFECT ON PARENTS

The decline in the family size of married couples in industrialised nations has been one of the most important aspects of social change over the last century, not least in its effect on the life chances of women in these countries. This can be seen by contrasting the typical life patterns of women born in the mid-nineteenth century with that of a woman born around the time of the Second World War.

A woman born in Victorian England in 1841 had a life expectancy at birth of about forty-two years, a figure which reflects the high infant and child mortality of the time. One in seven would die in their first year of life, and by the age of fifteen less than 70 per cent would still be alive. In towns, death rates amongst the poor would have been even higher, with up to 40 or 50 per cent dying in the first five years of life. For illegitimate children the chance of death in the first year of life was highest of all.

For the lucky two-thirds who survived to their late teens and became the potential mothers of the next generation, future life expectancy was about forty years, much of which would be taken up by child-bearing and infant care. A woman who survived to the age of forty-five would be likely to have married in her early or mid-twenties and to have produced at least six children, a third of whom would have died before reaching their late teens. A typical poor mother with five or six living children could have experienced ten or more pregnancies and would have spent the bulk of her reproductive period either pregnant or caring for a young baby. If she reached forty-five, she could look forward on average to a further twenty years of life, but with only a 60 per cent chance of reaching the age of sixty-five. If she had married a man of twenty-five, there would be a fifty-fifty chance of her being widowed before her sixty-fifth birthday.

If we contrast this picture with the life of a woman born during the Second World War, we find a very different story. Initial expectation of life would have been nearly seventy years and the chance of dying before the age of fifteen less than one in twenty. At this age, future life expectancy would be over sixty years, and death during her reproductive period most unlikely. Marrying in her early twenties, she could expect to have two or three children, all of whom would stand a good chance of surviving to adulthood. These children would probably have been born in the first ten years of marriage and today she would be in her mid-thirties, probably back at work, with her spell of pregnancy and nursing of infants behind her. When her children are on the point of leaving home, by the time she is forty-five, she will be able to look forward to an average of thirty-five more years of life, with a high probability of survival beyond retirement for both herself and her husband.

The differences in the typical life pattern of two such women, separated at birth by some 100 years, can also be thought of in terms of a family life-cycle from marriage, through child-bearing and rearing, to the stage at which children begin to leave home and marry, leaving the parents eventually with an "empty nest", retirement and, finally, death.

For a Victorian wife, marriage would usually be followed rapidly by pregnancy and the period of child-bearing. Infant care would involve a long period, taking her well into her forties and overlapping with the care of school-age and teenage children. It would be common for her first grandchild to be born while she was still caring for young school-age children. The period of pre-retirement independence would be short and the departure of her last, dependent child likely to coincide with the onset of old age and widowhood, if the mother were fortunate enough to survive that long.

In contrast, a girl born in post-war Britain, marrying in her early twenties around 1970, might well delay having a family for two or three years and then have her two children in close succession, so that the period of child-bearing and infant care is a brief one. By the age of forty her children will be in their teens, and by fifty both may have left home, leaving her with some ten years or more of independence before retirement, during which her grandchildren are likely to be born. Prospects of a lengthy retirement are good and a substantial proportion of this is likely to be spent as a widow, if current differences in mortality for men and women persist and she has married a man older than herself. For any individual woman today, the story may be very different, of course. Many girls still marry at younger ages, often when pregnant, and some of these may have larger families. Even here, however, child-bearing may be over by the late twenties. In this case a substantial proportion of her adult life will involve responsibilities for herself, her husband and children of an older age-group only.

The main difference for the woman born into modern Britain is that only a small proportion of her adult life is spent in being the mother of young children. For two-thirds of her potential working life the mother of today is free from any commitment to the care of dependent children. One major implication of this change is the prospect for female employment, which has itself been a factor in determining the low family size preferences of most women in Britain today. In recent years, delays in starting a family have usually involved, or been caused by, female work-force participation; part-time employment also has become increasingly common for women whose children have reached school age or older; and most women return to employment as they reach the stage at which their children leave home.

This pattern can be seen in the increase in the number of married women working, both part-time and full-time, since the Second World War. In 1955, there were about 3 million married women in the work force. By 1965, this had risen to 5 million and in 1975 there were over 6 million. Married female employment now accounts for more than two thirds of the female work-force, concentrated in the 25–49 age-group, which accounts for half of the total women employed. According to the 1971 British Census, the proportion of women who were economically active fell from 70 per cent at marriage to 35 per cent or less for marriages of three to nine years duration. It then rose steadily until over half were working at marriage durations of fourteen years or more. At all ages, a large majority of childless women work, while for those with children the proportion economically active rises from 14 per cent at the start of marriage to 40 per cent for marriage durations over ten years. The mean family size of economically active women is smaller at all stages, largely due to the high proportion of the childless amongst them.

Motherhood and employment are no longer seen as incompatible in our society. Women are returning to work earlier in their marriages for many reasons: to supplement a husband's inadequate wages, to gain some financial independence, to get money for the purchase of "luxury" goods, and also for companionship and to escape the isolation of the home (especially as children grow up and require less constant attention). Concern expressed in the 1950s over "latch-key" children has lessened and today there is more emphasis on the positive aspects of mothers working, and the advantages to pre-school children of an alternative to the home situation, leading to a demand for more play group and nursery facilities.

At the same time, the earning capacity of many women remains low, despite "equal" pay and the Sex Discrimination Acts. This affects particularly the life chances of the growing number of single-parent families. Furthermore, even though it is now accepted that a woman's place is no longer in the home, female socialisation has not fully caught up with this, so that for many women, early socialisation is still largely a preparation for marriage and motherhood and does not fully recognise that work outside the home is likely to take up a larger part of adult life than being mother to dependent children.

EFFECT ON CHILDREN

Changes in family size have implications for children as well as parents. In developing societies, a majority of births are third order or higher (*see* Fig. 44). In developed societies, most children are brought up in families where they have at most one or two siblings. Nevertheless, the total number of children currently being raised in families of four or more remains substantial (*see* Fig. 45). What are the implications for a child of being brought up in a large family in a low fertility society?

Bossard and Boll, in a study of American families with six or more children, suggested a number of characteristics of what they call the "large family system". They see parenthood in such families as "extensive" rather than "intensive", eliminating anxiety and possessiveness—but also stimulation, with the children being left to fend for themselves from an early age. The task of socialisation and discipline often falls to the group, and especially to older siblings, so that nagging and protective parents are rare. This is seen as advantageous in eliminating some of the neuroses of the small family system.

Large families are more likely to experience the loss of a parent whilst the last child is still young. There may be recurrent domestic crises with each birth, which can entail the admission to care of some of the older children, or impose added strains on those old enough to help. Large families are more subject to economic pressures, often have to face hostile attitudes from outside, and consequently stress the importance of "sticking together".

The large family system is also likely to generate role specialisation and a strong group and familial awareness. Conformity is valued

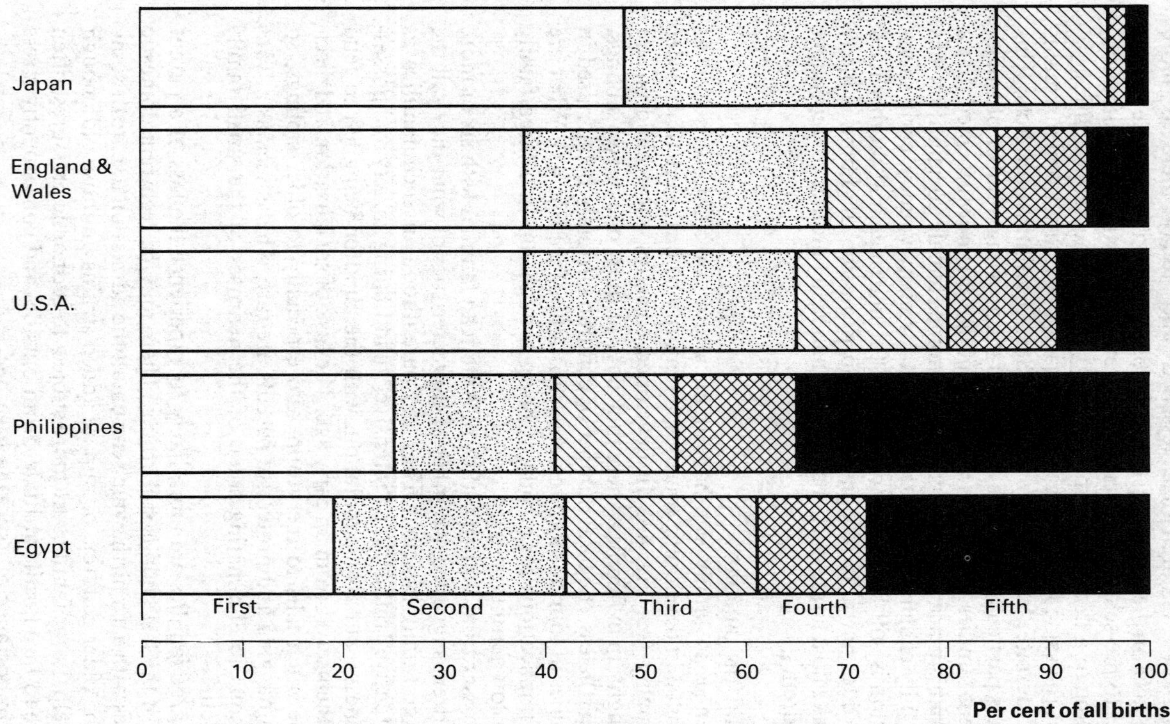

(*Source:* Berelson, B. *World Population Status Report*. Population Council, New York 1974)

Fig. 44. *Birth order in selected countries (1966–69).*

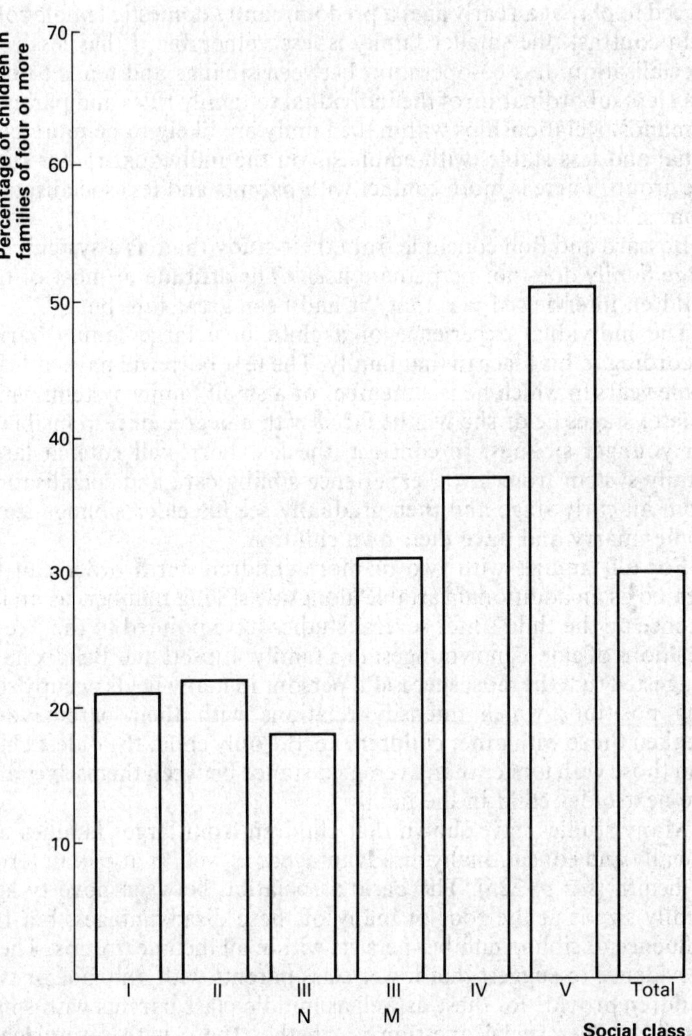

(*Source:* Davie, R., Butler, N. and Goldstein, H. *From Birth to Seven*. Longmans, London 1972)

Fig. 45. *Percentage of children (aged seven) in families containing four or more children by social class (Great Britain, 1965).*

above self-expression, listening prevails over talking, and co-operation and "doing one's bit" is vital. One result of this is that daughters, especially the older ones in the family, are likely to learn (and be forced to play at an early age) a predominantly domestic female role.

In contrast, the smaller family is less vulnerable. It has less role specialisation, less co-operation between siblings and tends to display less subordination of the individual to family rules and parental demands. Relationships within the family are likely to be more personal and less stable, with emphasis on the individual rather than the group. There is more contact with parents and less socialisation from siblings.

Bossard and Boll conclude from their study that, as a system, the large family does not perpetuate itself. The attitude of most of the children interviewed was that "it had been great fun, but ...".

The individual experience of a child in a large family varies according to his place in that family. The first born will have at least some years in which he is a member of a small family system, while at later stages he or she will be faced with a degree of responsibility for younger siblings. In contrast, the last born will enter a large family system from birth, experience sibling care and socialisation from an early stage and then gradually see his elder siblings leave home, marry and have their own children.

For all families with two or more children, birth order can be treated as an additional variable alongside sibling number, as an influence on the child's life; several studies have pointed to the "key" positions of eldest and youngest in a family. Lipsett and Bendix have suggested that the most successful persons in many fields occupy sibling positions which intensify relations with their parents and weaken those with other children, i.e. the only child, the oldest child and those with longer than average distance between themselves and the next older child in the family.

Many studies have shown that children from larger families are socially and educationally disadvantaged, as well as at risk in terms of health (*see* p. 225). The basic association between poverty and family size is at the root of many of these disadvantages, but the influence of sibling number persists within all income groups. There is evidence to suggest that lower class parents with only one or two children provide for these as well as middle-class parents with small families. The crucial question is whether those with several children would have been able to provide a better life for them if they had had fewer. Will reducing family size, or increasing birth intervals, actually reduce the disadvantages associated with larger familes?

It is possible that those parents who limit their families are in some sense qualitatively different and so better able to provide a good home, but it seems more plausible to suggest that many of the disadvantages faced by the child in a large family result from the size of family and consequent economic problems, rather than from parental fecklessness. Meanwhile, priority should go to helping those children already born into large families, especially where they are being raised in poverty. There can be little doubt that reducing the deprivation they experience in childhood will be an important step towards maximising the chances that, when they grow to adulthood, they will choose to plan a smaller family for themselves.

It would be misleading to leave the topic of the impact of family size on the child without noting the possible disadvantages of small families. The only child has long been seen as suffering a particular sort of disadvantage—materially favoured (but subject to parental over-indulgence and excessive protectiveness), lonely, selfish and missing out on the socialisation provided by sibling interaction. The widespread belief in this is reflected in the expressed preference of most married couples for at least two children—though much less markedly, let it be said, in their actual reproductive behaviour.

The French demographer, Alfred Sauvy, has argued that similar problems, though on a lesser scale, exist for the child with only one sibling. He sees a family of three, four or five children as the social optimum, a view shared also by Bossard and Boll, whose study of large families we considered earlier. Sauvy considers that three children is the minimum at which couples should aim, on the grounds that such a group is necessary to ensure the renewal of population: "Below this figure quantity and quality decline together: life revenges the insult directed at it." Fortunately, an increasing number of couples in both developed and developing countries seem prepared to ignore such advice, finding little to worry them in the prospect of a population that has ceased to grow.

In a field where new insights are certain to develop and new philosophies arise, one outcome seems likely to remain beyond dispute. As numerous studies indicate that many higher order births are unplanned and unwanted by the parents (*see* Fig. 46), there is every reason for society to pay special attention to extending birth-control choices to the underprivileged with large families, as one component in improving the lot of parents and existing children.

BIRTH TIMING

Just as the motivation to use birth-control arises both from a desire to limit the total number of births and a concern over their timing

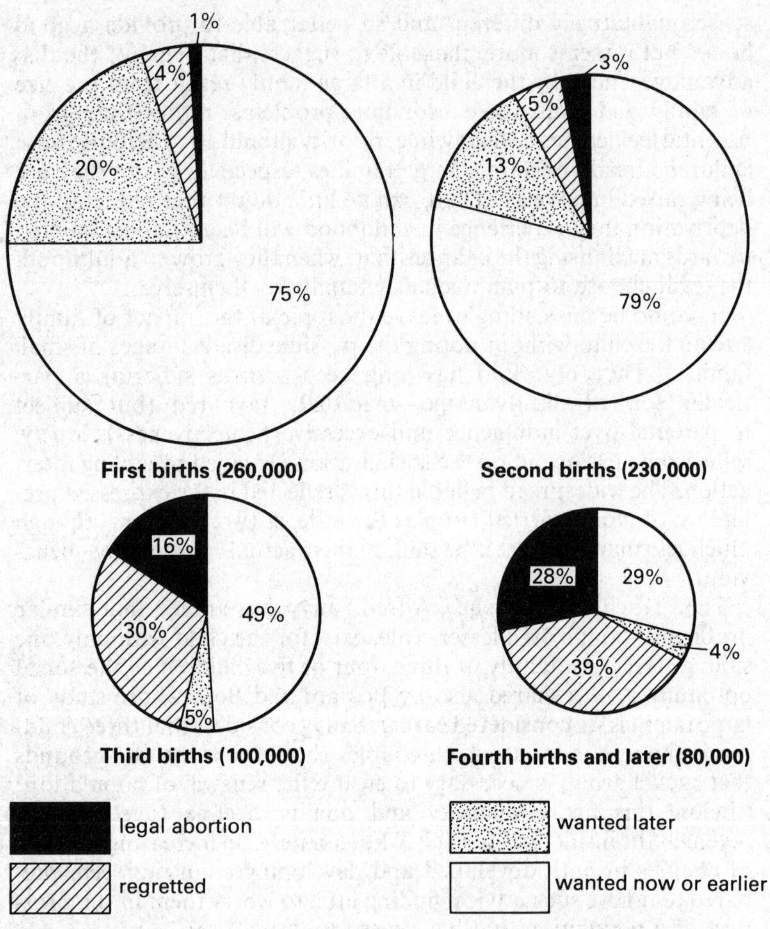

(*Source:* Thompson, J. "Fertility and Abortion Inside and Outside Marriage." *Population Trends*. 3, 8 1976)

Fig. 46. *Wanted and unwanted conceptions: annual births and abortions for England and Wales married women only (1973).*

and spacing, so the individual consequences of fertility patterns relate not only to the number of children a woman has, but also to the timing of their arrival. Likewise, a child's life chances are affected not only by the size of his family and the position he holds in it, but also by the age of his parents, whether he was born in or out of wedlock and whether his birth was wanted or unwanted.

TEENAGE PREGNANCY

Biologically, the late teens and early twenties represent the time of maximum coital activity. While the risks of delivery are high for a woman who conceives soon after puberty, they fall to a low level by the ages of eighteen or nineteen and do not rise again significantly until the thirties. In a modern society, most teenagers are still undergoing education and the trend to prolong education into the twenties is still rising. The conflict between biology and social constraints is obvious. For many it has an unhappy outcome. In 1977, in the U.S.A., approximately 1 million girls aged fifteen to nineteen conceived a pregnancy (*see* Fig. 47). This figure represents one in ten female adolescents, and one in four of those who were estimated to be sexually active.

For much of the post-war period there has been a rising i[illegible]dence of teenage pregnancy in Western societies, and the [illegible] mar-

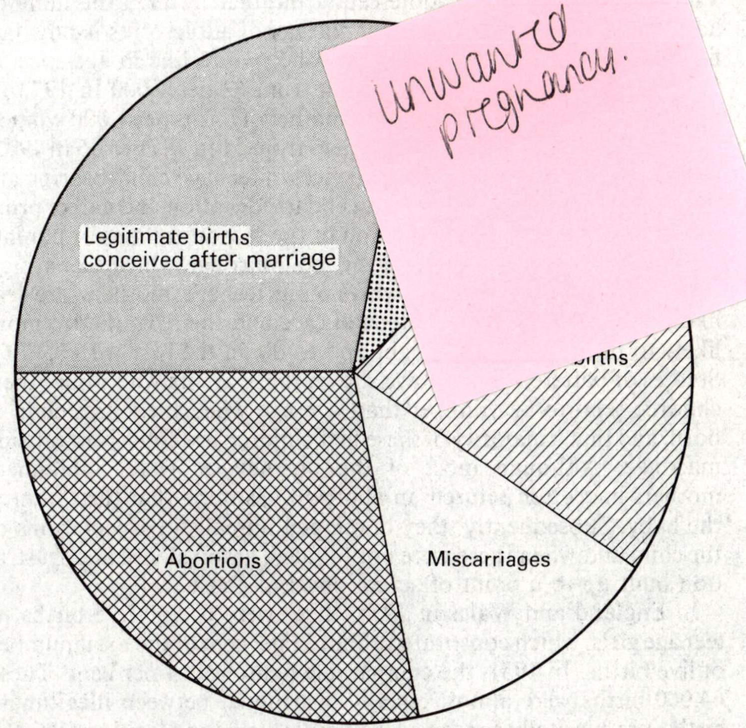

(*Source:* Jaffe, R. in Bogue, D. (ed) *Adolescent Fertility*. University of Chicago 1977)

Fig. 47. *Estimated outcome of teenage pregnancies in the U.S.A.* (*1975*).

riage fell to lower levels than had been common between the two World Wars. The incidence of venereal disease rose, patterns of premarital intercourse changed and vigorous public debate has revolved around the need to make contraceptive and abortion services available to the young unmarried, as well as around the factors that may be associated with these changes.

However, society often continues to debate a problem at the time when trends are being reversed. It now seems that, with a remarkable degree of homogeneity, levels of adolescent fertility are beginning to fall throughout the Western nations. In the United Kingdom it reached a peak in 1971 and in the U.S.A. in 1972. The fall is due both to an increased use of contraceptives and an increased resort to abortion, at a time when the proportion of young people who are sexually active is probably still rising. Although guesses are difficult, it is thought that in the U.S.A. in 1966 there may have been 3 million sexually active adolescents, and that by 1975 the number had risen to 4.5 million. The total number of adolescents is now falling in the U.S.A., but there has also been a decline in age-specific fertility rates for the under twenties, from 62 per 1,000 in 1972 to 56 per 1,000 in 1975. In Britain the number of births per 1,000 women aged fifteen to nineteen has also fallen, from 51 in 1971 to 36 in 1975.

The social and personal consequences of teenage child-bearing are many. For the girl, it can mean an end to education and career prospects, and a premature assumption of the responsibilities of parenthood, either as a single mother or in a marriage which has a high probability of later breakdown. Young teenage mothers are less likely to receive adequate antenatal care and their babies are more likely to be of low birth weight and to die in the first week of life. Studies of battered babies have shown that parents who injure their children tend to be younger than average when their first child is born, and that a majority of these first children are conceived outside marriage. Although most of the pregnancies were unplanned, mothers had often refused an abortion, claiming that they wanted the baby. Subsequently, they developed unrealistic expectations of the child and when these were not fulfilled, ambivalence and frustration built up to a point of actual physical abuse.

In England and Wales in 1975, there were 64,000 live births to teenage girls, which constituted about 11 per cent of the total number of live births. In 1951, the comparable figure was 4 per cent. These 64,000 births were almost equally distributed between illegitimate births, pre-maritally conceived legitimate births and legitimate births conceived after marriage. Although a majority of the births were legitimate, most conceptions occurred outside marriage and much interest has centred on the problem of extra-marital pregnancy in teenagers. Table 33 shows the changing pattern of outcome to such pregnancies, ignoring miscarriages and any illegal abortions.

The process by which single girls reach these various outcomes of pregnancy have been explored in America by Rains and in Scotland by Macintyre (whose study *Single and Pregnant* offers many interesting insights into the pregnant girl's perception, and subsequent handling, of her situation). Not all conceptions were "unwanted" and for many of those already planning to marry the event did not represent a great crisis in their lives. In her contact with parents, professionals and others, the pregnant girl is shown to be concerned

TABLE 33: EXTRA-MARITALLY CONCEIVED LIVE BIRTHS AND LEGAL ABORTIONS TO UNMARRIED WOMEN, AGED UNDER TWENTY, ENGLAND AND WALES, 1968–1975 (IN UNITS OF 1,000)

Outcome of Pregnancy	1966	1968	1971	1973	1975
Illegitimate Birth	21	22	22	21	21
Pre-maritally conceived					
Legitimate Birth	37	35	35	29	22
Legal Abortion	—	3	16	23	24
Total	58	60	73	73	67

(*Source:* Registrar-General's Statistical Review of England and Wales for the year 1968; *Population Trends.* no. 5, H.M.S.O., London 1976)

with negotiating a moral character: is she to be seen as a promiscuous "bad" girl, a "nice" girl who has made a mistake, or a "normal-as-if-married" girl who has conceived earlier than intended? For those with the latter perception of themselves, the offer of an abortion carried the implication that they were "bad" girls, while for others professional assumptions that they would marry pre-empted discussion about abortion; for the remainder, some doctors appeared reluctant to offer abortion out of a wish to punish. Actual outcomes depended on a range of factors, from the girl's own wishes to the possibility of marriage to the putative father and her luck in relation to doctors. All too often, those professionals involved in helping had only limited knowledge of the range of factors involved, or made grossly oversimplified assumptions about the girl's "definition of her situation".

ILLEGITIMACY

An illegitimate birth is just one of several possible outcomes of extramarital pregnancy (*see* Table 33). Any understanding of patterns of illegitimacy must recognise this and start with a consideration of sexual activity outside marriage (*see* Fig. 48). Becoming an unmarried mother is the result of a series of interdependent events, starting with forays into extra-marital sex, continuing with an unwanted pregnancy and terminating in the birth of an illegitimate child, and may be avoided at any one of several stages. The level of illegitimacy in any society is, therefore, dependent on the proportion of women of child-bearing ages who are unmarried, the proportion of these who are sexually active and the extent to which they are using contraception, and, finally, on how many of those who do conceive reach alternative outcomes through abortion or marriage.

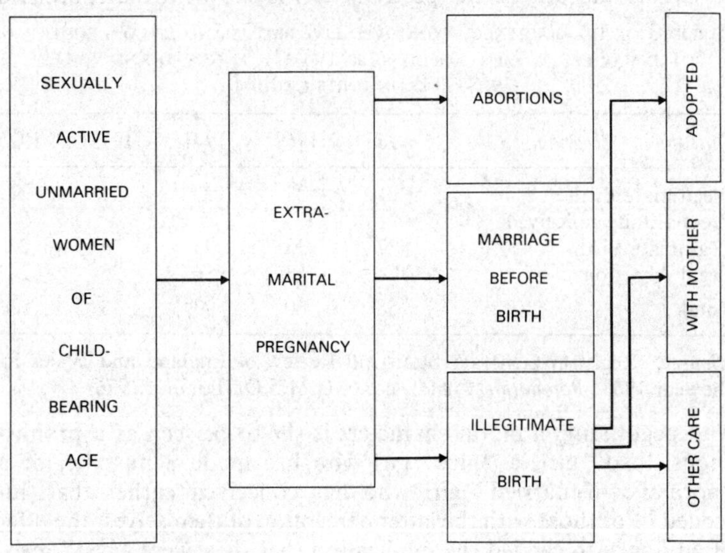

Fig. 48. *Pathways to illegitimacy.*

Patterns of illegitimacy vary considerably across the world (*see* Fig. 49). The highest levels, whether measured by the illegitimacy ratio or a general illegitimate fertility rate (*see* p. 33), are found in the Caribbean countries, where marriage is typically late and a proportion of women never marry; there are other countries, however, such as Eire, where illegitimacy levels remain low despite late marriage and a substantial number of women remaining single. Very low levels of illegitimacy are often associated with universal early marriage (*see* p. 60). However, Japan offers an interesting example of a country where barely 1 per cent of teenagers are married, but illegitimacy is very rare, as a result of limited pre-marital sexual activity and easily available abortion. The importance of the latter can be seen in the decline in the illegitimacy rate from 13.5 in 1940

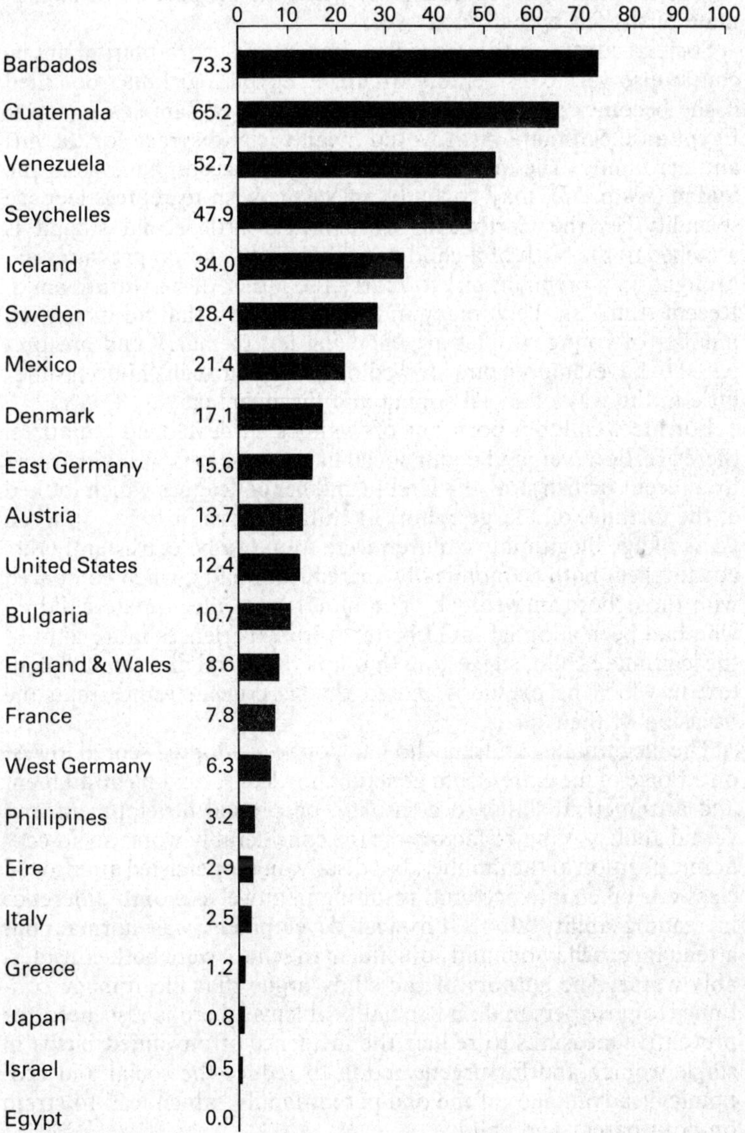

(*Source: U.N. Demographic Year Book 1975*)

Fig. 49. *Illegitimate births as a proportion of total live births in selected countries* (1972–73).

to 1.6 in 1964, the major fall occurring in the years after the liberalisation of abortion in 1948 and 1949, when the proportion of illegitimate births fell by half in six years.

Societal attitudes towards illegitimacy and extra-marital intercourse also vary considerably. In upper Egypt, a girl may be killed if she becomes pregnant, and even in educated families in lower Egypt an illegitimate birth would mean social disgrace for the girl and her family. The practice of female circumcision here, as in the Sudan (*see* p. 53), may partially reflect the wish to repress teenage sexuality. In the Caribbean, by contrast, little social stigma is attached to the birth of a child out of wedlock and no pressures are brought on a pregnant girl to marry the father of her future child. Recent trends in illegitimacy in Sweden suggest that an increasing number of young couples are choosing not to marry and are prepared to have children outside wedlock, and that such children suffer little in the way of social stigma and disadvantage.

For most children born out of wedlock in developed countries, there are, however, still major social handicaps, as is well illustrated by a recent British study by Crellin and her colleagues which looked at the fortunes of a large cohort of children born in 1959. At seven years of age illegitimate children were found to be consistently disadvantaged, both economically and educationally, when compared with those born in wedlock. The minority of illegitimate children who had been adopted fared better, with experiences more akin to the legitimate child, suggesting that it is the social and familial context in which he or she is reared that is crucial, rather than the occasion of their birth.

The illegitimate children who had not been adopted scored lowest on a range of measures from general knowledge, reading attainment and arithmetical skills, to creativity, perceptual development and verbal ability. A major factor was the considerably worse socio-economic position of the families, but disadvantage persisted after social class was taken into account, resulting in a twelve-month difference in reading ability alone. Physical development was normal, but attendance, behaviour and adjustment in school were both considerably worse. The authors of the study argue that illegitimacy continues to pose personal and social problems; there is also need for preventive measures to reduce the incidence of unwanted births in single women and for urgent action to reduce the social and economic disadvantages of the one-parent family, which lead to strain on both parent and child.

Recent increases in illegitimacy in developed nations The post-war period has seen major increases in illegitimacy levels in the U.S.A. and Britain. In the U.S.A. the illegitimacy rate rose from 7.1 per

1,000 in 1940 to 21.8 in 1960 and 24.1 in 1968. In England and Wales, the rate rose from 5.9 in 1940 to 10.3 in 1960 and 22.7 in 1968. Rates have fallen in both countries during the past decade, but the proportion of illegitimate births (the illegitimacy ratio) has remained at a high level, because marital fertility has been falling as fast or faster than extra-marital fertility.

In Britain, these increases were accompanied by a rise in the number of pre-maritally conceived legitimate births, emphasising the over-all increase in extra-marital conceptions. These increases cannot be explained in terms of a greater number of women in age-groups at risk, and seems rather to reflect a growth in pre-marital sexual intercourse (especially amongst teenagers). Cutright has suggested that part of the rise in conceptions at earlier ages may be due to a fall in age at menarche, but it seems more fruitful to look for answers in the changes in societal attitudes towards sexuality and illegitimacy in the post-war decades, which were accompanied by ambivalent attitudes towards the provision of birth-control to the unmarried.

In 1968 there were 70,000 illegitimate births in England and Wales and 75,000 pre-maritally conceived legitimate births. By 1975, the numbers had fallen to 54,000 and 40,000 respectively, while the number of legal abortions to single women had risen from 10,000 to 61,000. A key factor in the initial decline may have been the easier availability of legal abortion following the passing of the 1967 Abortion Act. However, the number of extra-maritally conceived births has continued to decline in recent years (when there has been little change in the total number of terminations) which suggests that increased use of contraception amongst the unmarried has been an additional factor. The fall in illegitimate births has been accompanied by a decrease in the proportion of these offered for adoption, from about one in five in the years before 1968 to less than one in ten since 1975. This suggests that those girls who do not want to keep their child are increasingly choosing to have an abortion, rather than surrender it for adoption. However, this trend has continued despite a levelling off in numbers of abortions, so that another factor is probably a greater willingness to accept unmarried parenthood. The more rapid fall in pre-marital conceptions may likewise reflect increased resistance to pressures to marry if a girl decides to keep a child. For this reason, we should be cautious about predicting further falls in illegitimacy. The stabilisation of illegitimacy ratios in recent years suggests that future trends may be determined as much by changing attitudes to marriage as by increased use of abortion and contraception.

By 1975, the illegitimacy ratio in England had risen to 91 per 1,000 (or 9 per cent of all live births) from a low point of 47 in 1955. There had been fluctuations in the ratio in the past (*see* Fig. 50). Both World Wars were associated with sharp increases in illegitimacy, largely at the expense of pre-nuptial conceptions, but earlier long-term increases had been associated with a general rise in extra-marital conceptions, as in the 1960s. Thus Stone writes, "The number of prostitutes plying their trade, the number of brides led to the altar when already pregnant and the number of bastard children born, all rose together in the eighteenth and early nineteenth century and it is reasonable to assume that these three phenomena are all interconnected."

The eighteenth century saw great secular changes in sexual attitudes and behaviour, which Shorter has described as a "sexual revolution", comparable to that experienced in post-war Britain. By the late eighteenth century, almost all brides below the social élite were probably experiencing sexual intercourse with their future husbands before marriage and well over 40 per cent of first legitimate births were occurring within eight and a half months of marriage. Bastardy ratios rose from under 2 per cent to over 5 per cent, and these figures are probably on the low side, as many illegitimate births were not recorded in the parish registers.

UNWANTED PREGNANCY

Both teenage child-bearing and illegitimacy are seen as problematic, partly because they reflect unwanted conceptions. The high incidence of abortion in many societies is further evidence of the existence of many unwanted pregnancies, although we should perhaps stress that abortic [illegible] extent of unwanted pregnancy and pr [illegible] g the unwanted birth.

Great difficul [illegible] or enumerate unwanted pregna [illegible] of a continuum of "wantedness" [illegible] ne mother "doesn't mind". The [illegible] nd unwanted pregnancy is als [illegible] obably the result of a more-or- [illegible] hat a pregnancy may be "miswant [illegible] for both mother and child. Attitudes towar [illegible] y over a period of time. The "wanted" pregnancy ca [illegible] ld who is later rejected and it has been pointed out that the [illegible] gest child in a family is often the most loved, although statistically it has the highest probability of being unwanted at conception. Madeleine Kerr, in her study *The People of Ship Street* describes the common pattern of

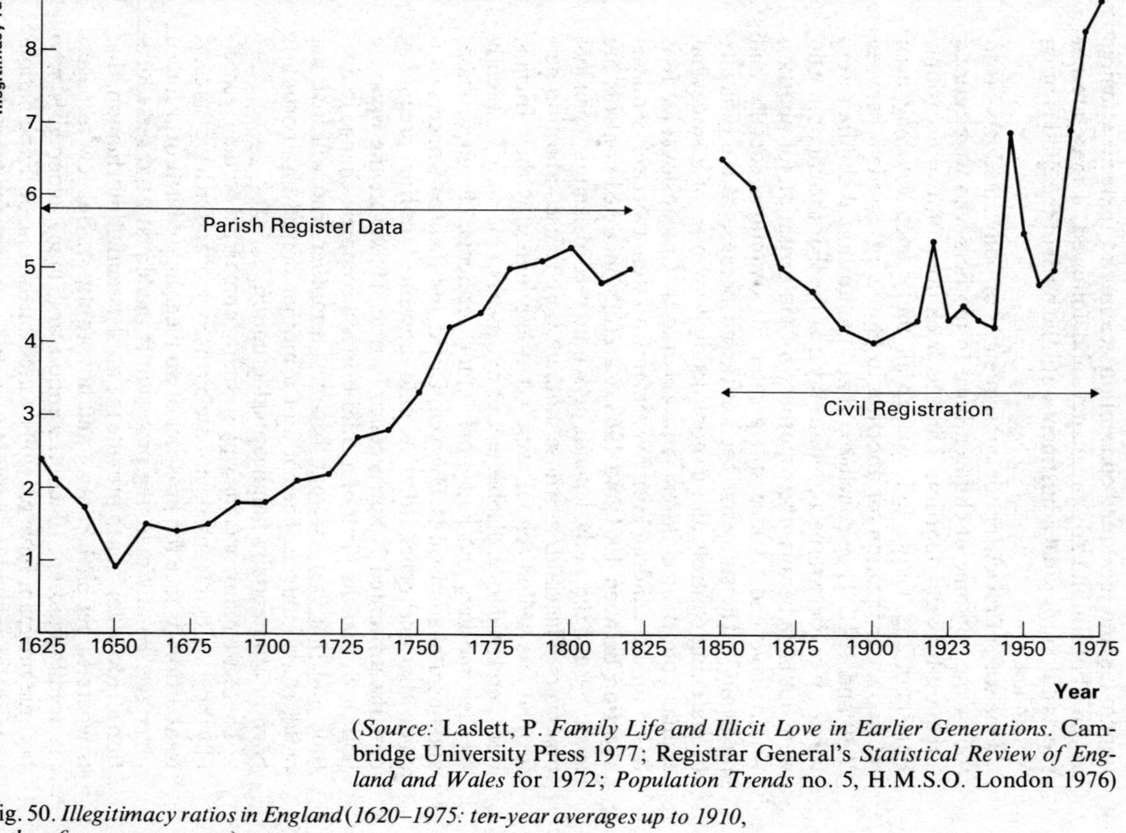

(*Source:* Laslett, P. *Family Life and Illicit Love in Earlier Generations.* Cambridge University Press 1977; Registrar General's *Statistical Review of England and Wales* for 1972; *Population Trends* no. 5, H.M.S.O. London 1976)

Fig. 50. *Illegitimacy ratios in England (1620–1975: ten-year averages up to 1910, then five-year averages).*

unplanned and unwanted conception, leading to frequent attempts at self-abortion in early pregnancy, and followed, if these are not successful, by gradual adjustment until the birth of the child is often welcomed.

One way of reviewing the consequences of "unwantedness" is to follow the outcome of children born to mothers who were refused a request for legal abortion. This has been done on two occasions. Forssman and Thuwe followed up all the women who had been refused an application for abortion in Göteborg, Sweden, between 1939 and 1941. They concluded that "the unwanted children were worse off in every respect . . . one may assume that the children who were not born because their mothers got authorisation for abortion would have had to face still greater disadvantages socially and medically". The study has been criticised because of the difficulty of matching controls and a more detailed analysis of a somewhat similar cohort of children is proceeding in Czechoslovakia. It is based on 233 children born to women who were twice refused legal abortion between 1961 and 1963. Carefully matched controls are available and the study depends on school records and independent observers. The children whose mothers were refused abortion performed less well at school, were rated less highly by their friends, were perceived to be disobedient or hyper-excitable more frequently by their mothers and had more minor accidents, chronic diseases and hospital admissions. Dytrych, David and their co-workers conclude that the belief "that a child unwanted during pregnancy remains unwanted is not necessarily true. However, the opposite notion . . . that the birth of a child brings a complete change in attitude and that every woman becomes a mother who will love her child, is also untrue. The child of a mother denied an abortion is born in a potentially handicapped situation."

There are many reasons why so many unmarried women, especially those in their teens, do not use birth-control and so have to resort to abortion or face the prospect of an illegitimate birth or a forced marriage. Family planning provision is inadequate and sex education all too often fails to provide the most essential information, that is where to get birth-control and how to use it. But few teenagers are totally ignorant of contraception and many older girls who become pregnant have previously used birth-control. Explanations in terms of individual pathology cannot account for more than a small proportion of current extra-marital conceptions and are ill-equipped to account for recent increases. It seems more promising, therefore, to treat many unwanted pregnancies as the result of more or less concious risk-taking of the sort described by Kristin Luker (*see* p. 106).

A central factor in the decision not to use contraception seems to be the social and cultural meanings attached to the use of birth-control outside marriage. Many single girls see it as an admission of their active role in extra-marital sex, which conflicts with their preferred interpretation of their actions in terms of spontaneity and romantic love. Especially at the point of transition between heavy petting and sexual intercourse, a lack of concern about birth-control allows a girl to evade recognition of what she is doing and sustain an image of her lost innocence. If she is lucky and does not become pregnant at this stage, she may convince herself that "it won't happen to me", until biology eventually proves her wrong. Risk-taking may be further sustained by a belief in possible benefits from pregnancy, in proving fecundity or defining a relationship, but these tend to disappear once pregnancy is confirmed, so that abortion is often sought instead. Many of these attitudes are supported by society's continuing belief that sexual relations outside marriage are morally undesirable, which manifests itself in ambivalence over providing easy access to birth-control for unmarried teenagers. It seems likely that a more open recognition of sexual activity before marriage would encourage wider use of contraception.

CHILDLESSNESS

Nothing more vividly demonstrates the importance of fertility to the individual than the reaction by, and to, those who do not have children. The Bible has several references to the plight of barren women, for example Sarah, Rachel, Hannah and Elisabeth, whose sterility was eventually removed by God. Rachel's desperate appeal to Jacob—"Give me children, or else I die"—is often quoted as an indication of the agony of the childless wife, made more bitter in this instance by her husband turning to a servant to bear a son. When she does conceive, her cry, "God hath taken away my reproach", sums up the stigma of infertility in Old Testament times.

The barren woman is subject to derision, condemnation or pity, according to society's view of the reasons for her condition. Worthless to her family and her husband, she can become totally devalued in her own eyes. Childlessness may be a reason for divorce, or for a husband taking another wife—in extreme cases the woman may be driven to suicide. In traditional societies, the fault is almost universally laid on the woman, although there are some instances of married women who have not conceived being allowed to receive lovers. In some cultures the severity of the sanctions suggest a belief that the childless woman wishes to avoid motherhood, is barren through personal fault such as adultery, or has in some ways displeased the gods. Often there can be no defence—the only escape is to become pregnant. Even where there are no specific sanctions, there is still an absence of the rewards of motherhood in terms of status within the community, and many infertile women in developed societies feel socially disadvantaged, quite apart from any personal feeling of loss.

The importance attached to avoiding childlessness can be seen in the widespread existence of fertility rites (*see* p. 1). Prayers for subsequent fertility are found in puberty and initiation rites as well as marriage ceremonies. Likewise, most societies have developed beliefs about how to cure infertility. This may involve prayers to the deities, carrying "lucky" dolls, or visits to sacred places (particularly wells, springs or rivers, reflecting the awareness of rain and water as having power to regenerate the parched and barren earth). In India, sterile women visited the temples of Siva, where they would press their naked body against the huge lingam (or phallus) of the god's statue. Other beliefs involve primitive "medicines"—the mandrake sought by Rachel, pig's teeth, frogs and spiders. In an old Hungarian custom, the childless wife was struck with a stick which had been used to part mating dogs.

The extent of childless marriages, whether voluntary or involuntary, varies considerably both from society to society, and over periods of time. Amongst the Hutterites, only 3 per cent of women remain childless at the end of their reproductive years. In most Western societies, the comparable figure is about 10 per cent, although much higher proportions are found in some countries such as West Germany. It is rare, however, for more than one in five marriages to be childless in any society, even after ten years of marriage.

In England and Wales, the proportion of women with no children after twelve years of marriage fell from 13 per cent for marriages of 1953 to 8 per cent for marriages of 1960, while for those marrying in the inter-war years it had been over 15 per cent and as high as 22 per cent for lower middle class couples marrying in 1925. These high rates must have resulted largely from conscious decisions to avoid or postpone child-bearing. In the U.S.A. the proportion of married women who remained childless rose from 8 per cent for those married in the latter half of the nineteenth century to 15 per cent in the first quarter of the twentieth century and approached 20 per cent in the period between the two World Wars. In the post-war years the proportion remaining childless fell back sharply, but has risen, at least for shorter marriage durations, in more recent cohorts.

Both voluntary and involuntary infertility are important to our understanding of levels of childlessness, although the boundaries between the two are not always clear.

VOLUNTARY CHILDLESSNESS

In all communities social pressures towards child-bearing are powerful, and a large majority of married couples say that they want at least some children. Yet at various times, the proportion who do not have children has been as high as 20 per cent, greatly in excess of those who say they want no children and more than can be accounted for by involuntary sterility.

In times of economic stress, married couples often delay child-bearing and this can lead to permanent postponement of having a family. Many may have always wanted a family and end up childless as a result of continuing economic pressures, or because of a life-style which increasingly becomes incompatible with parenthood. Many will claim that they could not afford to have children and see their decision primarily in terms of avoiding the costs of children. In other instances, a decision to try for children late in married life may reveal difficulties in conceiving.

In recent years, however, there has been evidence that an increasing number of couples in Britain and America choose to remain childless for positive reasons and come to such a decision early in marriage, if not before. Stress is laid on the rewards of not having children and the advantages of an adult-centred life-style. Whether the number of such couples is increasing or not, there has been a new readiness to assert their preferences, leading to the formation of groups for the "childfree", and the appearance of books with titles such as *The Baby Trap*.

An increasing number of childless men and women are seeking and obtaining voluntary sterilisation, underlining the finality of their decision never to have children.

Veevers' study of voluntary childlessness in Canada found that about a third of the couples had decided before marriage that they would have no children; for the remainder, childlessness resulted from continual postponement of child-bearing, culminating in an explicit decision that they would never have children. Many wives stressed that they felt they could attain adult status and a real social identity without children. A large proportion had a strong commitment to work, and saw a career as providing a more realistic means of self-enhancement and self-fulfilment than parenthood, and the presence of children as a positive hindrance. It was more important to gain success for themselves, rather than through their children, or in a domestic role.

Others stressed that not having children meant a closer relationship with their partners, resulting from the greater availability of time to spend together and a deeper emotional involvement. Alongside this, there was often an emphasis on independence, and the greater freedom to pursue adult activities, to travel, take risks and seek new experiences. The great stress laid by many couples on egalitarian sex roles fitted well with such rationales, but may have been a result, as much as a cause, of childlessness. Personal factors such as unhappy childhood experiences, or an awareness that their parents had stayed together only for the children, had also influenced their decisions.

Some couples mentioned more altruistic motives, such as concerns about overpopulation or food and energy shortages; some of these may have been *ex post facto* considerations, providing a socially acceptable rationale. Many such couples stressed their "liking" for children, their involvement in work with children and their contact with friends' children, often expressing an interest in possibly fostering or adopting in the future, perhaps as a reassurance that their decision not to have a family was not irreversible.

There will always be a minority of couples who choose not to have children of their own, because of an awareness of the risk of having a handicapped child or passing on a hereditary disease, but most of these would not class themselves as "voluntarily" childless and many seek to adopt at an early stage.

INVOLUNTARY CHILDLESSNESS

Single women are expected not to have or to want children, and the "problem" of childlessness, as traditionally defined by society, is confined to the married couple. The involuntarily childless may have had children and lost them. More common are situations of genuine infertility, where no live birth has been experienced, from either an inability to conceive, or failure to carry pregnancies to full term.

Most couples embark on marriage in the expectation of having children and a majority try for a baby within the first few years of marriage, quite apart from the substantial number who are pregnant at marriage. Potential fertility is usually taken for granted. Natural children, by definition, have parents who are not sterile, so that infertility is usually outside the experience of their own parents. Consequently, the discovery of any difficulty in conceiving can be a bitter shock to the couple. They have to learn to accept their infertility and handle it in relation to themselves and other significant people in their lives. There can be much uncertainty as to when it should be discussed as an issue and when external action should be taken. In a society which employs contraception, where many people choose to delay conception for several years, there is the added problem of handling the reactions of parents and those others who will be unsure about the reasons for the couple not having children.

A study by David Kirk of childless women who subsequently adopted, found that they described their feelings on discovering their infertility in strong terms—despair, bitterness, frustration. They felt forlorn, desolated, useless and found their daily lives full of constant reminders of their condition, so that some avoided shopping because they saw so many young mothers with prams or toddlers. The husband's reaction tended to be more muted, couched in terms of disappointment rather than deprivation.

The childless couple is not only deprived of children but also of an appropriate cultural script. They are not fulfilling the expectations of society, but equally have no means of knowing how to handle the situation (because they had nothing in their socialisation process which taught them how to do so). Many couples never seek professional help with their infertility, either resigning themselves to being childless or living with a hope that they will eventually conceive. For those that do, treatment is often disappointing. Many couples endure years of "investigations" without any cause being established or any solution found.

In many parts of the world the "blame" is automatically assigned to the woman. We have also met doctors in this country who still believe that a man should not be told if he is at fault. In fact, in about a third of those cases where a cause is established, it is the husband who is responsible and the first step in investigations should involve a semen analysis. In a typical ejaculation there should be about 300 million sperm; if the count falls below 120 million fertilisation of the ovum is unlikely. Male infertility often presents an intractable problem. Treatment may involve the use of testosterone, human gonadotrophins or clomiphene, but none have been outstanding successful. Sometimes, it may be practical to pool a number of ejaculates with poor sperm counts and artificially inseminate the wife with her husband's semen. Mechanical, as opposed to hormonal, problems can be easier to treat, as in the case of a blocked *vasa deferentia* or *hypospadia*, when the semen is ejaculted at the base of the penis and so outside the vagina. For the lucky, the problem may reside in testicular cooling (normal sperm formation does not occur at body temperature). Here wearing different clothes or operating on a varicole may cure infertility. When the husband has proven infertility the wife may consider artificial insemination by a donor, or, more simply, have intercourse with another partner, yet maintain her marriage.

If the husband's sperm count is normal and coitus with intravaginal ejaculation seems to be occurring regularly, the focus of investigation turns to the woman. A post-coital test will show whether sperm are able to survive in the wife's cervical mucus, but perhaps the commonest cause of female infertility is a blockage of the fallopian tubes. It can be demonstrated by X-ray, blowing gas through the tubes, or direct inspection through a laparoscope. A solution to the problem can be sought by repairing surgery. Results, although improving, are often disappointing and involve the further hazard of increased risk of ectopic pregnancy (where the conceptus attaches itself in a place other than the lining of the upper uterine cavity).

The other major cause of infertility in the woman is a failure to ovulate, often signalled by amenorrhoes or irregular menstruation. This may relate back to other diseases, such as anorexia nervosa, in which case fertility returns when the primary condition is remedied. When failure to ovulate involves a hypothalamic or pituitary cause, the use of a drug called clomiphene and of human pituitary F.S.H. can be considered. However, multiple ovulation and therefore multiple pregnancies are a risk of the so-called "fertility drugs".

Where investigations are inconclusive or direct treatment unsuccessful, a couple are faced with the problem of what further steps they can take to overcome their childless state or adjust to it. For many, the decision will be to accept the situation—for others the need for children may be met through fostering or adoption.

ADOPTION

In almost all human societies arrangements exist whereby adult members of the society can assume permanent parental rights and responsibilities over children, or other adults, who are not biologically their own offspring. Whatever its form, adoption involves three major parties: the person who is adopted, the "biological" parents (one of whom at least is usually losing rights over the child), and the adopters (who are taking on those rights and concomitant responsibilities). In any society, where adoption is practised, there will develop a set of rules, legal or otherwise, about who may adopt and who may be adopted and also a set of social pressures as to who should relinquish a child for adoption and who should seek to adopt.

In the West today, adoption is accepted as the neat and sensible solution to the problems of two groups of people; childless couples and children without families. The popular view of adoption is probably even narrower—that it concerns a married couple unable to have children adopting an illegitimate baby whose mother cannot keep him. However, in Britain in 1975 such adoptions accounted for less than one in six, and two-thirds of cases involved were couples one of whom was already the legal parent of the child.

Cross-cultural and historical studies of adoption reveal a wide variation in incidence, and also in the nature of the institution and its social functions. Traditionally, the main advantages of adoption concerned the adopters in guaranteeing the continuance of ancestral worship and the perpetuation of the family name or in enabling childless couples to leave their possessions to a person where there are no natural descendants. The children adopted were not necessarily unwanted and would usually be older, even adult, and often relatives. There was little pretence that natural parenthood was being replicated and links with the biological parents would often be maintained. Adoption could also be seen as a means of maintaining the freedom of the unmarried girl, or of unburdening the divorced woman so that she could seek a new partner. Meeting the needs of the child was at most a secondary aim.

Until recently, many European countries had laws markedly different from today, e.g. that adopters should be beyond child-bearing ages, that the adoptee must have reached the age of majority, that only one adopted child should be permitted to a couple (to provide an heir), or that any subsequently born natural children should have priority in inheritance.

In contrast, in contemporary Western countries adoption has increasingly become an institution concerned with providing a stable and happy home to children deprived of this. The "Hurst" Committee studying adoption in Britain (1954) wrote:

> The primary object at which all should aim in the arrangement of adoptions is the welfare of the child and adoption should, therefore, be approached as a means of finding the right home for a child rather than of satisfying would-be adopters.

A similar view has been expressed in more blunt terms by the Deputy Director of the Association of British Adoption Agencies:

> no couple has a right to a child but every child has the right to have parents.... Our first duty must be to the child. We cannot accept responsibility for meeting the problems of infertility.

The 1975 Children Act in Britain increased the rights of foster parents to adopt and weakened the rights of biological parents over children in statutory care. But in the U.S.A. Mandell argues that "child-welfare" adoption is still oriented towards providing children for childless middle-class couples. Interest in finding homes for older, handicapped and coloured children has grown only because of a dramatic decline in the availability of white babies.

In Britain, the number of illegitimate babies placed for adoption has declined rapidly in the last ten years. This is partly due to the 1967 Abortion Act; one good effect of this outcome has been the placing of a greater proportion of handicapped children and children of mixed parentage for adoption.

PARENTS

Adoption in the West today is firmly established as one of the solutions to the problems of biological infertility, albeit a solution sought only by a minority of the involuntary childless. Adoption practice often supports this concept by encouraging early placement, matching adopter and child, guaranteeing anonymity and providing a new birth certificate. This contrasts with adoption in other times and places, where there has been little pretence that it was other than very different from natural parenthood.

Adoption work has traditionally been focused on the needs of the adopter, while seeking at the same time to select only those who will make good parents. Adopters are expected to have a stable marriage, be not too young and not too old, and to have reasonable housing and adequate income. The wife is expected to give up work and to want to be a "proper mother". For many years, childlessness was seen as the only natural motive for adoption and applications to adopt from those able to have children of their own was viewed with suspicion, or seen as unfair, given the shortage of adoptable babies. Recently, however, there has been a growing interest in the needs of older "difficult to place" children, who are seldom sought initially by the childless couple, and a recognition that, if the needs of the child really are of paramount importance, the infertility of the would-be adopters is relevant only in so far as it is seen as being likely to enhance motivation and ensure a successful placement.

Recently there has also been increasing pressure from couples with children of their own who wish to offer a permanent home to a deprived child. It has been linked to a new category of potential adopters in Britain—those foster parents who have cared for a child for many years and who now have the right to seek to adopt without the natural mother being able to remove the child. Support for such a right arose from concern over "tug-of-love" cases in which children were removed—apparently against their wishes—from foster homes where they had spent most of their lives.

Adoption can be seen as a socially acceptable means of shedding responsibility for the care of a child. As such, it stands alongside abortion or infanticide as a solution to the problem of unwanted pregnancy and, as in the case of these alternative "solutions", it is the subject of much societal ambivalence. The adoption of "legitimate" children is seen as less acceptable than that of "illegitimate" ones and more understanding is extended to the girl who cannot, rather than will not, keep her child. The recent shortage of adoptable children has given rise to a new debate about the preferability of adoption over abortion, the former being seen by some as less selfish, in that it preserves the life of the foetus and provides joy for a childless couple.

It is becoming increasingly clear that, where there is adequate support for the single girl who wishes to keep her child and easily available abortion for the girl who does not want a child and is unable or unwilling to marry the father, very few will choose adoption as a solution. Thus in Sweden the number of babies available for adoption is minimal.

Where a child is legitimate, attitudes tend to be even more inconsistent. A married couple are expected to want and care for their children and it is thought undesirable and unnatural if they offer a baby for adoption. Nevertheless society retains the right to take away those children if parental functions are not fulfilled adequately, so that most adoptions involving the placement of legitimate children arise from a prior decision by society that the parents have failed in some way.

THE ADOPTED CHILD

Adoption is a cure for the ills of an illegitimate child, in that it provides a stable home and removes the stigma of illegitimacy, providing the child with a new identity and a new birth certificate undistinguishable from that of the legitimately born. Yet it is a "cure" that now applies to only one in ten of all illegitimate children in Britain; although many of the remainder will also be brought up in stable, two-parent families, as a result of their mother's subsequent marriage or co-habitation (a substantial number are born into a stable union). Indeed, it is important to stress that the vast majority of single parent families at any one time arises from the breakdown of marriage through death, divorce or separation, rather than illegitimacy.

The "success" of adoption for those illegitimate children whose mothers cannot keep them is now well documented. A follow-up study of illegitimate children in England and Wales showed that after seven years those adopted were faring much better on a range of social and educational measures than those who were not, and were much more like the general run of legitimate children. This is a tribute to the care with which adoption has been handled, but also of course reflects the favourable socio-economic position of most adopted children. It would, however, be an illusion to see adoption in such cases as unproblematic. There is some evidence of higher rates of referral to child guidance clinics of adopted children, and in recent years much attention has been focused on the right of the adopted child to know about his natural parents. This right (which has long existed in Scotland) has recently been extended to all children adopted in England and Wales. Although only a small minority of adopted children try to contact their parents, this has aroused concern amongst many biological parents about the possibility of being confronted by the child they had surrendered many years before.

Many older children, some illegitimate, some legitimate, often sibling groups or coloured or handicapped children, remain in institutions or long-term foster care and are in desperate need of a more permanent substitute home. In Great Britain there may be between 6,000 and 7,000 such children in care under the age of eleven. These experience little or no parental contact and are unlikely ever to be able to return home. The true challenge for a welfare-oriented adoption policy is how far the needs of these children can be met.

If adopters are to be found, society will need to abandon many traditional assumptions, such as the parental characteristics in terms of age, infertility etc., or the placement practice, with its assumptions of no payment to adopters and a complete break from the natural parents.

For a long time it was assumed that the placement of older children was bound to fail, based largely on the lack of success in long-term fostering, but a number of recent studies, involving older and coloured children, suggest that adoption can be very successful. The problem lies partly in finding a decision-making process that will not leave children to spend their life in an institution. On the other hand, neither must it so override the rights of biological parents that many, already suffering the deprivations of poor housing, low income and broken marriages, are further deprived of any right to part with their child temporarily without the risk that a court may decide that the substitute care is "better" and should therefore be made permanent.

In America, the question of inter-racial adoptions is acute. Black children deprived of a normal life tend to stay in institutions rather than be placed for adoption. The root problem in adoption revolves around placing the children of the poor with couples drawn predominantly from middle-class and respectable working-class backgrounds. If adoption works, do we need to bother about the reasons for families breaking up, or hardship to biological parents already victimised by poverty and poor education? Goldstein has written that "each child placement should be seen as an occasion for protecting future generations of children by increasing the number of adults to be who are likely to be adequate parents ... a real opportunity to break the cycle of sickness and hardship bequeathed from one generation to the next".

Yet the need for adoption arises out of the misfortunes and failings of biological parents and these in turn are sometimes rooted in the injustices of society. It would be a fatal mistake to ignore the need to remedy such injustices because adoption also meets the needs of other, more privileged, members of society who are able to provide the good home the poor cannot.

Even bigger issues are raised in relation to inter-country adoptions such as those of Korean and Vietnam war orphans by Americans, which have tended at times to become almost a requirement of radical chic. In Sweden, where adoption of native-born illegitimate children runs at about 100 a year, 1,500 foreign babies are adopted each year, mainly Korean. The adopters are enthusiastic, as are the intermediaries; here is a solution to world population problems—too many children in the Third World and too many childless in the West. To many developing countries, however, it is seen as yet another form of charity which ducks the real issues, a sophisticated extension of imperialist traditions. Yet individual lives are saved and happiness brought to the adopters. It seems too neat and tidy—an international class system perpetuating the right of adopters to have perfect children, while the handicapped of their own race, or the children of the immigrant coloured population, may remain in institutions.

CONCLUSION

One of our aims in this chapter has been to remind readers—and, indeed, ourselves—that the study of population and fertility is ultimately about people. The births that demographers measure are the children that make up our families; the result, wanted or unwanted, of their parents' lovemaking, and themselves the parents of the future generation. It is not enough to complain that there are too many or too few, that people are pollution or that we need more for our work-force. Our concern must also be with the quality of human life and a recognition that this is often closely linked to the patterns of fertility we have been exploring.

We have tried to show how parents, and especially mothers, are affected by their experience of child-bearing. We have tried to show that gaining increased control over reproduction has been of great importance to those women and can enable them to play a much wider part in society and develop a much wider experience of life. We have also shown that the lives of many women are still marred by their experience of unwanted pregnancy, the fear of which can destroy sexual happiness and the consequences of which may last a lifetime. For this reason alone, we see it as a matter of great importance to provide for all women the right to choose whether they wish to bear a child. To achieve this involves not only the provision of knowledge about contraception, but also genuine opportunities to obtain and use birth-control, with free access to safe legal abortion. Choices must be extended to the unmarried as well as the married. At present we are still a long way from achieving for most women that "fifth freedom" of which Sir Dugald Baird spoke, the freedom from the tyranny of unwanted pregnancy.

We have also looked at the implications for children of being unwanted, having many siblings or being born too soon after a previous child, and at the diminished life chances of the illegitimate child. One of the most important consequences of declining fertility has been that society has come to recognise more and more its responsibilities towards those children who are born. Likewise, parents have come to face the fact that they choose to have children. Awareness of this can lead to great problems for those children who are not wanted. Adoption practices have moved away from concerns over "blood ties" to the need for good parenting—as defined in social (and sometimes class) terms and often to the neglect of the natural mother.

In less developed countries, the population is also, as Dom Moraes stresses, "a matter of people". Recognition of this is essential if the problem of too rapid population growth is to be solved, for ultimately it is the people who will resolve it or not, by their actions. A population problem does not disappear because a government decides it wants more people, if those people are ill-fed and ill-housed; nor it is solved by compulsory sterilisation, if people still feel that they want and need more children. We are left with dilemmas; in Moraes's words, "... though every single individual born is desirable people in the mass can be lethal without them wanting to be". It is to this and other implications of fertility for society that we shall turn in the next chapter.

SELECTED REFERENCES AND BIBLIOGRAPHY

Benet, M. K. *The Character of Adoption*. Jonathan Cape, London 1976

Bogue, D. (ed) *Adolescent Fertility*. University of Chicago Press, Chicago 1977

Borland, M. *Violence in the Family*. Manchester University Press, Manchester 1976

Bossard, J. H. S. and Boll, E. S. *The Large Family System*. University of Pennsylvania Press, Philadelphia 1956

Bryant, J. H. *Health in the Developing World*. Cornell University Press, Ithaca 1969

Cheetham, J. *Unwanted Pregnancy and Counselling*. Routledge & Kegan Paul, London 1977

Chester, R. and Peel, J. *Equalities and Inequalities in Family Life*. Academic Press, London 1977

Crellin, E., Pringle, M. K. and West, P. *Born Illegitimate*. National Foundation for Educational Research, London 1971

Cutright, P. "The Teenage Sexual Revolution and the Myth of an Abstinent Past." *Family Planning Perspectives*. 4, 24 1972

Davie, R., Butler, N. and Goldstein, H. *From Birth to Seven*. Longmans, London 1972

Dytrych, Z., Matcejcek, Z., Schüller, V., David, H. P. and Friedman, H. C. "Children Born to Women Denied Abortion." *Family Planning Perspectives*. 7, 165 1975

Forssman, H. and Thuwe, I. "One Hundred and Twenty Children Born After Application for Therapeutic Abortion Refused." *Acta Psychiatrica Scandanavica*. 42, 71 1966

Goldstein, J., Freud, A. and Solnit, A. J. *Beyond the Best Interests of the Child*. Free Press, New York 1973

Humphrey, M. *The Hostage Seekers*. Longmans, London 1969

Kerr, M. *The People of Ship Street*. Routledge & Kegan Paul, London 1958

Kirk, H. D. *Shared Fate*. Free Press, New York 1964

Lehfeldt, H. "Wilful Exposure to Unwanted Pregnancy." *American Journal of Obstetrics and Gynecology*. 78, 661 1959

Lipset, S. M. and Bendix, R. *Social Mobility in Industrial Society*. University of California Press, Berkeley 1959

Macintyre, S. *Single and Pregnant*. Croom Helm, London 1977

Moraes, D. *A Matter of People*. Andre Deutsch, London 1974

Morley, D. *Paediatric Priorities in the Developing World*. Butterworths, London 1973

Newill, R. *Infertile Marriage*. Penguin Books, London 1974

Omran, A. R. *The Health Theme in Family Planning*. Carolina Population Centre 1971

Peck, E. *The Baby Trap*. Bernard Geis Associates, New York 1971

Pohlman, E. *Psychology of Birth Planning*. Schenkman, Cambridge 1969

Rains, P. M. *Becoming an Unwed Mother*. Aldine, Chicago 1971

Sauvy, A. *General Theory of Population*. Weidenfeld & Nicolson, London 1969

Schofield, M. *The Sexual Behaviour of Young People*. Penguin Books, Harmondsworth 1968

Seglow, J., Pringle, M. K. and Wedge, P. *Growing Up Adopted*. National Foundation for Educational Research, London 1972

Shorter, E. *The Making of the Modern Family*. Collins, London 1976

Stone, L. *The Family, Sex and Marriage in England, 1500–1800*. Weidenfeld & Nicolson, London 1977

Titmuss, R. M. *Essays on the Welfare State*. Allen & Unwin, London 1958

Veevers, J. E. "Voluntarily Childless Wives: An Exploratory Study." *Sociology and Social Research*. 57, 356 1973

Williams, J. M. and Hindell, K. *Abortion and Contraception*. P.E.P., London 1972

Wray, J. D. "Population Pressures on Families; Family Size and Child Spacing." In *Rapid Population Growth; Consequences and Implications*. Vol. 2, Johns Hopkins Press, Baltimore 1971

Chapter 10

Society and the Economy

The facts of world population growth are well known: the familiar upward curve of the graph has been reproduced in many places. It took the whole of human history and prehistory for the global population to reach 1,000 million by about 1800. The population doubled again in just over a century, reaching perhaps 2,000 million in about 1920. The next doubling took place in a generation and the 4,000 million mark was passed sometime in the mid-1970s.

Statistics, however, can be too remote to grasp; they may frighten or merely dim with repetition. It can be useful to express the world's death and birth rates not in thousands of millions, but like the ticking of a small clock with a very short pendulum (*see* Fig. 51).

Even if global fertility now declines relatively rapidly, the world will still reach 6,000 million by the turn of the century. It must be emphasised yet again that because of the rapid population growth which has taken place since the Second World War, the population of the world is now biased towards the earlier age-groups and global population will go on growing well into the twenty-first century (*see* Fig. 2).

Most of the population growth will take place in the developing countries which, with current rates of expansion, will double their population in about thirty years (*see* Fig. 52) while the developed world will take 75–100 years to double its population (*see* Fig. 6). Indeed, if the current slackening of birth rates in developed countries continues they will never double their populations again.

FOOD

The relationship between food production and population growth has been a matter of concern since Malthus uttered his famous "law", that populations grow geometrically, while food supplies increase arithmetically. Ultimately, predicted Malthus, population is bound to outstrip food production and so be curtailed by hunger and famine. The fact that Malthus's prediction has been refuted by two centuries of history and the arrival of new agricultural technologies has led many people to believe that food production can always be kept ahead of population growth. From 1950 to 1970 there was a steady increase in *per capita* food production, despite rapid rises in population, and developments such as the Green Revolution seemed to indicate that such progress could be maintained and improved. However, bad harvests and continual population growth in the 1970s have partly undermined previous optimism.

The real concern over food is felt not in the West but by the bulk of mankind today, whose lives are still dominated by a constant battle to obtain enough to survive (*see* Figs. 53 and 54). Underdeveloped nations are not always succeeding in the desperate struggle to keep food supplies growing as fast as their numbers (*see* Fig. 55).

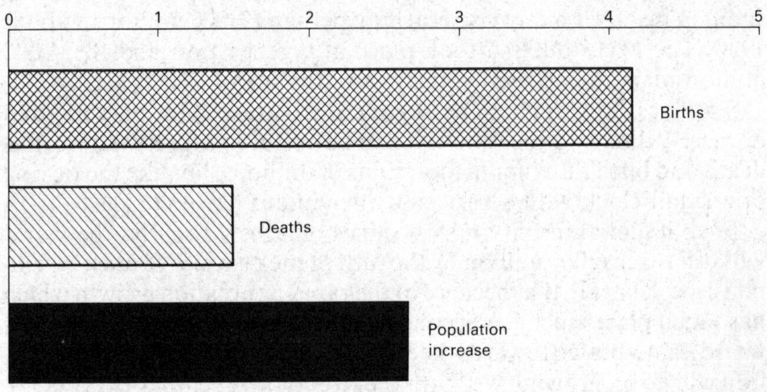

Fig. 51. *World events per second (1971 rates).*

As food production falls, it is the poorest countries and the poorest families within those countries which feel the worst effects, not only because they are in a weaker position to gain a share in what food is produced, but also because their share is already so small that any decline has a more devastating effect. Apart from drought areas, there are probably no places where population has actually passed the capacity of land to support it, but periodic famine and widespread malnutrition still arises in many places as a result of agricultural neglect, poverty and natural disaster.

In developing countries, urban families often spend 80 to 90 per cent of their disposable income on food, while a Western family may spend less than a fifth of their income on food. Therefore a rise in

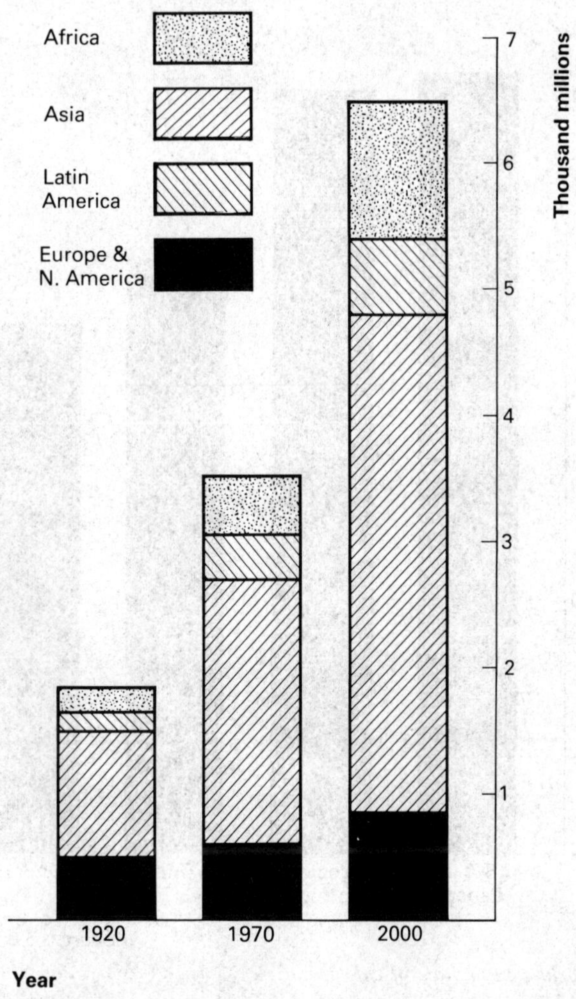

(*Source:* I.P.P.F. data)

Fig. 52. *World population growth (1920–2000).*

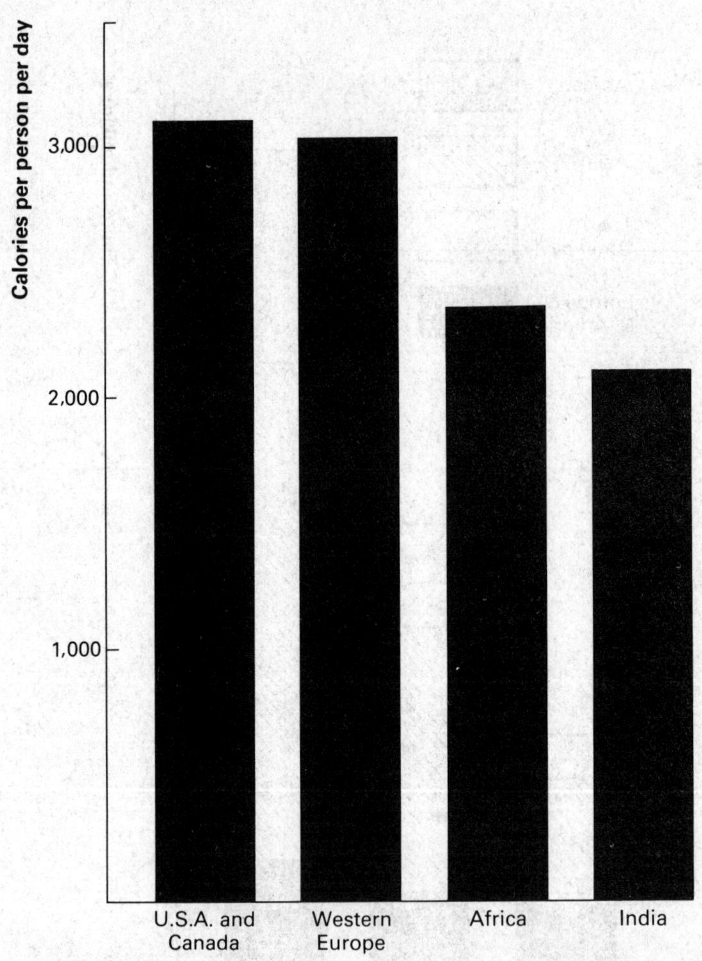

(*Source:* Sai. F.T.)

Fig. 53. *World consumption of calories.*

stable prices that may well only annoy the second, can leave the first hungry.

IMMEDIATE PROBLEMS

The ability to reach the high agricultural production of say the Netherlands or Japan requires a capital investment beyond the reach of poor nations and is more energy-intensive than the waning supplies

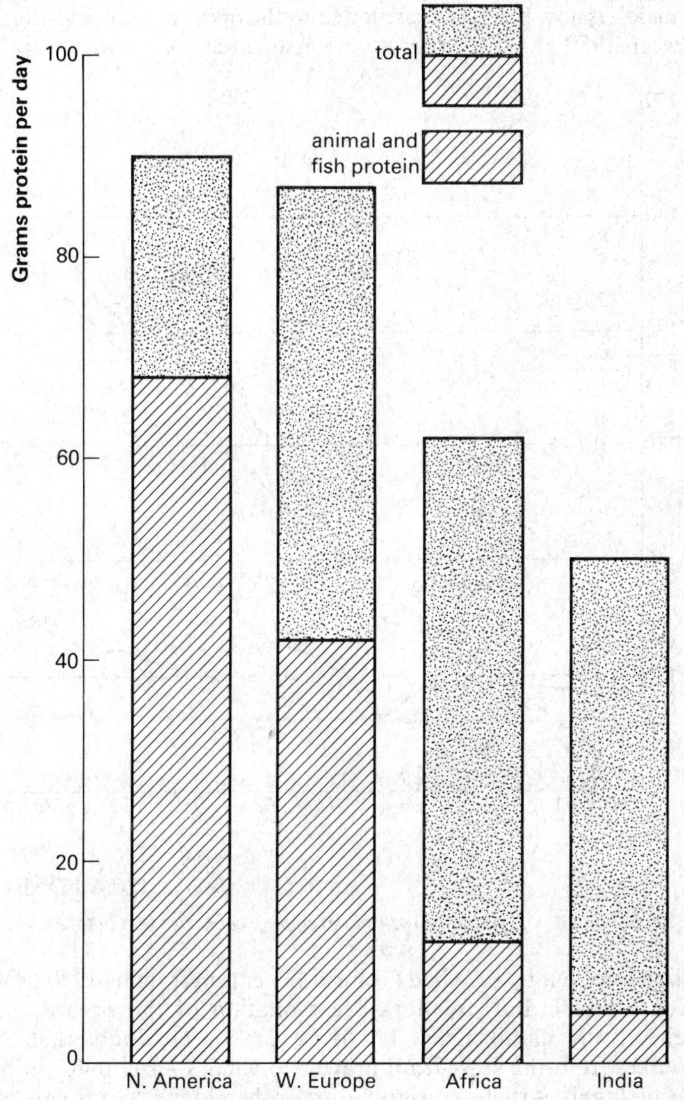

(*Source:* Sai. F.T.)

Fig. 54. *Protein consumption.*

of petroleum could support throughout the world. A number of warning signals are being sounded at present.

Fish, which is a major source of protein in many developing countries, is now being overexploited to the point of reducing yields. Between 1950 and 1970 the world's fish catch rose from 21 to 70

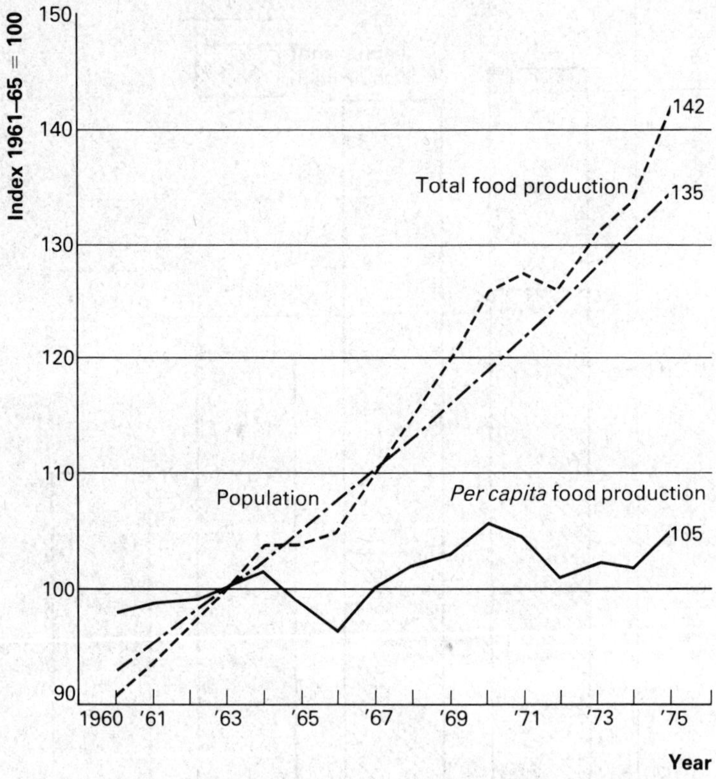

(*Source:* U.S.A.I.D. data)

Fig. 55. *Food and population growth in developing countries (excluding China).*

million tons, but by 1974 had declined 11 per cent from its 1970 peak. Given a less brutal, free-for-all exploitation of the oceans, fish catches could climb again, but there can be no doubt that the resources from the sea—from prawns to whales—are finite. In the case of highly structured agriculture, other limits to growth are visible. Since the Second World War, global fertiliser consumption has increased exponentially, with a doubling time of a mere ten years. Total use by 1970 was five times higher than in the 1940s. As the manufacture of artificial fertilisers requires large amounts of energy we cannot assume that this essential ingredient of modern agriculture will necessarily become available to meet world needs.

Production and pollution are closely linked. The run-off of agricultural chemicals into fresh water is becoming a problem and, for example, has been one factor in the 100-fold decline of fish catches from Lake Ontario. About 100,000 tons of D.D.T. was released annually into the world's environment in the 1960s, and even if use of this insecticide reaches a plateau now, levels in many animals will remain raised until nearly the end of the century. (There is so much mercury in the Mediterranean that Adriatic fishermen retain enough in their bodies to kill a cat.)

But as a more cautious attitude to pollution arises in the developed world, the immediate physical needs of the developing world continue to encourage risk-taking and short cuts. In the end it is Third World agriculture which is going to demand most fertiliser and the greatest weights of pesticides. When balancing starvation next year against possible damage to the global ecosystem in the twenty-first century, the developing world will make exactly the same choices in technology as the West has already made, and for even stronger reasons.

Bangladesh, with current population growth exceeding 2 per cent a year, high population density and one of the world's lowest G.N.P.s is already facing the Malthusian check of starvation. For example, a poor harvest in 1972 brought the already grossly inadequate food intake as low as 340 grammes of cereal a day. Although vital statistics are inaccurate for most of the country, in the Matlab Bazar research data has been carefully recorded for many years and here the death rate jumped to 21.4 per 1,000. At a national level there may have been something approaching half a million extra deaths that season (*see* Fig. 56). In 1974–5 death rates rose again, this time to 19.8. Bangladesh and, increasingly, other parts of the Indian subcontinent, are dependent after a bad harvest season on donations of U.S. and Canadian grain. One year those reserves may fail as well.

Starvation does not necessarily mean emaciated bodies dead beside the paddy-field. Spurts in death rates begin with rising infant mortality and more old people dying. And, as has been shown in Bangladesh, it is the poor who die most (*see* Table 34) although, officially, no-one ever dies from overpopulation.

In less extreme situations, the immediate effect of food shortage is on the quality of life of a population rather than on its size. Unless there is extreme scarcity most adult human beings do not die of starvation in this event, but rather suffer in health and vitality and

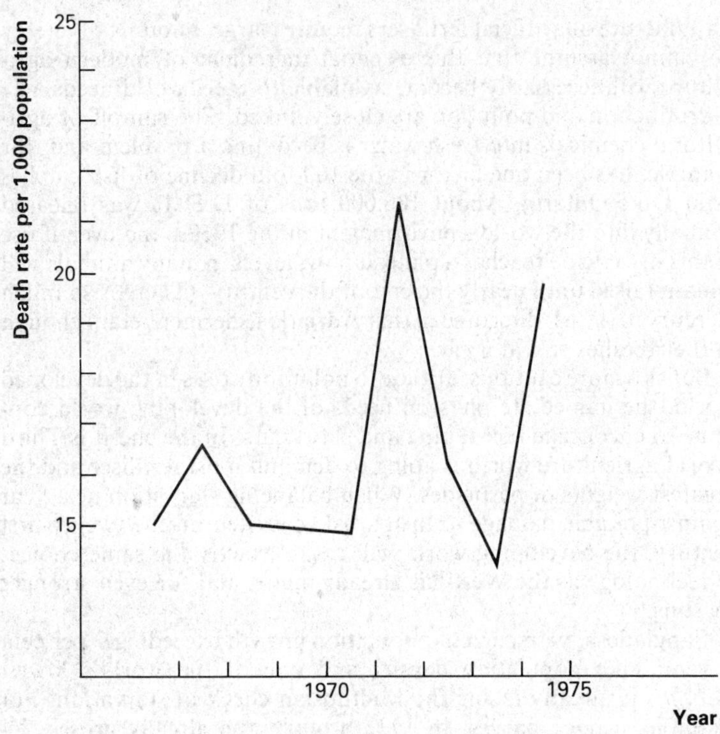

(*Source:* Cholera Research Laboratory, Dacca, Bangladesh)

Fig. 56. *Rising death rates in Bangladesh* (*Matlab Bazaar 1966–75*).

in their ability to work and play. Even as long as global supplies of food match population growth, large sections of the population within specific countries will experience serious shortages of food. Rich countries may donate food surpluses, but these do not necessarily reach the poor and hungry; if they do so it is at a cost to foreign exchange or involves growing dependence on the powerful. For most nations, future security depends on their ability to satisfy their own needs and this presents intractable problems for many areas where, especially on the Indian subcontinent, the most economically cultivable land is already in use, and the climate varies from year to year.

It is clear, therefore, that even if there is no long-term shortfall in world food production, the problem of providing adequate food for the millions of the world is one of distribution and purchasing power. The events of the early 1970s show clearly the need for world co-operation to avoid catastrophe, resulting from a succession of

TABLE 34: DEATH-RATE AND POVERTY (BANGLADESH 1975)

Size of land Holding (hectares)	*Death rate per 1,000*
None	35.8
0.01–0.20	28.4
0.21–1.20	21.5
1.21+	12.2

(*Source:* Brown, L. R. "World Population Trends; Signs of Hope and Signs of Stress." *World Watch Paper 8.* Worldwatch Institute, Washington 1976)

harvest failures at a time when there are only limited supplies available. The grain which the U.S.A. sells to offset the poor agricultural record of the U.S.S.R., or which it gives away to feed the Indian subcontinent, only amounts to 6 per cent of the world's production. As pressure on supplies increases, more and more grain will be eaten directly, less fed to cattle and the cost of meat in the West will continue to rise in the foreseeable future. At present the cattle being prepared for Western tables eat as much grain as all the human beings in India and China.

While the industrialised nations worry about the price of steak and while in many developing countries supplies of basic grains are still adequate, chronic malnutrition persists because poor families simply lack the means of purchasing sufficient food. When a country attempts to tackle such problems by stimulating food production and distributing food to the poor, it can face major economic problems from concentrating its efforts on this area and still only managing to maintain people at subsistence level, while having simultaneously to abandon other important goals. Lack of food is not caused solely by high rates of population growth, but few would doubt that a reduction in such rates would immensely aid efforts to ensure that all are adequately fed (*see* Fig. 55).

The basic need of the less developed countries is for an improvement in their agricultural technology and so in their ability to provide for themselves, by making the best use of the natural resources of the land. The U.S.A., with 8 million people employed in agriculture, produces 240 million tons of food a year, while India, with over 360 million farm workers, only produces slightly over 100 million tons of food. The developing world must produce better conditions for market, as opposed to subsistence, agriculture. This in turn depends on over-all socio-economic development, as well as the dissemination of new knowledge and technology. Such developments, especially if they bring an increase in *per capita* income and a more equitable income distribution, as we saw earlier, may be a necessary condition for substantial reduction in population growth rates.

Much of the world has enough food to provide sufficient calories for daily living, but is short of protein. Plant protein can be used to feed people, but to get the maximum benefit from it the cellulose walls of the cells must be broken up. The resulting protein-rich material demands alterations in eating habits which are notoriously difficult to make, but may in the end be achieved. Currently, leaf protein can be fed to cattle, and pilot experiments are taking place in human feeding. "Meals for Millions" in the U.S.A. has devised an appropriate technology, using a hand-operated machine that cost only $50. In Kenya an edible leaf protein is being developed.

In several ways the problem of protein malnutrition is similar to the problem of fertility regulation—a technology already exists that can largely dispose of current problems, but it is not in use. In the case of family planning, it is partly a problem of decision makers who shy away from the controversy which sex-related issues generate and partly a problem of social adaption and acceptance of new technologies. In the case of leaf protein this second factor is perhaps even more important.

However, there is a paradox here in that the earth's maximum carrying capacity for human beings will require a high level of agricultural technology across the globe, which in turn calls for a universally high level of social and economic development. This happy combination would be likely to ensure a cessation of population growth before the maximum carrying capacity of the land is reached The problem is that progress in economic development is also being inhibited by high rates of population growth. Can the vicious circle be broken?

INCOME

High rates of population growth produce a tangle of interlocking economic problems whether the economic structure of a society is capitalist, communist or anything else. Countries with economies as divergent as those of Brazil and China are appreciating the relationship between population growth and economic development.

Population size of itself has an economic impact (*see* Table 35). A large population is associated with economies of scale (although industrialised nations such as Switzerland do not seem to be at a disadvantage in the modern world). A large population provides a broader base for developing educational, scientific and managerial skills, which tend to raise output per head. But these advantages can be offset by the diminishing returns obtained as more and more labour is applied to fixed natural assets. Technology affects the "law of diminishing returns". The record of economic development in the West over the past century testifies to the resilience, flexibility and creativity of scientifically based industries and the ability of technology to cope with larger total populations than was once thought possible—even if it is an achievement that has been bought at the cost of pollution and some human suffering.

These generalisations, however, are secondary to the adverse effects of rapid population growth. If rates can be controlled then total numbers present a less insuperable problem. The relation between growth and economic change has been analysed from many points of view. From the viewpoint of the impact of fertility on the welfare of the individual in society we have found the arguments

TABLE 35: INCOME AND POPULATION GROWTH IN THE 1960S

	Per cent	
	Developed countries	*Less developed countries*
Total income	4.4	4.0
Population growth	1.3	2.6
Income per head	3.1	1.5

(*Source:* Taeuber, I. B. "Manpower Resources of Asian Countries in the 1970s." *Second I.P.P.F.W.P.R. Conference*. Tokyo 1970)

of James Meade, the Nobel Prize-winning economist, among the most illuminating. Meade is particularly concerned with low income countries with high population growth rates. He contrasts the problems facing "Fertilia"—a model nation with a high population growth rate—and "Sterilia"—a nation with a stable population. "Fertilia" is at a greater disadvantage if it is densely populated like Bangladesh or Java, than if it has a high population growth rate but still has some empty spaces like China or Brazil.

When the population is dense, land and capital are scarce, commanding high rates and interest, but wages will be low because labour is plentiful. The industries which develop will be those, such as textiles, which are labour intensive, but require relatively modest capital. High profits and low wages may encourage saving and foreign capital may even enter "Fertilia" to exploit certain opportunities, and help to create additional employment opportunities. Unfortunately, both these trends will increase the gap between property owners and wage-earners. As has occurred in Mexico and the

Philippines, the gulf between rich and poor will widen and eventually, all other considerations apart, the chasm may grow so great that it becomes socially unacceptable or politically disruptive. If, to avoid this latter stage, wage rates in "Fertilia" are maintained at a level more congruent with dignity and opportunity for the bulk of the population, the incentive to expand employment will disappear and unemployment will grow. Most developing nations already live with unemployment rates (up to 25 per cent) which are almost unthinkable in the West, even at times of economic depression. If underemployment is measured, then the situation becomes sadder. For example, in the 1960s, unemployment in Mauritius grew at 12 per cent a year, representing a level which, population-wise, would have been equal to the chronic unemployment of 1.75 million working

TABLE 36: PERCENTAGE FIXED CAPITAL FORMATION REQUIRED TO MAINTAIN CURRENT LEVEL OF PER CAPITA INCOME

	Nigeria	*U.K.*	*U.S.A.*
Annual population growth-rate (%) 1965–70	2.5	0.5	1.1
Investment of gross domestic product necessitated by population growth	7.5	1.5	3.3
Actual rate of fixed capital formation 1966–8	12.3	19.0	16.7
Percentage of fixed capital formation consumed by population growth	61.0	7.9	19.8

(*Source:* International Bank of Reconstruction and Development)

adults in Britain. One of the multiplying disadvantages of high unemployment is that it makes it doubly difficult for women to enter the work-force, although the opportunity for employment outside the home is one of the strongest correlates with declining fertility.

Problems of employment are not limited to capitalist economies. Commentators on China point to the overmanning of factories and farms. Perhaps it is more humane to overman the production line than to leave able-bodied men to beg on the pavement, but it is the lesser of two evils, not a solution to the basic problems associated with rapid population growth. Although the birth rate of China is falling the present adult population was born at a time of rapid population growth.

While "Fertilia" is struggling to provide employment, without further widening the gap between rich and poor, it has some other problems that are not present at all in "Sterilia". A growing population must be supplied with its complement of capital goods (*see*

Table 36). India should build a new school every half hour, if it is to meet the demand for education represented by her population growth. Housing, schools, hospitals, roads, and all the goods and services for the extra people maturing in a growing population must be financed from savings within the community, or through the palliative of overseas aid. If the population of "Fertilia" grows at 3 per cent per annum, 12 per cent of "Fertilia's" national income must be invested just to maintain services at the level existing in the previous generation.

Lack of capital is often associated with its misuse. One of the paradoxes of developing countries is that there may be under-utilisation of the investment already made in those services which appear to be most in need. Steel mills run at half capacity and the state airline is half empty; often they are in the wrong places, or at the wrong times or inappropriate in some other way. An expensive ambulance may lie unused because spares are unavailable. Maternity beds may be empty all the year round, although women are dying in childbirth a kilometre away, because tradition (or poor quality of service in the hospital) deters women from coming for delivery. Family planning clinics may be poorly used.

The total number of children and old people in the population of "Fertilia" will be higher than that in "Sterilia" and each worker in "Fertilia" will be supporting more dependants than his cousin in "Sterilia" (*see* Fig. 57). The problem of employing women outside the home will be compounded because mothers in "Fertilia" are looking after more children than their friends in "Sterilia". A high burden of dependency makes saving more difficult in "Fertilia" and yet as we have just seen "Fertilia" must save more than "Sterilia" even to stand still.

Every force combines to pull the knot of economic problems tighter. While the leaders of "Fertilia"—be they communist, socialist or capitalist—strive to maintain employment while keeping wages above subsistence level (and while they struggle to maintain national and personal saving to provide the capital for the goods and services required by an expanding population) they also have to transform their industries more actively than their neighbours in "Sterilia", with its stable, or near stable, population. Even if industry can expand to meet the growing needs of "Fertilia" it must also change because the natural resources are inelastic. New lines of production must be continuously sought which use lower ratios of land and natural resources to men and man-made capital resources.

It is not difficult to categorise real countries as "Fertilias" and "Sterilias" (*see* Fig. 58). The inescapable logic of economic forces is preventing developing countries with high population growth rates

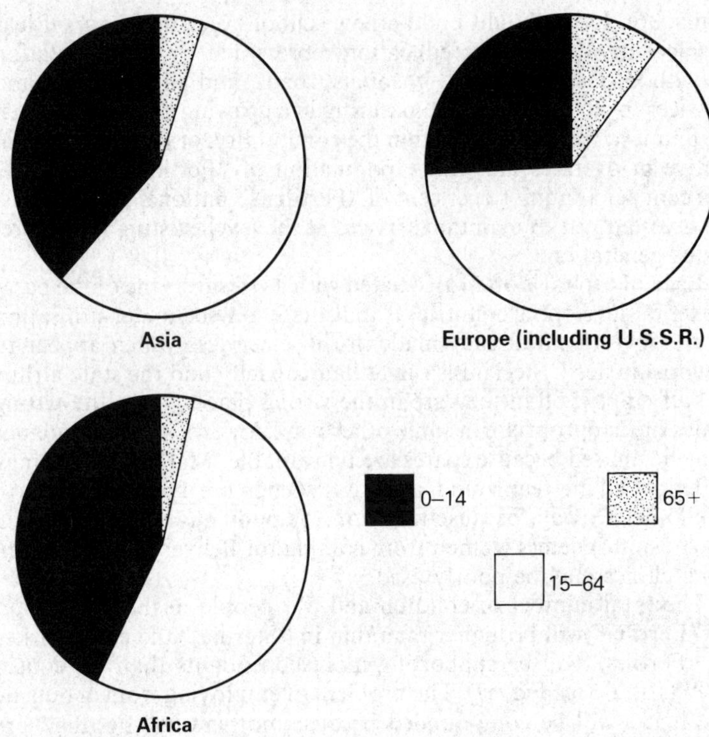

(*Source: World Population Prospects, 1965–2000 as Assessed in 1968*. United Nations 1970)

Fig. 57. *Dependent population in selected continents.*

from progressing towards the living standards of those with stable or slowly growing populations. When Britain entered the Industrial Revolution, the birth rate was 35 per 1,000 and the population growth rate in the nineteenth century rarely exceeded 1 per cent per annum. The birth rate in Pakistan is near 50 per 1,000 and many large countries still have population growth rates over 2.5 per cent. Sometimes, even dramatic leaps in technology fail to keep pace with the growth in people—the High Aswan Dam increased the cultivable area of Egypt by 40 per cent, but the population rose by that amount during the years it took to plan and build the dam and for Lake Nasser to fill. Between 1955 and 1975, the G.N.P. of the Philippines expanded by 88 per cent but the *per capita* income only rose by 25 per cent. The labour-force increased by 15 per cent; one-third of these were illiterate, one-eighth of the adults was unemployed and an even greater number underemployed.

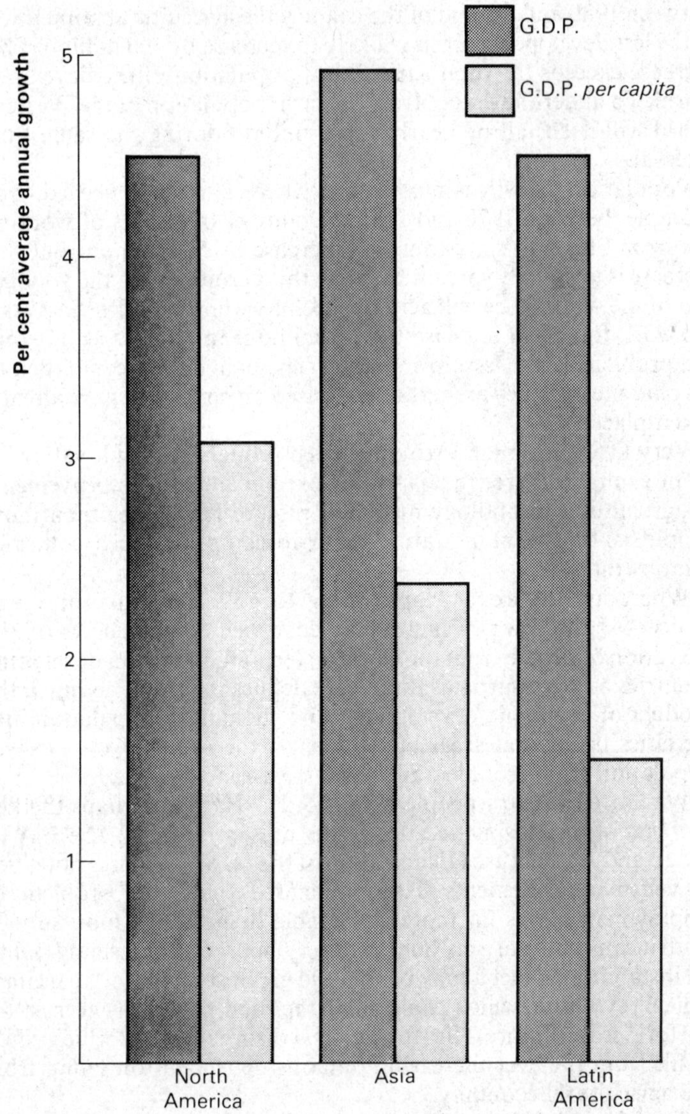

(*Source:* International Bank of Reconstruction and Development)
Fig. 58. *Growth of Gross Domestic Product and per capita income* (*1960–67*).

EMPLOYMENT AND URBANISATION

Between 1980 and the end of the century the agricultural population of the less developed nations is likely to increase by 300 million. This increase exceeds the total agricultural population of the developed world. To underline the contrast the farm population of the Western world will itself fall by nearly a 100 million during the same time interval.

Population growth is most rapid where it is least needed. For example, between 1970 and 1985 the number of Asians of working age from fifteen to sixty-four will increase by 500 million. But this increase is unequally spread. In Japan the recruitment to the younger end of the work-force will actually decline, while in South East Asia the work-force will increase by 325 million. In Africa (*see* Fig. 59) the problem is no less formidable. These figures are not demographic guesses, they are certainties based on births that have already taken place.

Very little fertile land remains to be brought into cultivation; it is one capital resource that is largely fixed in amount. Improvements in agricultural technology may well require less rather than more people, as the shrinking farm labour-force in developed countries demonstrates.

Where are the extra people going to go? They have only one choice—to the towns. Hauser has described some aspects of the migration of people from the countryside to the towns in developing countries as "over-urbanisation". He defines it as "not so much the product of economic development and the pull of population into the cities from rural areas but rather ... the result of the push of population from troubled and insecure areas".

What are the extra people going to do? Here is perhaps the key problem of the closing decades of the present century. The F.A.O. (Food and Agriculture Organisation of the U.N.), which is not given to vehement statements has commented that "the problem of employment looms far more intractable than that of food supply. With it can come not only human misery but social unrest and political instability. In fact it may be that the greatest threat to the technological revolution which could solve the food problem—at least for the foreseeable future—lies in the social disorganisation which could result from the ever increasing millions dependent on living from the agricultural economy."

The biggest migration in human history is already taking place. Hundreds of millions of people are leaving a traditional village way of life, which in many ways has changed little over 4,000 years, to enter the exploding cities of the contemporary world. In the past

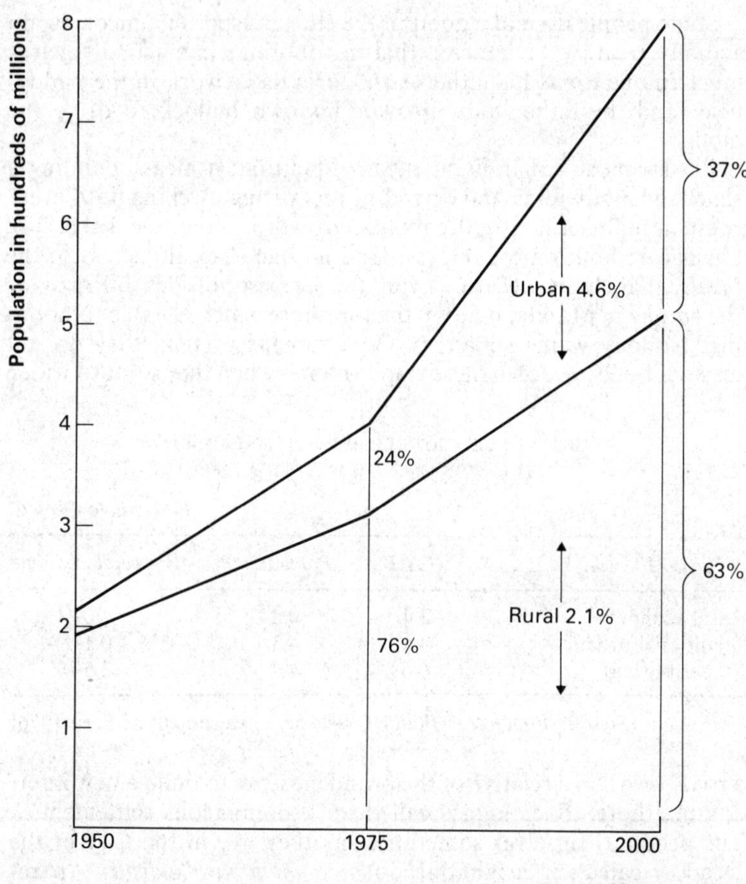

(*Source:* I.P.P.F. data)

Fig. 59. *Urbanisation* (*Africa 1950–2000*).

fifteen years nearly 600 million people—approximately the population of India— have become city dwellers for the first time. By the end of the century they are likely to be joined by another 1,500 million people—equal to the total world population in 1900—who will either be born into cities or come from the continued migration from the countryside. In 1950, the Brazilian population was 64 per cent rural; by 1970 it was 56 per cent urban. In Pakistan between 1951 and 1961 the urban population rose by 4.5 million: 42 per cent was by natural increase, 32 per cent by migration from the countryside into established towns and the remainder due to the creation of new urban areas.

Some people do make good in the cities; disposable incomes are actually greater which means that the doorman can actually get as much in one tip as his father earns for a day's work in the paddy-field (and the father must provide his own bullock to drive the plough).

But for most, urban living means squatting; it means building a shack, or subdividing and extending an existing dwelling until every room contains a family. Economic growth is slow (*see* Table 37). Shacks are built on the poorest land no one else can use, as in the *favelas* that climb precariously up the steepest hillsides in Brazil, or the *barong* in Manila, built on the foreshore which is liable to flooding. Nobody wants squatters. Governments pretend they do not exist, or bulldoze down these fragile homes when they want to widen

TABLE 37: RELATIONSHIP BETWEEN ECONOMIC AND POPULATION GROWTH BY SECTOR (PERU)

Percentage Growth

1950–1975	*G.N.P.*	*Population*	*Per capita income*
Rural economy	2.4	0.8	1.6
Traditional urban	4.6	4.5	0.1
Modern urban	6.6	4.4	2.5

(*Source: Population Policy Guideline*. Government of Peru 1976)

a road, or when a relative of the president seeks to build a new international hotel. Sociologists call them "spontaneous settlements". The people themselves sometimes say they live in the City of the Dead or call their neighbourhoods *colonias paracaidistas* ("parachutists' neighbourhoods").

Squatter areas can contain immense numbers of people. A *favela* in Rio, which you may pass in a car in less than a minute, often contains more people than all the high-rise buildings in the next fifteen minutes' drive. There are over a million and a quarter squatter homes in Seoul, South Korea. In Ankara, two in three homes are of this type; in Manila a million people or more live in the Tondo and Pasay and they are only two of the squatter settlements in the city. 100,000 people live in slums in Dar es Salaam (one-third of the total) and half the population of Guayaquil (Ecuador) are squatters. 70 per cent of the families in Calcutta live in one room or less.

Life in squatter areas can be harsh. We have known of property developers who start fires in squatter areas and municipal authorities who delay the arrival of the fire services. The rule of law does not extend to squatter areas and no one leaves their homes unattended. Tempers are short in crowded conditions. One of the few people to observe slum life objectively has been the Filippino anthropologist, Landa Jocano, who lived in a squatter area for five years. He found that neighbours had five major husband/wife quarrels a month with screams and blows and wailing and cursing. There were daily misunderstandings.

In Jocano's immediate neighbourhood in his Manila slum, two-thirds of the able-bodied population was unemployed. Among those fortunate enough to be employed, the largest single group (105 out of 507) were prostitutes. In many Oriental and African cities, and especially in the cities of Catholic developing countries, prostitution is a major route by which wealth is transferred from the wealthy to the less fortunate. Many prostitutes support children, or other relatives, and some have husbands, boyfriends or protectors. All pay rent and buy food and clothes—they are a major economic group. Incidentally, a great many family planning programmes specifically exclude this group of sexually active young women from their help.

Governments, institutions and even academics do not want to know about the squatter life. When the World Bank met in Manila in 1977, the government literally built wooden walls round the squatter areas to that the distinguished visitors would not see them, as they sped in their cars from the airport to their air-conditioned hotels.

But a slum is not an accidental collection of packing-case homes on some insanitary swamp in Asia or dangerous hillside in Latin America. A slum represents a finely balanced social system, with roots that extend back into the traditional villages that so many families have just left, and branches that reach into the wealthy oases of city life. It is a delicately-tuned economy that runs at the maximum rate its small resources allow. The smells and the shouting can be forgotten in the smiles of the children. The most remote relative can share the family's meal and everyone will shift over at night to find one more space on the floor. A family that lives in one room may have a television set or a hairdryer.

Modern medicine also finds its way into squatter life. Pharmacies do a brisk trade, even though many of the drugs purchased may not give value for money. Many mothers will have their deliveries in hospital, even though they may be two in a bed and be discharged a few hours after delivery. People will use their small disposable income to go to private doctors (who are remarkably accessible in shanty-towns), but private doctors are nearly always omitted from governmental and non-governmental family planning programmes. On the whole, the poor urban population, which is most influenced by the modern way of life and more eager to plan their families than their rural cousins, receive poor family planning services. Abortion (illegal in Latin America) becomes a major variable in fertility control in modern Third World cities, just as it was in the urban areas of the U.S.A. and Europe in the nineteenth century.

CALCUTTA

Calcutta is the archetypal urban slum. Mark Twain said the climate "was enough to make a brass door-knob mushy"; Winston Churchill declared he was glad he had seen it because "it will be unnecessary for me to see it again" and Geoffrey Moorhouse called it "a definition of obscenity". Calcutta has long been the centre of one or other Malthusian problem. It was host city to the Bengal famines of 1770, 1783, 1866, 1873–4, 1892, 1897 and 1943. In the latter 3 million people died. Calcutta has been the centre for civil and religious strife, as after "Partition" in 1946.

There are over 38,500 people per square kilometre (four times the density of New York); over 400,000 men are unemployed and perhaps 100,000 people, who have neither shack, hovel or *bustee*, live, sleep, copulate, give birth and die on the pavements. There are 400,000 lepers in Calcutta. But perhaps the depressing spiral of problems consequent on excessive population growth is best illustrated by the daily comedy of the public transport system. The double-decker buses are so overloaded that passengers stand upstairs as well as down and cling to any toehold on the exterior. The conductor can rarely collect all the fares and may give up altogether, sitting on the front mudguard shouting to the driver and passengers. Less than 400 trams carry a quarter of a million passengers each day. An average of ten are derailed each day due to poor track and worn out vehicles. The transport system makes horrendous losses and it is impossible to raise the capital to renew it. And if it was possible to improve the transport system it would still become bogged down in the streets, where pedestrians push one another off the uneven pavements, where sacred cows still wander and where rickshaw men run ten to twenty miles a day between the shafts of their vehicles and earn no more than one U.S. dollar for their effort. A single bridge connects Calcutta (9 million) with Howrah (600,000) and it can take an hour to push across it. But if the money could be found to build a second bridge, would it be best spent on such a project or on building a sewer? There is no sewage whatsoever in Howrah at the present time.

Urban poverty on the scale found in Calcutta erodes language, alters perspectives and unbalances the best of human intentions. The middle class becomes defined as those who live in rooms 2.5 m by

1.5 m. Mother Teresa's famous *Nirmal Hriday* gives succour to the dying, but opposes modern contraception and abortion and misses out the rest of human life between conception and death.

There are many reasons for the sad history of the world's most unhappy city. It ceased to be the administrative centre of India when the Imperial capital was transferred to New Delhi on 1st April 1912. The jute trade is being overtaken by artificial fibres and the harbour is situated on a river which has changed course and really no longer exists. But underlying all other problems is the problem of population. Calcutta drains excess population from West Bengal, Bihar, Orissa and Assam—all rural states with only sixteen other towns that even exceed 100,000 in population between them. Calcutta is largely the result of rural-urban migration from an area containing approximately 100 million people. There is no doubt the developing world is going to create a great many more Calcuttas.

In a sociological sense Calcutta is a large number of villages compressed into a small space. The way of life of the people, their kinship ties and their technology are in many ways closer to rural than urban life. In this way, Calcutta is different from Mexico City, and poles apart from Chicago; in comparison with the ghettos of North America, it is a safe place to work and live, despite the poverty.

EDUCATION

In the last analysis, the prime resource of a nation is not the oil under its continental shelf or the iron in its mountains, it is the education and training of its people. Japan, with few natural resources, has made herself the third richest nation in the world. By contrast, India is blessed with a range of natural resources, and a large enough population to bring about any imaginable economies of scale; but the bulk of her population is not trained, organised or practised in living with, and contributing to, a modern industrialised community. So despite having 14.6 per cent of the world's population and 2.4 per cent of the world's land area, India only commands 1.5 per cent of the global income.

Population growth puts enormous strains on educational systems battling to reduce illiteracy. One of the arguments that persuaded the Ghanaian Government to adopt a population policy, was the realisation that if population growth in the 1950s and 1960s could have been halved, then the investment which was actually made in education would have been sufficient to bring every child into the classroom—but as it is, this dream remains unfulfilled in Ghana as in most other developing countries.

ENERGY

For much of the world's population, energy involves heat for cooking the day's inadequate meals: with growing numbers, firewood must be gathered from increasingly remote areas, as in Nepal. As the trees are destroyed, flash floods become more common and soil is eroded. In India most meals are cooked on dried cow dung, denying the land precious fertiliser.

For the exploding urban areas of the world, energy means fuel for transport, for a tiny minority energy is the power to drive the air-conditioning, the coal to smelt the steel and the gasoline in your personal automobile. 42 per cent of the energy used in the U.S.A. goes into transport, which in one way or another accounts for a remarkable one-sixth of the G.N.P. of the country. As Loraine has pointed out, "there are more licensed U.S. drivers than registered voters; for every baby born in America in 1976 two cars were produced".

The global use of oil increases by 8 per cent a year. In the United Kingdom, the importation of oil increased twelve-fold between 1946 and 1973. Before the world's population doubles yet again, the majority of the readily recoverable crude oil in the world will have been used up. The pace of use is so rapid that the world seems unlikely to adjust to current demands and future changes without major economic and political upheavals—changes which may indeed be catastrophic for sections of the population in developed and developing countries. By 1970, the world had used one-eighth of estimated petroleum reserves; by 1979, it will have consumed one-quarter and by 1988 one-half of all the liquid fossil fuels. The much publicised North Sea Oil reserves represent no more than 2 per cent of the global total.

Therefore the global use of energy is only tangentially related to current population growth. Until a few years ago, the moderate increase in population in developed countries represented a greater potential increase in energy consumption than the more rapid rates in poorer countries.

Most of the world's oil reserves lie in the Middle East. The U.S.A. has been an oil importer since the late 1960s. Japan is totally dependent on foreign reserves and the U.S.S.R. may need to be an oil importer within the foreseeable future. The economies of most developing countries have been built around relatively cheap supplies of imported oil. Nigeria, Iraq and Iran (and possibly China) are populous developing countries which may be able to husband their oil resources for several decades into the future. Indonesian reserves may run dry in as brief an interval as fifteen years. There are many alternatives to oil as an energy source, although they are more expensive. In Britain, coal output has fallen since the Second World War, but could be increased again. At present rates of use, the world's coal reserves would last for 2,500 years. Coal is a polluting fuel and the prevention of pollution, in turn, puts up the cost of energy. The burning of oil and coal raises the carbon dioxide concentration in the atmosphere and this is thought to increase by an average of 1.5 parts per million each year and by the year 2000 may be 30 per cent higher than the estimated content in 1860. This apparently modest rise may well be enough to change some of the major climatic patterns in the world, making the grain-growing areas of North America drier but perhaps bringing some rain to the fringes of the Sahara.

Coal and oil shale can be made into petroleum, but the cost per barrel is more than ten times that of the price of oil at the well-head in the Persian Gulf at the present time. The ecological consequences of vastly increased coal mining and the use of oil shales are formidable.

Uranium, like fossil fuels, is only found in finite amounts. Nuclear energy programmes are not contributing the share of energy that it was once hoped they would and are running into increasing technical and political bottlenecks. In the United Kingdom, nuclear power plants only produce one-tenth of the nation's electricity. The handling of waste materials is still controversial technology. Every nuclear power plant that is built raises the probability that the control of atomic weapons will become increasingly fragmented, raising the possibility of their use in local or global wars. A great many countries, from Brazil to Israel, now have the potential to make (or have already manufactured) atomic weapons. In 1974, India demonstrated with the explosion of its first atomic bomb that the "peaceful" use of nuclear energy could be easily switched to more threatening ends.

If nuclear fusion, rather than fission, can be perfected, then a solution to the world's energy problems will be in sight. The raw materials for fusion are isotopes of hydrogen found in the sea and there is no polluting radioactive waste. The principle is the same as the hydrogen bomb, but the technology to tame nuclear fusion has yet to be perfected. If and when it is, the world will have at its disposal, in Loraine's vivid phrase, "the equivalent of 500 Pacific Oceans of high grade fuel oil".

Fossil fuels consist merely of stored solar energy. The world's consumption of oil in the 1980s will represent withdrawing from the geological bank, each year, capital assets that took approximately 5 million years to accumulate. By 1980, the waste heat generated from burning fossil fuels will amount to about 5 per cent of the total solar energy absorbed at the ground in the U.S.A. Although solar energy can make local and important contributions to the world's problems, it is not going to make a major contribution in the short term. Unfortunately, the capital costs of collecting solar energy are high and although the amounts of energy that can be collected are very applicable to Third World societies in tropical countries, it is unlikely that they could afford to use them. Hydroelectric energy, which is merely a short term storage of the sun's power, only supplies 2 per cent of the world's energy needs and a great many of the obvious resources are already in use. Brazil has launched an ambitious scheme to replace petroleum with alcohol derived from the fermentation of plant products. It is a potentially realistic solution applicable to a large tropical country which still has a relatively low density of population: but a similar technology in a country like the Philippines might involve some competition with land currently given over to growing food.

Mankind is at a turning point in its profligate use of natural resources. Profound adjustments in the amount and type of energy consumption are inevitable in the coming decades. The problems which exist are partly the result of population growth in the past. The problems that they will create will throw new stresses which are difficult to predict on the world's ability to accommodate the population growth currently taking place.

One thing is certain: exponential growth of the sort which has taken place in the current generation cannot continue into the next, in either rich or poor countries. Currently, the U.S.A. invests approximately 10 per cent of its output and achieves an annual *per capita* growth in income of 2 per cent. In the brief years before the year 2000, the average American family, if current economic growth rates continue, will be 80 per cent richer than today and the G.N.P. of the country 170 per cent larger. However, such changes may well press at or beyond the limit of the environment to absorb the pollution or to supply the means to sustain an economy of such a size.

Growth in the rest of the world, including developing countries, will transform the formidable problems (posed by the expansion of the U.S.A. and other developed economies) into what may be an insoluble problem for the planet as a whole. The G.N.P. of some developing countries grew by 4 per cent a year in the 1960s. When economic and population growth are viewed together, the total world output would multiply four times by the year 2000, or eleven times the present U.S. output and income. On this assumption the annual consumption of materials would have to rise to 173,000,000,000 tonnes of steel, 610,000,000,000 tonnes of coal and the consumption of 60,000,000,000 barrels of oil, much of it going to an estimated 110,000,000 motor vehicles.

But such predictions can be dangerous. The world growth in material goods may slow. The doubling of electricity consumption each decade, which for example has been the characteristic of developed countries in recent years, need not go on for ever. Countries like Japan may discover what the United Kingdom has already demonstrated—that the optimistic forecasts of economists are not always met. The only certainties for the future are that the unpredictable will become a major variable.

Perhaps the most immediate policy that needs to be adopted, now that the era of cheap fuel has passed for ever, is to conserve energy and natural resources with great care. The U.S.A., with 6 per cent of the world's population, consumes 40 per cent of the available global resources. It also wastes more energy than is used by two-thirds of the world's population.

CONCLUSION

Demographic change is an unforgiving master. Much that has been written on population points to future doom. But in truth, changes of horrendous proportions have already occurred: the die that will determine the way of life for thousands of millions of people has been cast. The hundreds of millions who will be seeking employment at the end of the century are already born. Many who should be at school, have no school to go to. Hunger could have been largely banished from the world if population growth since 1950 had been less. The opportunities for individual economic progress which existed at the end of the Second World War, have been largely eroded by the population growth that has taken place.

Cities are going to get larger and more numerous. Problems of squatter settlements will worsen. In the past, urban problems were solved, but the miracle that transformed the slums of mid-nineteenth century Europe and North America into the cities of today (whatever their defects) are not destined to be repeated in the developing world. Urban Europe grew by 1.5 per cent per annum in the last century, but the cities of today grow three, four and sometimes five times as rapidly. In 1851, unemployment in Britain ran at 6–7 per cent; today in the Philippines it is 13 per cent or more and over 25 per cent in parts of Africa.

There is another outstanding difference between nineteenth century cities and those of the contemporary developing world. 100 years ago, urban death rates were consistently higher than rural, while today this pattern is reversed. Cities no longer kill to the extent they did in the past. However inadequate the sewage and piped water supply, communicable diseases are controlled.

The long-term future is perilous, if not bleak. By the end of the century, Third World cities will not only have to deal with rising food prices but sudden dramatic increases in fuel costs as world petroleum resources are exhausted. And a slum needs fuel just as much as a modern Western city, yet it will lack the capital for more expensive forms of transport and industrial application. For the burgeoning squatter populations of the developing world, the road ahead has a fork in it: will they become crowded, busy, polluted Tokyos, where nevertheless life has some promise of quality, or Calcuttas which, like a cancer, grow at the edges and decay in the centre, destroying even the quiet dignity of life associated with a traditional village?

A traditional village society is characterised by a simple agricultural technology and low literacy rates. Mouth to mouth communication is more important than in complex societies and family relationships are usually the basis of economic and organisational decisions. On the whole, emotional commitment towards relatives, perhaps also neighbours, is stronger than in an industrial society, but conversely, the sympathy and commitment towards the community as a whole is lower.

By comparison, a modern industrial society has a complex structure with a very high division of labour, and is not only literate, but places high value on science and education. It is cosmopolitan in its social relationships, and individuals in their working and social lives create links with a variety of people from many backgrounds. Consequently, economic decisions are more rational than in a traditional society. The emotional links, for example to aged parents, are less than in a traditional society, but the empathy felt by people for the poor and sick of society as a whole may be greater.

Unhappily, the gap between the rich and poor sections of the world continues to grow. A question mark now hangs over some of the more optimistic forecasts of the 1960s. The increase in the price of oil, inflation and the economic problems of the 1970s (most of them aggravated by moderate population growth in developed countries after the Second World War) will hurt developing countries most. The gaps between the rich North and the poor South may widen from the current embarrassing $2,000 a year *per capita* to an obscene $7,000 a year at the end of the century. The implications of this chasm between rich and poor are frightening.

If a total inventory of the world's resources is made out and the global national product is divided by the world's population, average *per capita* income works out at approximately $800 a year or just over $2 per person per day. This is just about enough to buy the average North American a poached egg and a cup of coffee for breakfast. There is, on the one hand, a manifest need to attempt a more equitable distribution of the world's wealth, both by raising the flow of aid from rich to poor countries up to and beyond the 1 per cent level recommended by the Pearson Commission report, and by more advantageous terms of trade to developing nations. But, on the other hand, it is cruelly false to imagine, along with those whose arithmetic appears as weak as their theological or political theory, that the world's problems can be solved by merely dividing the material resources available for the banquet more equally between the guests who continue to join the table.

The remaining decades of the twentieth century are going to be ones of rapid change in almost all spheres of life for nearly all the people on Planet Earth. In some ways developed and developing countries face equally difficult but essential adaptations. Developing countries are controlling their fertility with increasing rigour but still have a long way to go. Family planning schemes have not helped as much as they might and have often omitted the over-the-counter sale of contraceptives and the option of abortion, which observation shows are usually the starting point for family planning in poor countries. If family size is to fall from six or seven children to two or three in the coming generation it will demand great changes in social and emotional expectations.

Equally in the developed world, economic changes are now taking place which are as far-reaching as any alterations in family size will be for the developing world. As the era of cheap petroleum comes to an end, as society appreciates that natural resources are finite and there is increasing competition for raw materials during a decade of unprecedented global inflation, so society is beginning to appreciate that, just as the developing world has to achieve zero population growth within the foreseeable future, so the developed world will ultimately have to live with the reality of zero economic growth.

SELECTED REFERENCES AND BIBLIOGRAPHY

Brown, L. R. *In the Human Interest*. W. W. Norton, New York 1974

Cassen, R. "Population and Development: A Survey." *World Development*. 4, 785 1976

Jocano, F. Landa. *The Slum as a Way of Life*. University of the Philippines Press, Quezon City 1975

Loraine, J. A. *Syndromes of the Seventies*. Peter Owen, London 1977

Meade, J. "Population Explosion; The Standard of Living and Social Conflict." *The Economic Journal*. 77, 235 1967

Meadows, D. H., Meadows, D. L., Randers, J. and Behrens, W. W. *The Limits to Growth*. Universe Books, New York 1972

Mesarovic, M. and Pestel, E. *Mankind at the Turning Point*. Dutton & Co., New York 1974

Moorhouse, G. *Calcutta*. Weidenfeld & Nicolson, London 1971

Report of the Commission on Population Growth and the American Future. Signet, New York 1972

Stevas, N. J. *The Agonising Choice*. Eyre & Spottiswoode, London 1971

Wilsher, P. and Righter, R. *Exploding Cities*. Andre Deutsch 1975

Chapter 11

Family Planning in Developed Countries

The demonstrable ability of Western communities to control their fertility preceded the intellectual ability of the community to understand what it was doing, and has frequently run counter to the philosophies and politics which society itself professed to follow.

THE PIONEERS

Evidence for the voluntary restriction of fertility in pre-industrial Europe has been discussed in Chapter 7. However, it was only in the early nineteenth century that writers first began to describe the practice and extol the virtues of birth-control practices. Perhaps the greatest of these was Francis Place, born in 1771 into what today's social worker would call a "problem family". At the age of nineteen he married a girl two years younger, and although the couple eventually had fifteen children (of whom five died early) and suffered great economic hardship, it was a happy union. When Place was fifty-two, and long after the birth of his last child, he launched a campaign of public propaganda for contraception through a series of printed leaflets which became known as the *Diabolical Handbills*. They were widely distributed in London and the North of England. Addressed "to the Married of Both Sexes of the Working People and Similarly the Married Sexes in Genteel Life" the author noted the use of coitus interruptus and advocated vaginal barrier methods:

> A piece of soft sponge about the size of a small ball attached to a very narrow ribbon and slightly moistened (when convenient) is introduced previous to sexual intercourse and is afterwards withdrawn, and thus by an easy, simple, cleanly and non-indelicate method, in no way injurious to health, not only may much unhappiness and many miseries be prevented, but benefits of an incalculable amount be conferred on society.

The ideas of the British movement were taken to America by Robert Dale Owen, who went to the New World at the age of twenty-four and in 1831 published *Moral Physiology—or a Brief and Plain Treatise on the Population*. The book was adorned with a frontispiece depicting a mother abandoning her child and lamenting: "Alas that it should have been born." It discussed the sponge, condom and withdrawal, but the book's importance lies largely in the influence it had on an American, Charles Knowlton, who in 1832 published anonymously a book called *The Fruits of Philosophy*. Knowlton recommended post-coital douching, giving details of various formulations such as "liquid Chloride of Soda, a pint of water, four or five great spoons full". Both Place and Knowlton had their disciples and the ripples which they caused in society continued to spread in ever larger circles throughout the nineteenth century. *The Fruits of Philosophy* was printed several times on both sides of the Atlantic.

Two courageous free thinkers—Charles Bradlaugh and Annie Besant—set up the Free Thought Publishing Company to publicly challenge the fact that a minor Bristol printer had been sentenced to two years imprisonment, with hard labour, for selling Knowlton's *Fruits of Philosophy* in an edition said to be interleaved with obscene pictures (probably anatomical diagrams of the genitals). Bradlaugh and Besant provoked a test case by republishing the same book in a new cheap edition, informing the police of their action. The case of *R.* v. *Charles Bradlaugh and Annie Besant* ended in their acquittal following an appeal to the High Court. At the original trial, the jury had found that the book was "likely to deprave public morals", but exonerated the defendants from any corrupt motives in publishing it. The judge interpreted this as a guilty verdict and imposed a sentence of six months' imprisonment, a fine of £200, with £500 recognisance of good behaviour for two years. A stay of execution was granted when they pledged not to republish the book, and the appeal was granted subsequently on the grounds of a technical error in the indictment.

The details of the trial and the book were secondary to the revolution in public attitudes which the publicity surrounding the trial brought about. Birth-control, it has been said, was "thrown onto the breakfast tables of the English middle classes". There was an explosion in printed literature about family planning. Sales of *The Fruits of Philosophy*, previously less than 1,000 a year, rose to over 100,000 in the three months preceding the trial and continued at a high level thereafter. Mrs. Besant subsequently produced her own book, *The Law of Population*, dedicated to "the poor in our great cities and agricultural districts, dwellers in stifling courts or crowded hovels, in the hope that it may point a path from poverty and may make easier the life of British mothers". In earlier versions she advocated the use of the sponge, but later editions favoured two new methods, the cervical cap and soluble pessaries. The manufacture of spermicides and condoms and vaginal occlusive devices grew rapidly. In 1879 the Malthusian League was founded and its journal

The Malthusian began publication. It was perhaps an accident of statistics and social history that the birth rate in Britain fell in every year from 1877 to 1918, but certainly the Bradlaugh/Besant trial marked a turning point in social and demographic attitudes, and there was a marked improvement in contraceptive practice in the latter part of the nineteenth century.

Annie Besant subsequently became a religious mystic, moving to India in 1880. One of the main roads in Bombay is named after her, but unfortunately her family planning message was not transmitted to this part of the then Empire. Bradlaugh became the first free-thinker Member of Parliament and was persistently re-elected by his constituency in Northampton, even though his right to take his parliamentary seat was for many years resisted because of his refusal to swear a religious oath. Indeed, many of nineteenth century intellectuals who promoted birth-control were Humanists. One such was John Stuart Mill, who advocated birth-control through the columns of the radical paper, the *Black Dwarf*, and who had been arrested at the age of seventeen for handing out birth-control leaflets in a market place.

Unfortunately, prosecutions for selling family planning works continued, and in 1878, Edward Truelove, a 67-year-old "rationalist" publisher, was sent to prison for four months for publishing Owen's *Moral Physiology*; while as late as 1892, a Newcastle phrenologist received a sentence of one months' hard labour for selling Dr. Allbutt's *The Wife's Handbook*, which had first been published in 1886 and contained a four page comprehensive review of methods of contraception from "coughing" (unreliable) and coitus interruptus (hurtful to the nervous system in many persons), to French Letters (a very certain check) and Rendell's soluble quinine pessaries—still in existence. For the most part the medical profession was implacably opposed to such ideas, with the *Lancet* praising the views expressed at an annual meeting of the B.M.A. about "beastly contrivances and filthy expedients for the prevention of conception". Dr. Allbutt, author of *The Wife's Handbook* (price 6d) was struck off the General Medical Register and his publication condemned as indecent by the Royal College of Physicians at Edinburgh.

The scientific analogue of the social campaigners is to be found in the writings of Thomas Malthus. Unlike Place, he had a happy childhood, contact with liberal thinkers, a good education and spent his life as an academic and a clergyman. He only had three children. "Perhaps" he wrote, "there is scarcely a man who has once experienced virtuous love ... who does not look back to that period as the sunny spot in his whole life." He was moved by the sufferings of the poor, especially during his travels in Scandinavia. He wanted greater equality for women than he found in his contemporary society.

Malthus's simple theory that population grows by geometrical increase while agricultural production expands arithmetically became indelibly etched on the thinking of subsequent generations and he was an important influence on Charles Darwin and Karl Marx.

It is one of the many paradoxes of the history of fertility control that Malthus' own attitudes have been so misunderstood and abused. Although neo-Malthusianism has become a dirty word in the twentieth century, like neo-colonialism, and is supposed to express an aggressive policy of population limitation, Malthus himself eschewed all policies of artificial birth-control. He was as pronatalist as Marx and Engels, writing "countries which unite great landed resources with a prosperous state of commerce and manufacture, and in which the commercial part of the population never essentially exceeds the agricultural part, are eminently secure from sudden reverses ... there is no reason to say that they might not go on increasing in riches and population for hundreds, nay almost thousands of years".

Francis Place in *The Principle of Population* (published 1822) among other things foresaw the famines that were to cut back the population of Ireland in the generation that was to follow. He felt that the Malthusian recommendation of moral restraint was absurd. He wrote to a correspondent "you and I—and Mill and Wakefield—mustering among us no less I believe than 36 children ... rare fellows we to teach moral restraint".

THE PRAGMATISTS

The spread of family planning practices in industrial nations has been discussed in Chapter 7. By the last quarter of the nineteenth century every method of birth-control now in use—with the exception of oral contraceptives—had been described, was manufactured, advertised and distributed. Condoms and spermicides were increasingly widely used. A range of intra-uterine devices and cervical pessaries was devised. A first human vasectomy was performed around 1893—although Sir Astley Cooper had been experimenting on dogs at the time Place was writing his handbills. Abortion, as we have seen, was illegal but well known (*see* page 202–4).

It was the human suffering of abortion that started Margaret Sanger (1883–1966) on her great family planning crusade, which was not only to change public attitudes in the U.S.A., but to lead to international action. She helped organise the World Population Conference in 1927 and was the force behind the foundation of the International Planned Parenthood Federation in 1952.

Sanger recounts in her biography how, as a young nurse in 1912, she attended a Russian immigrant family where the mother was suffering from a self-induced abortion. Timidly, Margaret Sanger asked the doctor to give the woman contraceptive advice. "Any more such capers, young woman," said the doctor, "and there will be no need to send for me . . . you want to have your cake and eat it too? Well it can't be done. Tell Jake to sleep on the roof." Three months after this pathetic episode the woman died in the presence of Margaret Sanger, from another criminally induced abortion.

Marie Stopes, Margaret Sanger's great British contemporary, came into the realm of birth-control through a different but equally personal route. Her first marriage was unconsummated and such were the attitudes of the time that, seeing something was missing from the marriage, she had to take herself off to the British Museum in an attempt to discover what normally happened in the marital bed. From this bitter experience she made a second, happier marriage with Humphrey Verdon Roe (a founder of Avro, the firm that ultimately was to build the Lancaster bomber during the Second World War). Her burning desire for women to enjoy equality and sexual pleasure in marriage inevitably drew her into the need for sexual freedom and contraceptive practice.

Unlike the pioneers of the nineteenth century, Sanger, Stopes and those who joined them (and those who quarrelled with them) went on to found clinics and attempted to create services that reached a whole range of social groups. "Clinics, clinics and more clinics are needed: clinics all over the world," cried Marie Stopes; although she had to remain disappointed that her family planning clinic (which still exists in London) could not claim to be the first in the world. That honour went to the Dutch and to a Dr. Aletta Jacobs, the first woman to be medically qualified in Holland, who opened a clinic in 1882.

The movements and services which grew up between the two World Wars occurred when birth-rates in Europe had already fallen to low levels. Marie Stopes herself was not averse to describing the need for the white inhabitants of the British Empire to breed in terms that many might find offensive today. The dramatic decline of fertility in Britain has been documented in Chapter 7, and although fertility was higher in the U.S.A., the trend was the same. Society had largely solved the problem of fertility regulation before the family planning movement became a significant force at the service level. In retrospect, what the twentieth century family planning movement did in developed countries was to make public something that had been going on in private for two generations; it attempted to introduce more humane and, it was hoped, more effective methods to replace the primitive and sometimes brutal solutions which society had already evolved to solve a problem. It was in some ways a physical expression of the political emancipation which women were seeking and it was a movement which concentrated very much on female methods of contraception, for philosophical as well as for technical reasons.

In the world of conflict and paradoxes in which the early family planning workers lived, it is not surprising that they took a number of actions which were explicable in the situation that they found themselves, but were to hamstring the development of services a generation later. With very few exceptions, they disassociated contraception from any relationship with abortion. Stopes began her influential book *Birth Control Today* (1934): "This book deals with the *control* of conception solely. It does not discuss the destruction of the embryo after it has been formed, that is *abortion*, legally and philosophically quite a different process", and she goes on to say that women who ignore this distinction are "a danger to the human race".

Society forced the activists into a position which was counter to emerging observational data. Raymond Pearl writing a few years later, in 1939, pointed out that

> respectable white married women, those who practise contraception as part of their sex life, by their own admission resort to criminally induced abortion about *three times* as often proportionately as do their comparable non-contraceptor contemporaries.

Almost alone amongst the early writers on family planning, the Americans Dickinson and Bryant in their *Control of Conception* written in 1932, were unusually direct about the role of abortion in family planning. "Some day," they concluded, "all fair reasons for interruption of pregnancy will be frankly faced in our country as they are now in Russia." They described very early abortion without dilation of the cervix, using a small curette and avoiding even the need for local anaesthesia. But the mainstream disassociated abortion and contraception, and the division which arose for valid political reasons between the two World Wars is still with us.

At the governmental level in Britain, the same political pressures which had suppressed rational thinking about abortion in the 1930s still, in the 1960s, prevented the N.H.S. filling the needs opened up by the 1967 Act. Unfortunately, the British Family Planning Association, ostrich-like, opted out of anything to do with termination of pregnancy, even after it had become legal. As a consequence new charities, the Pregnancy Advisory Services, had to be created and the established voluntary movement missed an opportunity and failed in an obligation.

In the U.S.A., Planned Parenthood, the heritage of Margaret Sanger, did discharge its duties as attitudes to abortion evolved, but the movement had to carry a different burden from between the war years. Margaret Sanger had very consciously brought physicians into the family planning movement, not because they were technically necessary for the vaginal barrier methods that she was able to offer, but because they brought a veneer of respectability to a frequently unpopular movement. This decision, combined with the natural American tendency to deify and overpay anything to do with the medically qualified, created and still creates problems inside and outside the U.S.A. Clinic services remain dominated by doctors, who are always expensive and often conservative. The cost of taking family planning services for a year to individuals amongst the so-called indigent in the U.S.A. exceeds the total *per capita* income of many developing countries.

But in the mid-1970s, as if to prove that the ashes of controversy from which the phoenix of family planning arose are still not cold, services in many developed countries have come under attack. Although the U.S. Congress earmarks very considerable sums of money to subsidise contraceptive services, legislation in 1977 removed the payment that was made previously to assist people with abortions. Once again this essential factor in fertility regulation is not equally available to all citizens. Likewise, in Britain, Australia and New Zealand counter-pressure has been brought on abortion services in particular and also on some of the other choices that are the hallmark of mature family planning services. And, as always, it is those who are most disadvantaged socially who suffer from society's inability to approach the subject of fertility-limitation with the objectivity it applies to other aspects of health and preventive medicine.

THE CONTEMPORARY PICTURE

BRITAIN

The number of births occurring in England and Wales has declined in comparison to the previous year every year since 1964. Following the passage of the Abortion Act the number of legal abortions increased year by year, the largest increase occurring in 1969/70. However, then the yearly increment began to fall and in 1972–3 and 1973–4 both the number of births in the country and the number of legal abortions declined (*see* Fig. 60). The age of marriage was roughly constant at this time and therefore these statistics demonstrate that the use of contraception and of sterilisation improved, allowing a more rigorous control of conception and some replacement of abortion by contraceptive practice.

In 1974, the National Health Service finally accepted responsibility for providing contraception and took over the majority of services previously run by the non-governmental Family Planning Association. The single most important consequence of this change

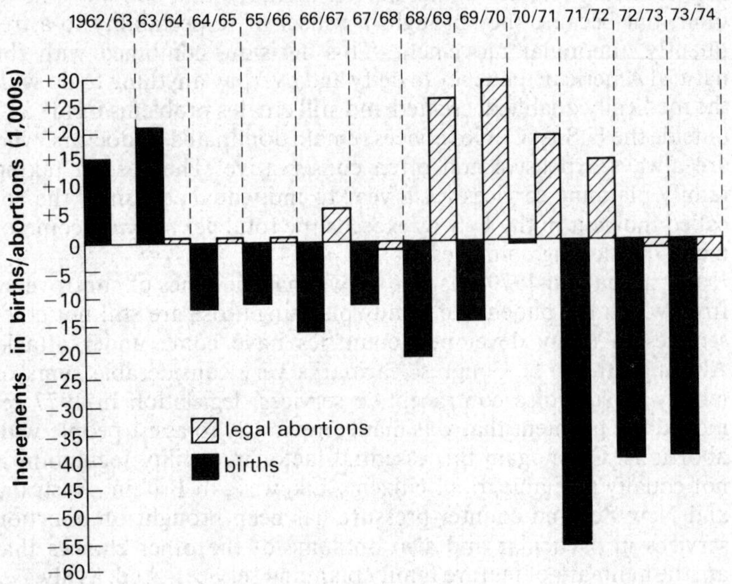

(*Source:* Potts, M., Diggory, P. and Peel, J. *Abortion*. Cambridge 1977)

Fig. 60. *Annual increments in legal abortions (England and Wales residents only) compared with changes in total number of births.*

was that general practitioners, who had been playing an increasingly important part in family planning, were now formally involved.

However, family planning could not shake off its controversial history. In all routine medical care general practitioners are remunerated by the size of their "list" of patients and only receive "item-of-service" payments for obstetric care and a few trivial items. However, it was felt necessary to pay an item-of-service fee in relation to family planning; £3.50 was given for writing oral contraceptive prescriptions and £10 for the insertion of I.U.D.s. It is impossible to say if this service would have worked equally well without incentives, but following their introduction, well over 90 per cent of general practitioners became involved in family planning. There was still a backlog of general practitioners who were not adequately trained in family planning, but on the whole, doctors in Britain have now woven the clinical aspects of family planning into their day to day work.

In 1975, following negotiations between the British Medical Association and the Department of Health and Social Security, a series of item-of-service payments were negotiated for hospital staff in relation to family planning. Again, the British tradition was to pay consultants a set rate and item-of-service payments had no precedent in the National Health Service. But having set out on the slippery slope in relation to general practitioners, the administrators were trapped and forced into accepting a "menu of payments" (a vasectomy £16.25, £8 additional fee if a general anaesthetic is given; tubal ligation £22; reversing a vasectomy £25). Predictably, no monetary award was offered for abortion, although this was the one aspect of family planning which is treated with great unevenness between different regions of Britain.

These administrative decisions are only explicable in the light of the controversial history of family planning. Within two or three years they have proved to be philosophically and tactically disruptive, and at times of economic stringency the National Health Service has been unable to meet the cost of the consultant's contribution to family planning. A number of local steps were taken: in some areas the payments ceased and, not surprisingly, surgeons stopped offering sterilisation; in other areas, family planning clinics were closed down to get money for sterilisation and in further areas numerical limits were set on sterilisation.

In the long run, these set-backs will probably sort themselves out. Currently, in the United Kingdom, a woman can obtain oral contraceptives free of charge from her general practitioner. G.P.s are not obliged to inform the parents of an unmarried girl and can use their judgment in relation to girls under the age of sixteen. The Pill is now the single most common method. I.U.D.s are freely available but still not a popular method in the country. The government has recently ruled that the doctor is not obliged to get the husband's signature before inserting a device. In many areas, female sterilisation is readily available, but there is still unevenness in service. Waiting lists for vasectomy can be long and charitable clinics offering sterilisation still play a useful role in the national availability of services. Abortion remains the most controversial and irregular service and it is a matter of circumstance whether a woman can obtain a free termination on the National Health Service, or must pay £70 for an operation through the charitable pregnancy advisory services or higher fees still for a private operation.

Theoretically, condoms and spermicides are available free of charge, but no way has been found of bringing these methods into the general run of the National Health Service. In 1976 barriers were still being placed in front of the London Rubber Industries Ltd, if it attempted to advertise its contraceptives both on street hoardings and on television. It succeeded, against tiresome opposition, in the first goal, but commercial television in Britain is still forbidden to take advertisements from undertakers, astrologers or contraceptive manufacturers. When a racing car with the brand name "Durex" painted on its body appeared on the circuits it required some dizzy work by television cameramen to keep it off viewers' screens! However, subsequently, in 1977 the same car appeared in street posters with the slogan, "Small family car".

Female sterilisation has had a long history in Britain and Sir Dugald Baird has described how he first offered tubal ligation after delivery to women between thirty-five and forty with eight or more children during the 1930s. Over the years the criteria have slowly been relaxed and most surgeons have recognised that arbitrary rules of age and parity are not useful when making decisions concerning sterilisation. However a shadow of former attitudes emerged, when ministerial guidelines distinguished between men under and over thirty in relation to vasectomy.

In Britain there is no statute law controlling sterilisation but until the 1960s vasectomy was felt by many surgeons to be in an ambiguous situation. However, following the pioneer work of the Simon Population Trust, the operation was popularised, largely through surgeons at the Marie Stopes Clinic, and a significant number of general practitioners were trained to do the operation during the 1970s. Again, part of the problem facing those engaged in family planning came from within the family planners themselves and the Family Planning Association leant very heavily towards limiting vasectomy to specialist surgeons. Fortunately, the Marie Stopes Clinic resisted this trend and together with the Kingston Contraceptive Clinic and some other non-governmental agencies offers an efficient self-sufficient outpatient vasectomy service (£35) in competition to free N.H.S. operation, where waiting lists in many areas exceed twelve months.

JAPAN

Japan is a country of paradoxes. It is illegal to prescribe the Pill for contraception, but abortion is readily available; it has the highest use of the rhythm method in the world, but no significant number of Roman Catholics in the population; three-quarters of all family planning users adopt the condom and yet male sterilisation is unknown; the I.U.D., which was partly a Japanese invention was only made legal in 1974. Japan has attained a net reproduction rate of unity since the mid-1950s (that is, the average family contains two children) and yet the population continues to grow by more than a million a year.

When Japan ended the Second World War, her crude birth rate stood at nearly 35 per 1,000. The nation's economy was shattered and a million men came back in defeated armies from an empire which, a few years earlier, had stretched into China and down to Indonesia. By 1954 the birth rate was 20; 10 years later it stood at 17.7 per 1,000 and the mean family size had fallen from nearly four children to only two.

The decline in fertility was one of the most rapid in the world. It left, and still leaves, a population with a large load of relatively young people, which explains the statistical paradox that, although the average family is just replacing itself, the population of the country is still growing. Just as world population will go on growing well into the twenty-first century, whatever happens to birth rates, so the population of Japan will grow from the present 115 million to 135 million in the year 2000 and 145 million in the year 2050.

Contraceptive practice in Japan has been followed in a number of regular surveys, mainly by the Mainichi newspapers, and has climbed from 20 per cent in 1950 to 60 per cent currently using some form of contraception in 1975. The same socio-economic pressures, the same urban/rural differentials and the same effects of education and income apply in Japan as they do in Britain or the U.S.A. However, the range of methods used is different. In 1969, 68.1 per cent of all contraceptive users had adopted the condom; the method became even more popular so that by 1975 a remarkable 77.8 per cent of all users were condom users. This is the highest single use of one method in any country and exceeds the popularity of the Pill in Europe and the U.S.A.

The positive reasons for the success of the condom has been an aggressive, imaginative and comprehensive marketing, where the Japanese Family Planning Association (J.F.P.A.) has made an outstanding contribution. J.F.P.A. was founded in 1954. It saw the need for fertility regulation, was aware that it had to be largely self-sufficient and saw the need to enter the community, rather than wait for people to come to its services. It created mobile teams which sold condoms on a door-to-door basis. Their success stimulated other door-to-door sales systems and, today, a number of manufacturers field up to 2 or 3 thousand part-time saleswomen who visit homes (at a time carefully chosen so that the husband is usually at work) to sell condoms. The saleswomen have a month's basic training, are expected to visit thirty houses a day (8.45 a.m–6 p.m.), and make a sale in at least five. They only get a commission. Of course, a great many men buy condoms directly, often from the pharmacy and cosmetic stores, which remain the main condom outlets and account for 60 per cent of the total trade.

The packaging of the Japanese condom is imaginative, sophisticated and designed to appeal to a highly diverse and segmented market. In the case of condoms sold to women, the packages simulate non-contraceptive domestic items, such as boxes of sweets, boxes of biscuits or cigarette cartons. This sales technique presumably avoids embarrassment at the point of purchase—although it may lead to confusion if a child thinks it is raiding its mother's larder!

J.F.P.A. made constructive use of local midwives, who were becoming increasingly unemployed because of the declining birth rate, but who proved to be appropriate condom sales ladies.

The practical approach of J.F.P.A. and its striving for self-sufficiency is probably the reason why the related organisation, Japanese Organisation for International Co-operation in Family Planning, is emerging as a unique donor agency for the Third World, pressing both a self-sufficient and a humanistic approach to family planning and linking such things as the provision of contraceptives to parasite control.

Use of the rhythm method in Japan exceeds the use of this method in any Catholic country and seems to fill the slot in contraceptive practice that coitus interruptus does in the Western world. The popularity of the method partly stems from the fact that it was a Japanese, Ogino, who in 1928 gave one of the first accurate descriptions of the time of ovulation. But the paradox is deepened by the fact that Ogino only recommended it as a fertility-promoting technique. A combination of the rhythm method and abortion can be a very satisfactory one and is simple, cheap and predictable in its results.

As noted earlier (*see* p. 129) Ota developed an effective intrauterine device as early as 1929, although it only became legal in Japan in 1974. Oral contraceptives are available for the treatment of irregular periods and used by a few per cent of women. Sterilisation is restricted to the mentally defective (the one group most British doctors would avoid operating on). For the rest it is available—if you pay enough: £120 for vasectomy and £200 for female sterilisation—only about 30,000 cases are performed a year.

The Japanese experience in abortion is often commented upon but rarely well understood. The reform of the abortion law was a response to the epidemic of illegal abortions then occurring and was not seen as an instrument of population control. It is certainly true that Japan reformed its laws at an earlier state in the demographic transition than any Western country. The legal abortions that have been performed in Japan almost certainly reflect a general pattern of induced abortion which, although difficult to document accurately where illegal, probably occurred in most or all Western nations at an earlier stage.

The number of registered abortions reached a peak of well over a million in the mid-1950s (1957: 1,122,000 abortions) and has declined every year since then (1974: 680,000 abortions). Over 95 per cent of abortions are now performed within the first three months of pregnancy and the death rate is low. Abortions are rare in hospitals and nearly all of them are performed in small clinics, by surgeons specially licensed for this procedure and charging about £60. The important fact about the Japanese experience is that the use of contraception has improved against a background of freely-available, early abortion. Muramatsu has estimated the relative roles of contraception and abortion in fertility control in Japan since the War: the ratio of births averted by contraception and abortion was 100:250 in 1955, yet fell to 100:100 by 1965.

Family planning in Japan has been marked by extreme self-sufficiency at the individual level and although between 1950 and 1968 the governmental contribution of the Ministry of Health and Welfare rose from 4 to 8 million yen this still only represented 0.5 cents (U.S.) *per capita*.

U.S.A.

The U.S.A. entered the period after the Second World War with a nationwide system of clinics run by Planned Parenthood, and offering predominantly female methods in a situation broadly similar to that in the United Kingdom. In 1970, the House of Representatives voted the first substantial moneys for family planning, making $382 million available for fiscal years 1971–3. The prime purpose of the legislation being "to assist in making comprehensive voluntary family planning services readily available to all persons desiring such services".

As the U.S.A. does not have a system of state medicine comparable to that in Britain, a substantial part of this governmental money is channelled through Planned Parenthood and other non-profit-making organisations.

During the 1960s oral contraceptives came to play a significant role in family planning in the U.S.A., as in most developed countries, although the response of the media to fears over oral contraceptives, injectables and I.U.D.s have been more extreme in the U.S.A. than in Britain. As already pointed out, the Food and Drug Administration (F.D.A.) has proved as much a political as a scientific body and, although its clinical and biological advisors have been of the highest order, its final decisions have been irregular or, as in the case of the injectable hormonal contraceptive Depo Provera, counter-productive. Sterilisation has proved even more popular than in the United Kingdom and the widespread use of vasectomy is several years in advance of Britain (*see* Fig. 61). In many parts of the States sterilisation is now the single most common method of fertility regulation and on the West Coast vasectomy vies with tubal ligation as the popular method.

The acceptance of abortion came later in the U.S.A. but was more dramatic. Whereas in Britain a significant number of abortions were performed following the Bourne case precedent of 1938, in the U.S.A. therapeutic abortion was at the rate of about 2 cases per 1,000 deliveries in hospital practice in the 1960s.

In the middle of 1971, rather to the surprise of all the principal actors involved, the New York State legislature repealed a restrictive law that had been in force since the early part of the nineteenth century. A number of states had passed reform legislation prior to the events in New York; Hawaii had repealed its law in February 1970, but limited its application to residents of the state. In the case of New York, abortion suddenly became available without limit—and even those sympathetic to abortion waited apprehensively to see how the law would be implemented. Remarkably, a group of free-standing clinics arose very rapidly, vacuum aspiration was almost universally used for first-trimester abortions, women travelled to New York from every state in the union as well as from outside the country. Prices were often in the range of $100 for out-patient procedures. One service performed over 100 operations a day from the middle of 1971 and completed its first 21,000 procedures without a known maternal death. Follow-up showed that on a series of more than 300,000 cases performed before the twelfth week of pregnancy the death rate was 1.9 per 100,000. The mortality after the 13th week was 17.4 per 100,000. Within New York State abortion became the great remover of previous social injustices. Prior to the change in the law the fertility rate for black residents was 2.85 as compared with 2.15 for whites. In the course of just eighteen months the total fertility rate for blacks fell to 2.1 and that of whites declined more modestly to 1.84. Yet abortion was not the only factor; analysis by Tietze of the birth and abortion statistics for New York State showed, beyond reasonable doubt, both that contraceptive practice improved in the year immediately following the repeal of the abortion law and that the overwhelming majority of the legal abortions replaced illegal operations. Indeed, nine-tenths of the effect of changing the New York Law appears to have been in transferring previ-

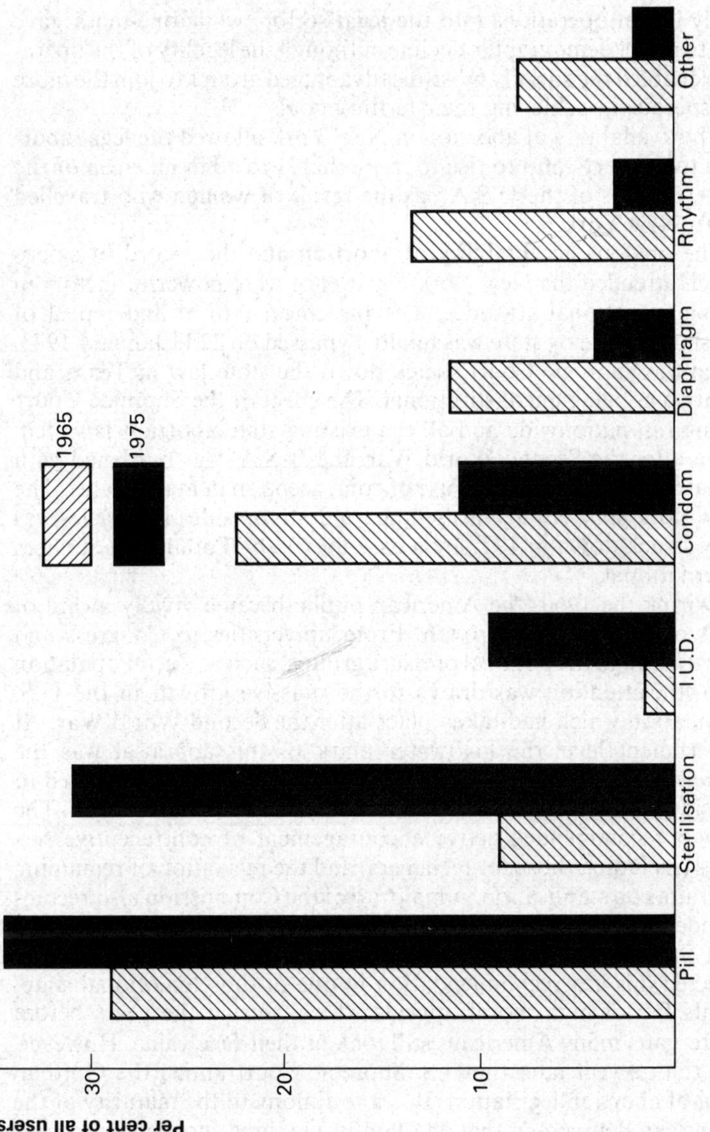

Fig. 61. *Modernisation of U.S. contraceptive practice.*
(*Source*: Population Reference Bureau 1977)

ously illegal operations into the legal sector; while one-tenth gave rise to direct demographic decline, although the legality of the operation enabled the socially most-disadvantaged groups to join the more prosperous in achieving their fertility goals.

The availability of abortion in New York allowed the legal abortion to delivery ratio to rise to more than 1 to 10 in nineteen of the eastern states of the U.S.A., as the result of women who travelled up to New York.

The obvious acceptability of abortion and the record of safety which attended the New York experience were powerful factors in changing national attitudes. The piecemeal reform and repeal of legislation state by state was finally bypassed on 22nd January 1973, when the Supreme Court struck down the state law in Texas and Georgia as being unconstitutional. The effect of the Supreme Court ruling ran nationwide and all the existing state abortion laws fell. Even after the Second World War, the U.S.A. was burdened with statute laws forbidding the use of contraception in many states. The New York State law against selling condoms outside pharmacies was only struck down in 1977 by a case moved by Population Services International.

During the 1960s the American public became vividly aware of their own population growth. From universities to Congress and down through the political pressure groups, such as Zero Population Growth, attention was drawn to the massive growth in the U.S. population which had taken place after the Second World War. At government level the highwater mark of this appraisal was the *Report on Population Growth and the American Future* submitted to President Nixon by John D. Rockefeller's Commission in 1972. The *Report* recommended active encouragement of contraceptive services (including those for teenagers) and the relaxation of remaining restraints on sterilisation. A majority of the Commission also recommended that "women should be free to control their fertility" and that State laws prohibiting abortion should be liberalised. Nixon rejected this last recommendation in one of those emotional statements full of high moral appeals which, during the years before Watergate, many Americans still took at their face value. However, less than a year later the U.S. Supreme Court untied the Gordian knot of abortion legislation. It is a testimony to the maturity of the American democracy that the family planning movement became so articulate, was listened to and in a remarkably short space of time saw its goals achieved.

The issue of the later 1970s is whether the goals will be reversed as a result of the political attack initiated by the "Right to Life" movement.

THE LAST STAND?

There are still some countries in the developed world where there continue to be major restrictions on access to all types of fertility control. Here family planning workers find themselves fighting battles not dissimilar to those described above for nineteenth century Britain.

In Spain, the penal code drawn up under Franco banned the dissemination, public display or offer for sale of anything intended to avert pregnancy. Despite this, the practice of birth-control has spread in recent years and by 1977 it was estimated that about a million women were "on the Pill", the majority being upper and middle class and living in the urban centres. Doctors are permitted to prescribe the Pill for "menstrual irregularities". As the country moves towards democracy following the death of Franco, the law is being changed, but abortion remains illegal and a growing number of Spanish women are travelling to England each year to seek a safe termination of pregnancy; and despite the change of regime the editor of the Madrid daily *El Pais* was recently put on trial for reprinting a *Sunday Times* article on contraception.

The outstanding example of continued official opposition to birth-control is Southern Ireland, where in 1978 abortion was still illegal and access to contraception surrounded by many restrictions. The 1935 Criminal Law Amendment Act, which remains in operation makes it an offence for any person to "sell, expose, offer, advertise or keep for sale, or to import into Saorstat Eireann for sale, any contraceptive".

Despite this, there has been a growing interest in contraception in Ireland, especially over the last fifteen years, and there has been growing pressure to reform the law. In 1969, with hopes of liberalisation dashed by the publication a year earlier of the papal encyclical *Humanae Vitae* (which prohibited the use of the Pill), a small group of doctors set up the first Irish family planning clinic. Located in Merrion Square in Dublin, and called the "Fertility Guidance Clinic", it avoided conflict with the law by not selling contraceptives, but offering them free of charge. The Pill was prescribed and sold, technically for regulating the menstrual cycle. A second clinic was opened two years later in a working class area in Dublin. Meanwhile, in October 1970, the Irish Family Planning Rights Association was formed to work for changes in the law and shortly afterwards a non-profit-making company, Family Planning Services Ltd., was formed to supply condoms, caps and chemicals free of charge by post, the "customers" then being invited to make a donation to the work of the company.

An important challenge to the law came in 1972, when a Mrs McGhee, a young married woman with a heart condition, brought an action in the High Court, claiming that the confiscation of a supply of spermicidal cream by customs officers, operating under the 1935 Act, was an infringement of her constitutional rights. She lost the judgment, but the case provided much publicity for the family planning movement and a year later the Supreme Court ruled in her favour, declaring that the ban on the importation of contraceptives was unconstitutional.

Attempts by private members to change the law in Parliament had been less successful and in 1974 a Government Bill was introduced which recognised the legality of importing contraceptives but sought to restrict this to licensed persons, and to make it an offence for the unmarried to purchase them. This conservative Bill outraged many reformers, but it was even more bitterly opposed by those who saw it as too liberal. The Bill was defeated, following what the *Irish Times* called a "prolonged and profoundly embarrassing debate", which ended with the Prime Minister, Mr. Cosgrave, voting against his own Bill. Thereafter nothing was done until the beginning of 1978, when the new government was preparing a Bill which would legalise contraceptives and remove the anomaly that allows anyone to import them, but bans their sale. The Bill is expected to put strict controls on the sale, possibly confining them to prescriptions or distribution by local health authorities. With some sort of liberalisation certain, the Catholic Church in Ireland has been extrolling the merits of "natural methods of contraception", especially the "Billings" method which determines the woman's fertile period, and clinics are being established to offer advice on such methods.

Those involved in the family planning movement in Ireland have many fascinating, and often amusing, stories to tell of their struggle over the past decade, not least in relation to the smuggling in of contraceptives when their importation for sale was banned. A worker with a boot-load of condoms was stopped in his car by the British army who thought he was carrying explosives or guns, and then by the Irish police, who were told he carried them for his own personal use; a woman with a case full of diaphragms successfully declared them as jam-pot covers. As recently as September 1978, at a time when Ireland's Minister of Health Charles Haughey was committed to introducing a Bill to legalise the sale of contraceptives, Family Planning Distributors Ltd. (the main suppliers of all contraceptives except the Pill) was faced with a major crisis following the seizure by Irish customs at Dundalk and Dublin of £5,000-worth of "contraceptive contraband", on the grounds that it was intended for illegal resale.

The demographic pattern of post-war Eire shows a marked contrast with the rest of Europe, with birth rates remaining consistently above 20 per 1,000 and none of the fluctuations that have marked the last thirty years in Britain and West Germany. In part this is due to a continued preference for large families and the low level of contraceptive use, but the situation is complicated because any tendency for fertility to decline as more women use birth-control has been countered by a fall in age at marriage, an increase in the number of marriages, and a substantial rise in the number of women in their twenties, as the rate of emigration from the Republic has slackened.

CONCLUSION

The American, British and Japanese experience with family planning and population growth since the Second World War lends support to a generalisation which probably applies to all industrialised nations, namely that where population size continued to increase, a substantial part of the growth was due to births resulting from unplanned pregnancies. As adequate means of fertility control became available, birth rates fell towards replacement level, leading in some cases to zero population growth. It has been the pace and form of family planning services which have lagged behind public need.

The establishment of realistic family planning services proved an uphill task in developed countries and even today has not yet come to a reasonable resting place.

The U.S.A. has perhaps made some of the greatest strides; legal abortion, access to contraception and elective sterilisation are available to all its citizens, both married and unmarried. The integration of family planning services in the N.H.S. in Britain is uneven, but better than previously. But in the family planning movement, the child that developed in the nineteenth and early twentieth century is still father of the mature services found today in the U.S.A., Britain and most other developed countries. Managers and decision-makers in the U.S.A. have been able to bring abortion services into the mainstream of family planning more effectively than in Britain but, by contrast, have been unable to move as far as Britain in the non-clinical approach to contraception. In Britain, medical leadership has been able at least to recommend non-physician distribution of oral contraceptives, while in the U.S.A. even such expert recommendation is unthinkable.

In continental Europe, the French abortion law was altered in January 1975. Like many late starters in family planning services, the French moved rapidly and in many ways overtook the situation in Britain. The French law permits abortion on request during the first ten weeks after conception and oral contraceptives are routinely available through the government health services. In Austria, which is 90 per cent Catholic, the abortion law was repealed in 1974 and similar changes took place in the German parliament, although the implementation of the law was blocked in the Constitutional Court. It will be interesting to see what happens in Spain which rescinded anti-contraceptive laws late in 1977.

Scandinavia, which has a reputation for liberal sexual attitudes, began a piecemeal reform of abortion laws before the Second World War, commencing with the remarkably far-sighted legislation in Iceland in 1934. By the late 1960s and early 1970s Norway, Sweden, Denmark and Finland had passed abortion-on-request legislation. Oral contraceptives were readily available and, in Sweden in particular, condoms are promoted in aggressive and amusing ways. However, Scandinavia has long been ambivalent towards sterilisation. While during the 1950s and early 1960s women seeking abortions (if they could afford it) would fly from London to Stockholm to get an operation, in the early 1970s, Swedish men (if they could afford it) flew from Stockholm to London to obtain a vasectomy, which was then illegal except for the mentally abnormal—the one group that Britain with its more liberal traditions of sterilisation has learnt to avoid operating on.

Paradoxes of this type are characteristic of family planning. In Eastern Europe, where most countries have had easily available abortion since the 1950s, sterilisation is almost totally unknown. It is not uncommon that a busy hospital may do 4,000 abortions a year, deliver 2,000 babies, yet do only two or three sterilisations. They are always on women and always for serious medical conditions. Whereas a conservative gynaecologist in Britain would be reluctant to perform an abortion, claiming that women regret the operation afterwards and ascribing to it a higher degree of physical risk than objective data suggests, he might perform sterilisation in an almost punitive way; so in Eastern Europe, a gynaecologist may find himself providing ready abortion services without many second thoughts and yet would be seriously challenged by the possibility of a sterilisation, again asserting that women regret the operation later and sometimes perceiving it as a physically dangerous procedure.

To continue the paradox, in Japan oral contraceptives are illegal (although used by a measurable number of women for "menstrual irregularities") and sterilisation is almost never performed, although abortion has been freely available since 1949.

An "Alice in Wonderland" attitude towards fertility regulation in developed countries is apparent at a world level. While every known method of fertility control is available and promoted in at least some countries, nearly every country has one or more arbitrary restricitions on methods which others use freely.

In Eire, although contraception and, needless to say, abortion are illegal, there is no statute law against sterilisation. Tubal ligation *de facto* is not available because institutions with operating theatres are dominated by groups opposed to family planning. However, there is nothing to stop courageous doctors offering male sterilisation in their surgeries and this has been done. So in a country where a man is not allowed to buy a contraceptive, or his wife to have an I.U.D. inserted, he can obtain a vasectomy.

Whatever the limitations of voluntary family planning organisations, in the paradoxical and confused world of fertility regulation, non-governmental effort has invariably been the pace-setter. In some developed countries, for example Britain, charitable family planning services became perhaps the largest non-governmental social service in the country. Even the control of venereal disease was absorbed into government services at a relatively early stage, but the aurora of controversy surrounding family planning made its absorption impossible.

A developed community can solve its fertility problems on a self-sufficient basis, without large subsidy from the government, if there is adequate commercial distribution in reversible methods and access to early fee paying abortion. At a time when the U.K. and U.S.A. are spending increased sums on family planning, the fact that the Japanese government only spends a few cents *per capita* on family planning is worth digesting.

In developing countries a similar evolution of voluntary action leading to eventual government intervention is now taking place.

SELECTED REFERENCES AND BIBLIOGRAPHY

Allbutt, H. A. *The Wife's Handbook*. London 1886

Banks, J. A. *Prosperity and Parenthood*. Routledge & Kegan Paul, London 1954

Besant, A. *The Law of Population*. Freethought Publishing Co., London 1877

Dickinson, R. L. and Bryant, L. S. *Control of Conception: An Illustrated Medical Manual*. Tindall & Cox, London 1938

Diggory, P. and McEwan, J. *Planning or Prevention?* Marion Boyars, London 1976

Hall, R. *Marie Stopes*. Andre Deutsch, London 1977

Institute of Medicine. *Legalised Abortion and the Public Health.* National Academy of Sciences, Washington, D.C. 1975

Knowlton, C. *The Fruits of Philosophy*. London 1841

Owen, R. D. *Moral Physiology*. New York 1831

Peel, J. and Potts, M. "The Sociology of Population Control." *Social Science & Medicine*. 7, 179 1973

Place, F. *Illustrations and Proofs of the Principle of Population*. London 1822

Report of the Joint Working Group on Oral Contraceptives. H.M.S.O., London 1976

Smith, M. and Kane, P. *The Pill off Prescription*. Birth Control Trust, London 1975

Westoff, C. F. "The Modernisation of U.S. Contraceptive Practice." *Family Planning Perspectives*. 4, 9 1972

Wilson-Davis, K. "The Contraceptive Situation in the Irish Republic." *Journal of Biosocial Science*. 6, 483 1974

Wood, C. and Suitters, B. *The Fight for Acceptance*. Medical & Technical Publishing Co. Ltd., Aylesbury 1970

Chapter 12

Developing Countries

Developing nations have moved from public apathy or antagonism towards family planning to government policies and national programmes in less than twenty years. Until 1956 the Thai Government offered bonuses for large families; the Prime Minister said he wanted 100 million people and the Ministry of Health had a Wedding Promotion Committee. Today Thailand has a population policy; the government spent $2.9 million on family planning in 1976, the Prime Minister frequently endorses the need for small families and the population, now at 43 million, is growing more slowly than previously. These changes, which have their parallel throughout Asia, parts of Africa and in an increasing number of Latin American countries, have occurred at a relatively earlier stage in the demographic transition than did the evolution of public approval and assistance to fertility regulation in the West.

To some extent, Asia had its population explosion thrust upon it: death rates in traditional societies fell precipitously after the Second World War in a way that few would have predicted. Malaria eradication, vaccination programmes, the sale of antibiotics and modest advances in transport and sanitary arrangements all contributed to this. Latin America, however, acquired its demographic problems partly by a wilful act of community self-mutilation. By the 1950s, most Latin American countries were partly urbanised and held the seeds of a modern industrialised economy, yet due to the political power of the Church the possibility that might have existed for effective family planning policies was thrown to the winds. While *Humanae Vitae* made no difference to the behaviour of individuals in their homes and abortions continued to rise among the middle classes, it denied desperately needed services to the poor.

Africa still has the opportunity to decide what type of community response it will make to demographic change and the signs are that it will do better than Latin America.

To the degree to which the post-war population explosion was foreseeable, Christendom has a particular guilt, because as colonial rulers it prohibited, rather than assisted, family planning and more recently some "Western experts" have not given the most rational or useful advice.

SUCCESSFUL PROGRAMMES

In a difficult and often disappointing subject perhaps it is useful to begin with some successes. Fertility can and will fall in advance of socio-economic development. Family planning programmes can alter trends in fertility, gain time and cut total numbers.

INDONESIA

Indonesia has come a long way in a short time. In 1968 the government spent $75,000 on family planning and in 1976 $15 million. Although access to the means to control fertility is still uneven, there have been some spectacular successes.

The island of Bali has 2.3 million people who are nearly all Hindus. As a minority surrounded by nearly 140 million Indonesian Muslims, Bali might be expected to be resistant to family planning. Yet between 1970 and 1976 the birth rate fell from over 40 to 27 per 1,000. In 1970 modern methods of birth-control were virtually unknown; by 1976, 53 per cent of married women in the fertile age-groups, and not currently pregnant, used some form of contraception; two-thirds of this number adopted I.U.D.s, one in five the Pill and the remainder condoms. Sterilisation is becoming increasingly common. The government programme has been particularly well developed under the leadership of Dr. I. B. Astawa.

In the islands of Java and Bali where the majority of Indonesia's population lives, it is thought that 25 per 1,000 eligible couples use contraceptives. In the outer islands, such as Sumatra and Sulawesi (Celebes), the figure falls to 7.6. It is estimated that at least 50 per cent of women who begin the Pill, 84 per cent of those would have an I.U.D. inserted and 42 per cent of those who adopt condoms continue with their respective methods for at least one year.

THAILAND

Thailand is a predominantly Buddhist country, although there are some Muslim areas in the south. The literacy rate and income are higher than in Indonesia. In recent years, one-third more couples have adopted family planning than the managers of services expected. In 1977, just under half a million women began taking oral contraceptives for the first time, over 100,000 had a tubal ligation, 15,000 men were vasectomised, 58,000 women adopted injectable contraceptives (Depo Provera), 67,000 used the condom and 75,000 had I.U.D.s inserted. Over one-third of eligible couples now use family planning and the total fertility rate has fallen from 6.25 in 1967–9 to 4.85 in 1970–4.

In some areas where family planning has been particularly intense the decline has been even more rapid. In 1974 Community Based Family Planning Services began to organise one distributor for every 500–1,000 people in the villages. The person selected had one day's training and he or she is visited once a month by a full-time supervisor who travels on a motorbike, or in a boat. The village distributor has no salary but keeps five U.S. cents from every cycle of oral contraceptives which they sell for 20 U.S. cents. The programme is under the imaginative and forceful leadership of Mechai Viravaidya who, among many other achievements, made the condom not only an acceptable contraceptive, but a symbol of family planning and of the fact that sex and humour should never be too far apart. Today the programme covers about 5 million people and has recruited 176,000 Pill users. Couples switch methods or drop out altogether, but the important end-point is that, in districts where the programme has been established for three years or more, the number of pregnant women in the community has fallen by 40 per cent. In other areas it has declined by 20 per cent, showing that family planning programmes are particularly successful at accelerating existing trends.

In the two northern provinces of Thailand, another older programme has met with equally measurable success. In Chaing Mai and the neighbouring province the average family size has fallen from 6.5 to 2.8 children over the past twenty years. The alteration is partly attributable to a realistic family planning programme centred on a single hospital and initially driven forward under the leadership of an American protestant missionary born in Thailand, Dr. Edwin McDaniel.

CHINA

Changes which have affected a few million of people in isolated areas of Asia seem to have extended to hundreds of millions in the Peoples' Republic of China. At first sight the Chinese programme appears unique, but on closer examination does not turn out to be as unusual as is sometimes believed.

First and foremost, the Chinese effort involves a realistic availability of all possible methods of family planning. The breadth of choice is unusual for a large developing country, though every item has been made available in one or more or the family planning programmes of other Third World countries. In addition women are discouraged from getting married before the age of twenty-five in the towns and twenty-three in rural areas.

Condoms and oral contraceptives are available at the household level and involve the barefoot doctor. China is the only developing country to manufacture oral contraceptives from the plant raw materials. Ingeniously, they have invented the so-called "paper pill". Instead of using a tablet formulation, which is rather like making currant buns and requires sophisticated equipment to get the right degree of mixing, the process involves dipping an edible paper sheet through an alcoholic solution of steroids, more reminiscent of mixing a cocktail.

Abortion is available and widely used. The vacuum aspiration technique of abortion originated in China. Male and female sterilisation are available.

Nationwide statistical data is not available, but detailed information has been produced in some localities. For example, the population growth rate in some of the more densely populated areas of the country is down to 1 per cent.

The Chinese do not call their activities family planning but "birth planning". In some areas "group planning" has evolved. This is a unique system, almost as fascinating for the reactions it arouses in Western observers, as for its intrinsic interest. Briefly, the larger units of Chinese administration, such as the municipality, determine the optimum birth rate for a locality. This is then translated at the commune level to the actual number of births possible. All the fertile couples in a production brigade sit together and select who will have children over the next year or more. There may even be a chart displayed in a public place, setting the target number of pregnancies.

To the Western mind, this system appears illiberal, threatening and incomprehensible: but group-planning of births is worth study. It assumes that couples have total control over their fertility—which indeed they do in any country where early abortion is available. It demonstrates that human beings can plan children with regard to community needs as well as family needs, in the same way that they plan to use their resources to irrigate a field or build a temple. It demonstrates a strong desire for human beings to conform in reproduction, as in much else. There is no coercion, in the sense that a woman who gets pregnant accidentally is not forced to seek an abortion, but there are strong social pressures. Stranger, less rational and perhaps even less desirable patterns of social conformity are found in other cultures: millions of healthy young men have lost their lives in brutal wars—is it odd for millions of young Chinese women, whose parents knew the reality of starvation, to volunteer not to have babies? In the war against fertility, as in other battles, altruism is possible. In one commune a group-plan for birth was drawn up before it was realised that, because one husband worked in another province, his wife might have to wait four years to conceive a child—

this was felt to be too long and another woman passed on her "chance" of a pregnancy to the wife concerned.

It is easy for the Westerner to forget that our own society has its own particular variety of group-planning. Most Western societies and all developing societies apply the strongest possible social pressures to restrict fertility outside marriage. The fact that illegitimacy is condemned in so many societies is so obvious that we hardly pause to think about it, but the sociology of the mechanisms which control it are, perhaps, not fundamentally different from those used to limit fertility within marriage in China.

As in many other developing countries, the Chinese have a strong preference for male children. In the commune system, cash payment is made according to work points, and boys work and earn points at the adult level from the age of sixteen. When sons marry, their wives bring additional points to their family. In an attempt to modify, but not overthrow, the old patterns of family structure, the government is encouraging men who marry girls who are the only child of the family, to join the family of their mother-in-law.

Nearly all decision-making is decentralised. At a managerial level it is notable that the programme has been implemented without the type of obsessive, time-consuming and frequently corrupted record-keeping which has been a feature of national programmes elsewhere in Third World countries.

OTHER EXAMPLES

Encouraged by a small but vigorous band of volunteers in the Planned Parenthood Federation of Korea and certain universities, the Government of Korea embarked on a national family planning programme in 1962. Intra-uterine devices were introduced in 1964 and their use pressed with remarkable vigour. Between 1964 and 1969 55 per cent of women in the 35–39 age-group had an I.U.D. inserted at some time. Unfortunately, I.U.D.s did not perform as well at a national level as when they had been used in well-controlled clinical trials. The harsh lesson was learnt (as in many other countries) that this method, which was initially seen as one that required a minimum of manpower, in fact responded closely to the degree of follow-up. Not only did discontinuation rates rise from 36 per cent at the end of twenty-four months in the clinical trial situation to over 50 per cent at a nationwide level, but discontinuation rates rose year by year, as devices were offered to less and less suitable clients and as rumours about adverse effects spread. With experience, it became apparent that I.U.D. insertions and expulsions eventually reached an equilibrium, like a mass reaction in chemistry.

However, the programme learnt from its failures and in 1968 oral contraceptives were added. More recently, improvements have been made in the availability of condoms, and sterilisation of both men and women is proving increasingly popular. Other developments have also helped. Between 1963 and 1969 over four million Pill cycles were sold commercially and oral contraceptives had been widely advertised in the Press, on the television and even on signs hung from lamp posts, which proclaimed "the eatable contraceptive" and gave a brand name. The mean age of marriage for women arose from 20.5 in 1955 to 23 in 1968 as a result of universal military service. The population growth rate in Korea fell from 3 per cent a year in 1961 to 1.7 per cent in 1977.

In Latin America, where public policies on family planning still lag behind private needs, results have been almost as remarkable as some from Asia. Between 1960 and 1970 the total fertility rate in Colombia fell from 7.0 to 4.2 children per woman and this was in significant measure due to the work done by the non-governmental family planning association PROFAMILIA. Under Dr. Fernando Tomayo and his colleagues the organisation set bold policies. Occasionally it clashed with the government and more frequently with the Church, but it won through because it was meeting existing needs.

FAILURES

INDIA

The scale of India's problems dulls the senses. This one poor nation has more people than the U.S.A., the U.S.S.R. and Japan put together, although its G.N.P. is no more than four times the budget of the municipal authorities of New York City. The single state of Uttar Pradesh has a population of nearly 90 million and is larger than any country in Western Europe. Many vivid illustrations of population growth have been devised: India has an excess of births over deaths of approximately one million every month, or an annual increase in population greater than the total number of people presently living in Australia. It is inescapable that rates of increase of this order of magnitude pose insoluble problems. For one or two—perhaps three or four—decades, it may be possible to feed these growing numbers, although the level of nutrition of the average Indian is already poor. An impossible amount of investment is necessary to house and educate the additional population with any degree of dignity. The necessary improvements in agriculture are likely to drive people from the land rather than create additional jobs.

The problem of employing the additional millions that will be added to the work-force in the remaining years of the twentieth century is staggering. The Taj Mahal took 20,000 men nine years to create. Contemporary India adds to her population a potential work-force that could build two Taj Mahals every twenty-four hours—the human manpower available using traditional methods of building is sufficient to string out Taj Mahals across the subcontinent like electricity pylons! Unfortunately, the growing population of India will not be educated or organised to produce anything as improbable as a row of Taj Mahals, as useful as a row of houses or as productive as a line of tractors. It seems inevitable that the excess population from the countryside will drift into the ever growing urban centres to live in the slums and on the pavements.

The logistic problems of family planning in India are enormous. 80 per cent of the population is divided amongst half a million villages, most of them remote from any satisfactory form of communication and rarely or never visited by medical personnel or any type of professional. Individually, the population problem is difficult to grasp: the religious philosophy held, the way of life and the extended family structure all mean that there is little immediate difference in the problem facing parents whether they have three or six children. Children are god-given and the social structure lays stress on the sexual potency of the man; the unhappy woman is pressurised by all around her, perhaps and most especially by her mother-in-law, to have more children.

Family planning was first promoted in 1951, when the annual addition to the population of India was approximately five million a year. Twenty-one years later it was estimated that a total of 7.4 million births had been averted by all the family planning effort. At that time the population growth was more than double what it had been in 1951. It was estimated that by 1991 26 million births might have been averted by the family planning programme. In other words, the best that could be hoped for from forty years of family planning effort appeared to be the equivalent of two years breathing space in the rate of population addition.

The Indian family planning programme has had more than a reasonable share of mistaken policies. It began in 1952 by trying to propagate the rhythm method, with a budget of £24,000 for what was then 360 million people. By the late 1960s, one-tenth of 1 per cent of the country's G.N.P. was committed to family planning, but services were supposed to be integrated with maternal and child health services which themselves were weak or non-existent, and numerically insignificant inroads were made into the growing numbers of fertile couples. One of the few successes was in the social marketing of condoms (*Nirodh*), but even here the dead hand of the civil service held back the business-like approach needed and the city-based obstetricians lacked the imagination to permit oral contraceptives to be distributed in a similar over-the-counter way.

Desperation over the failure of the programme led the Indian government to seek a more effective solution through wide-scale sterilisation. In the early 1970s mass vasectomy camps were established and in some parts of the country large incentives were offered. The operation was advocated and taken up with an almost religious fervour. More than 2 million male sterilisations were performed in 1972 and over 3 million in 1973. However, by 1974 this approach had been largely discontinued in the face of cuts in funds, doubts about the effectiveness of large scale camps and a growing number of cases of tetanus, some of which resulted in death.

The abortion law was reformed in 1972. Politically, this was a bold step, but in practice the law was hedged about with so many fine print regulations that in the next three years only a quarter of a million operations were carried out, while an estimated four million back-street abortions continued to take place each year.

In April 1976 the programme entered a new coercive phase. Through the incompetence and complacency of those who were supposed to provide services, the millions who for years had suffered lack of choice in controlling their fertility suddenly found themselves coerced into having sterilisations. Mrs. Gandhi urged the twenty-two Chief Ministers of the Union "to take all necessary steps" and Karan Singh (then Minister of Health and Family Planning) urged a "direct assault" on fertility. Monetary incentives were increased and in August 1975, Maharastra became the first of four states to pass a law which would have imposed fines and imprisonment on couples (with three or more children) who refused to be sterilised. This law never received the assent of the Indian President, but in practice compulsory sterilisation came into existence as local administrators, attempting to achieve the "targets" set for them, used police and bully squads to round up men for the operation.

Over 7 million sterilisations were performed during the "Emergency". Some, probably many tens of thousands, involved men sterilised against their will, but abuses were spread unevenly and most operations were undergone willingly. While men were beaten on the head and forced to have a vasectomy in Haryana, in other parts of India services remained inadequate to meet the existing demand. The total family planning programme also clearly remained inadequate, with oral contraceptives still excluded as a result of unrealistic policies set by specialist doctors.

The ultimate effect of the excesses of the emergency was to bring about the downfall of Mrs. Gandhi and to set back the cause of family planning by two decades. In March 1977, the Janata party ended thirty years of Congress Party domination in India, as the electorate rebelled against coercive birth-control. The new government of Moraji Desai quickly put an end to the sterilisation campaign and, although the wider family planning programme has not been dismantled, it has been stalled, numerical achievements are trivial and the country is back to slogans of self-control reminiscent of the 1950s.

The tragedy is not that the electorate rejected the family planning programme, but that most people in India still have not been offered any choice in family planning. Occasionally a badly organised government programme has passed through their village offering a "one-shot" solution—I.U.D.s in the 1960s, vasectomy in the 1970s—but the overwhelming majority of Indians have never been offered a realistic, mature set of options. Yet there are many experiences to suggest that the electorate which had the good sense heartily to reject compulsory birth-control, would have readily accepted genuine choices in fertility regulation, had they ever been offered.

SOME EXCEPTIONS

A few small family planning experiences in India stand out. They transmit a new message about the willingness of people to control their own fertility.

In July, 1971, in Ernakulam (Kerala, South India), vasectomy was made available on a massive scale but in a culturally appropriate way, amounting to almost a mass religious conversion. Through community organisation, large incentives (over $10 for each person being vasectomised plus food, clothes and sometimes additional leave and bonuses from the employer) and with massive publicity (including bands leading columns of men for the operation), 63,000 men came forward for vasectomy within a month. Shortly afterwards in Thanjavur District, another camp was conducted, this time with even greater thoroughness and with particular attention to the follow-up of patients. Within forty days 20,000 men were sterilised.

Pressure was certainly put upon men, but there was none of the justifiably angry reaction which followed forcible sterilisation during the "Emergency." The camps were not followed up for bureaucratic reasons: there is in many countries, and most especially within the Indian Civil Service, an unwillingness to move rapidly which verges on a fear of success.

Howrah is the poor end of Calcutta (see p. 280) and nowhere in the world are the suffocating effects of overpopulation more visible and the lack of education and economic progress more frustrating. In 1968, the Humanity Association under the leadership of Dr. Biral

Mullick offered oral contraceptives in three areas with a total population of 30,000. Out of 5,000 married women aged fifteen to forty-four, living in these underprivileged and problem-filled communities, 2,552 began taking the Pill and 1,700 (66.6 per cent) continued after four years. The slum dwellers and illiterate villagers persisted better than higher class women. They demonstrated that, if your husband is unemployed and you are near starvation, you may not want children—at least not this year. Perhaps if life is drab and routine, taking a Pill each day is more exciting and easier to remember than for a Western woman.

In 1972 the programme was stopped as a result of arbitrary, uninformed decision-making hundreds of miles away in Delhi. Supplies of Pills were forbidden and money cut off. Three years later it was possible to survey the women who had previously belonged to the programme; nearly one-third had managed to scrape together sufficient money to buy Pills from pharmacies at something over $1 a cycle—women in abject poverty were paying up to 10 per cent of their disposable income to buy contraceptives! One-third got by with other methods. Some had abortions. Nine-tenths would still have used the Pill had it been available.

Fortunately, late in 1977, after the catastrophe of the "Emergency", the programme was set up again and once more seems to be giving promising results.

OTHER COUNTRIES

The performance of massive and expensive family planning programmes has been disappointing in many countries. In Egypt, little progress has been made; Pakistan has had many setbacks; after some initial success the performance in Sri Lanka levelled out for many years; fertility in the Philippines remains high despite a national population policy and programme and Latin America has hardly begun to face its problems.

Both the Church and the military dictatorships of South America combined to delay overt family planning activities. On the one hand this created a situation where countries, if they wished, could learn from the mistakes of Asia. Therefore, the contraceptive distribution programmes in Colombia and Brazil which were implemented by non-governmental organisations in the late 1960s and early 1970s were amongst some of the most innovative and successful in the world. On the other hand, the unyielding impatience of demographic change does not tolerate such interruptions. By 1975, only an estimated 8 per cent of Mexican women were using any form of contraception and the average user was thirty years old and already had five to six children. With a broad-based pyramid, the population growth rate may still rise and perhaps approach 4 per cent by 1985. Mexico is likely to contain 150 million people by the year 2000 A.D. and perhaps 30 million will live in Mexico City.

Even in the mid-1970s, projects which are pure fantasy continue to be put forward and sometimes to be implemented. For example, in Guatemala, where only 3 per cent of women are reached by existing family planning programmes, the government has forwarded to the United Nations Fund for Population Activities (U.N.F.P.A.) a $900,000 programme for maternal and child health care and family planning, with a forecast for contraceptive supplies which would allow increased use by no more than an additional 1 per cent of fertile women. In Bolivia, where the political climate is even more difficult, there are only five family planning clinics for 5 million people: the country may well have more presidents in a year than it has contraceptive outlets.

Kenya, like Mexico, has a population growth rate of approximately 3.5 per cent per annum. It has had a government commitment to family planning since 1966, but the goal is only to cut population growth rate to 2.8 per cent by the year 2000. 46 per cent of the population is under the age of sixteen. At first glance, plans look promising and between 1974 and 1978 a $36 million budget has been set aside. However, it is to go to a programme linked to health services in a country where there are 8,000 people to every physician. The goal is to attempt to avert a mere 150,000 births and achieve a theoretical decline in the population growth rate of 0.25 per cent. An analysis of 1974 statistics shows that each clinic sees on average two new Pill users every three days and inserts one I.U.D. a month! Doctors receive two lectures on family planning during their six years of training, which includes a warning that oral contraceptives may affect those who wear contact lenses (hardly a common event in a poor country), but no comment on the relationship between steroids and lactation (although breast feeding is universal in the rural areas).

PROBLEMS AND OPPORTUNITIES

The clue to the highly uneven performance of family planning programmes in a wide variety of cultures lies in the programmes themselves: technical, managerial and policy mistakes have abounded.

In general, family planning has always begun with the least effective methods and programmes (*see* Table 38). This is because family planning always commences in a controversial atmosphere. The reversible methods of contraception generally become acceptable before sterilisation. Invariably, abortion remains the most threatening to politicians and decision-makers. The clinical, as opposed to

TABLE 38: PERCENTAGE OF WOMEN STILL USING CONTRACEPTIVE METHOD (AND PERCENTAGE PREGNANT) AT SELECTED INTERVALS AFTER FIRST ADOPTING THE METHOD

Number of months after adoption of method	*Pills*	*Per cent pregnant*	*I.U.D.*	*Per cent pregnant*	*Rhythm*	*Per cent pregnant*	*Condoms*	*Per cent pregnant*
6	63	3.2	80	1.4	68	13.8	35	6.6
12	48	4.6	70	2.3	55	19.4	25	12.6
24	29	5.3	55	3.0	36	27.0	13	14.6
36	16	5.6	42	5.5	20	33.4	—	—

(*Source:* Philippines National Program Data. Laing 1974)

the commercial, channels of distribution become part of the wrapping perceived to be necessary to make programmes respectable. Physicians, after all, are the only group whom society sanctions to enter the privacy of other people's bedrooms, so by inference, doctors are felt to be useful in deflecting criticism from family planning programmes. Therefore services often begin with a white-coated doctor sitting in a tiled clinic, offering I.U.D.s or prescribing oral contraceptives to a population still seeking to solve its fertility problems with abortion provided by traditional midwives and through the sale of herbal remedies by petty vendors. However, the non-prescription commercial sale of contraceptives and well advertised, clean, non-exploiting early abortion services are the last things which societies are permitted to receive.

What then divides the relatively few successful family planning programmes from the larger number of failures? The factors appear to be realism about fertility regulation methods and their limitations, a clear perspective about the way in which they fit together, practical insight into the resources available in a village or shanty-town, human leadership and the will to succeed.

RANGE OF METHODS

It is not generally appreciated that, even in countries with a government commitment to family planning and population policy, it is still extremely rare to find ready access to all methods of fertility control. In Malaysia, oral contraceptives are used by over 90 per cent of women entering the national family planning programme, but access to female sterilisation is limited, vasectomy has not been made available and abortion is illegal. In India vasectomy has been forcibly performed, abortion has been legal since 1971, but oral contraceptives have never been used.

Clinically and socially it seems as if the control of family size is difficult. Observation suggests that communities benefit from access to as wide a range of methods as possible (*see* Fig. 62). Whenever a new method of fertility control is added to those already present, there will be some degree of substitution of methods; but an additional number of people in society, who were not attracted by any of the previous options, will adopt the newly available method. What is true of methods is probably also true of patterns of distribution. If services are made available through clinics, a certain number of highly motivated couples will use them, but a substantially larger number will use contraceptives if they are conveniently available from neighbours, local storekeepers or clinic outreach workers.

Data from programmes and from measurement of contraceptive failure rates, demonstrates that the reversible methods of contraception are inadequate for a community to control its fertility within the goals now found in the West—and hoped for in the Third World. The journey to low fertility is always associated with abortion—whether legal or illegal—and sterilisation has been welcome wherever it has been made available. In China, all methods are available, from barefoot doctors distributing Pills in the paddy-fields to abortion in health centres. Interestingly, from the consumer's point of view, the availability of family planning in communist China looks remarkably like that in the capitalist U.S.A. One of the reasons for success in northern Thailand was that Dr. McDaniel noticed that women responded enthusiastically to the possibility of an injectable contraceptive. Initially it was difficult to obtain a regular supply and it would have been easier to offer no choice but oral contraceptives, but McDaniel persisted in trying to offer people what they wanted. With the passage of time he found that additional options were desirable and most recently female sterilisation has proved popular in the area.

In order to meet the shortage of medical personnel which has already inhibited this method of family planning in developing countries, nurse-surgeons are being taught female sterilisation, using minilaparotomy (*see* p. 134). Often where programmes of reversible contraception appear to have been successful, as in Korea, Bali or Taiwan, a look under the surface shows that abortion, even if illegal, has been readily available at a low price and with reasonable safety.

A rational and serious approach to family planning would begin by offering abortion and elective sterilisation. In a traditional society, breast feeding may space pregnancies as well as the use of Pills, I.U.D.s and condoms does in the West. The need is to deal with unwanted, accidental pregnancies (and abortion is already part

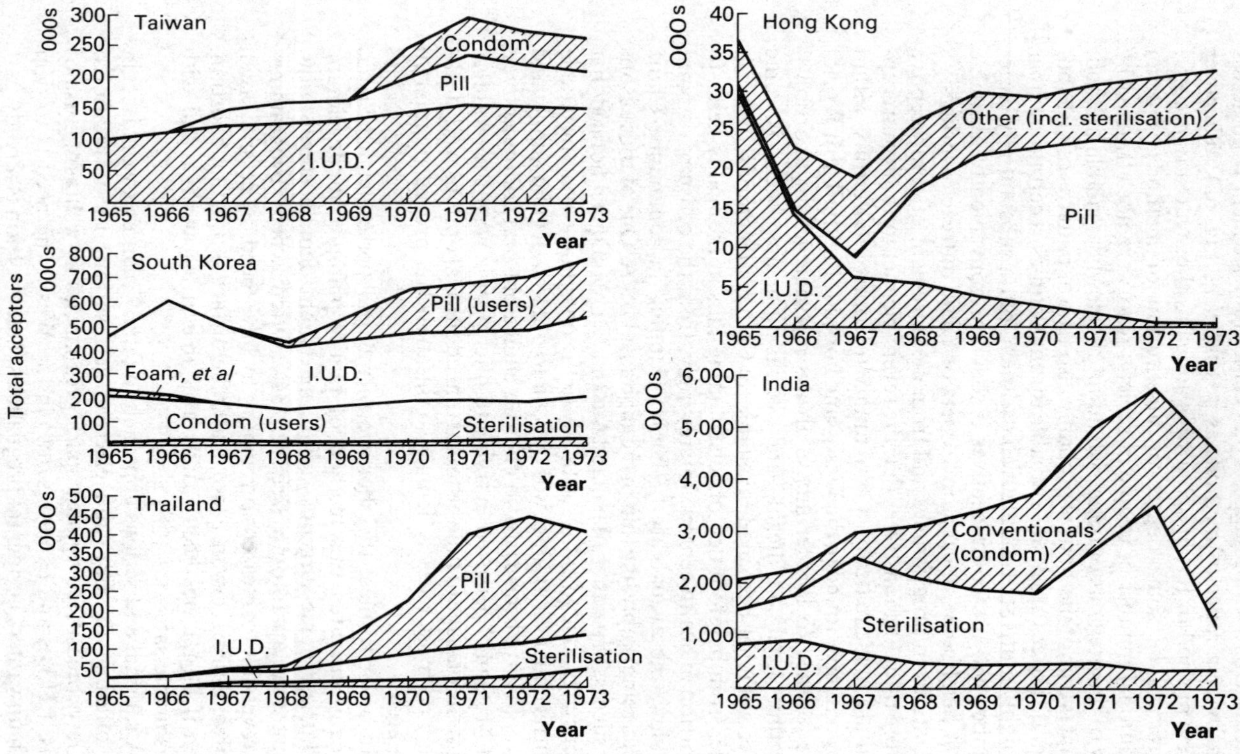

(*Source: Studies in Family Planning*. Population Council, New York)

Fig. 62. *Addition of "new" methods of family planning and total acceptors.*

of all traditional cultures) and to terminate fertility with the option of sterilisation. Again, it is remarkable that in northern Thailand women from the hill tribes of Burma trek many miles through the jungle to join the queues of Thai women seeking sterilisation, receiving the operation from people with a different language and a different culture, who offer to meet a universal human need.

Unfortunately, in the pursuit of family planning, unlike the problem of building an irrigation dam or erecting a steel mill, rational decisions are not made. A sequence of family planning methods rise to the surface of public use according to their political acceptability and not to their usefulness or acceptability to the bulk of the population. A great deal of money and effort spent in family planning programmes is not a direct response to the manifest needs of people to control their fertility, but a way of sidestepping those needs (particularly when they involve the options of abortion and sterilisation).

COMMUNITY INVOLVEMENT

Methods of distribution are as important as the physiological side effects of a method. The Western device of using doctors to make contraceptives less controversial also works politically in developing countries, but has backfired at the community level: it has restricted potential services and has overlooked the genuine potential of the community to help itself.

In developing countries, nearly 40 per cent of contraceptives are sold over the counter. Perhaps the single most important step which could be taken in the immediate future to improve family planning services would be to free oral contraceptives from the necessity of medical prescription. When the method was first introduced, it was reasonable to limit these physiologically powerful and relatively poorly understood drugs to medical prescription. However, with the passage of time, a great deal of information has become available. The rare potentially serious side-effects that may occur are not made any less frequent by medical examination. Where screening is possible it depends upon the patient's history and such simple factors as age. In nearly all developing countries the Pill is available over the counter to the middle classes, but national and international agencies abide by the fiction of prescription, discriminating against the poorest members of the community.

The traditional village has the one resource needed for family planning: a large supply of intelligent people. The training of village and shanty-town distributors has proved successful in Colombia, Thailand, Indonesia and the Philippines. Nowhere has it been attempted and failed.

In Bali the key to the successful programme has been the involvement of the village political and organisational structure. When the programme started, there were clinics and doctors trained in family planning. It was obvious that clinic-based services would always be inadequate. But by simplifying the programme auxiliary workers were trained in I.U.D. insertion and more than 2,000 villagers became depots for oral contraceptive distribution.

In Thailand, the village distributors have proved consistent and enthusiastic workers. Care has been taken to help raise their status within the village: they have been given certificates which they proudly display upon the wall and visits from supervisors and doctors, the extra money which they earn and the appreciation of the community, all combine to make them successful workers. Some have been taught additional skills such as parasite control. In the Philippines, the social structure of the "Iglesia ni Cristo" Church has become involved in family planning. This is an indigenous, evangelical, Christian denomination, known for its discipline. The theological leadership has espoused the cause of family planning and sermons are preached on texts such as "Blessed are the barren and the breasts that never gave suck" (Luke 23, verse 9), and oral contraceptives are available after the Sunday service. More than 100,000 women now take the Pill through this scheme and have the highest continuation of anywhere in the world. More recently, vasectomy was added to the choices of the members of Iglesia ni Cristo and mobile teams travel the Philippines offering the operation in church premises.

By contrast, many countries, such as India, have steadfastly avoided involving the community and refused to use auxiliary workers. The shortage of trained medical personnel in the developing world cannot be overemphasised. Not only are there few doctors, but most of those that are qualified are concentrated in the cities and especially the capital city. (*See* Fig. 63). The problem is further exaggerated by the loss of doctors to rich countries (*see* Table 39). If we put these two facts together we come to some stark contrasts: there are as many Indian doctors practising in the National Health Service in Britain as there are among the half-million villages in India. Everything that can be said of doctor–patient ratios is even more marked in the case of specialities, such as obstetrics. But often the biggest single problem facing a country is shortage of trained midwives. In Iran there are over 11,000 practising doctors but less than 700 fully trained midwives. To take an example from family planning, in 1966 the government of India decided to institute a core of 180 general duty, family planning women officers. By 1971, twenty-nine had been appointed. At the same time provision was

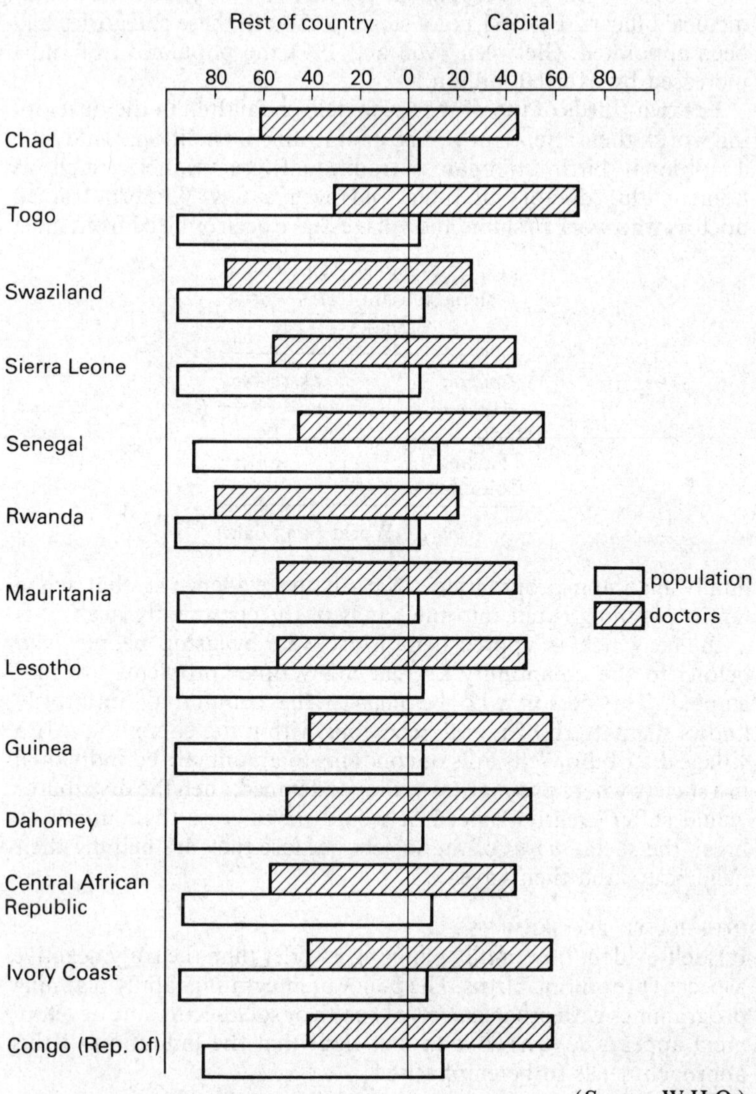

(*Source:* W.H.O.)

Fig. 63. *Diagram to show the percentage distribution of doctors and population between the capital city and the rest of the country* (*in the African region*).

made for fifteen gynaecological specialists and fifteen honorary medical officers. By 1971 not a single person in these categories had been appointed. (Between 1966 and 1971 the population of India increased by over 60 million.)

For two-thirds of the women who deliver children in the developing world, their attendant will be an untrained, traditional midwife. Traditional birth attendants, traditional practitioners, such as homeopathic doctors in India and even a few Western trained doctors who work in slums and villages have been omitted from most

TABLE 39: PERCENTAGE OF NEW MEDICAL GRADUATES WHO EMIGRATE

Country	*Percentage*
India	18
Thailand	67
Colombia	14

(*Source:* World Bank data)

family planning programmes. Yet all the evidence is that when family planning is put into the hands of the community itself, it is a choice which is appreciated. Moreover, by using people who belong to the community a great many other problems are pre-empted. The person who belongs to the community intuitively knows the pattern of moral behaviour within the community. If a village distributor sells Pills or condoms to an unmarried individual in a society where pre-marital sex is condemned, then the distributor would suffer greatly. Indeed, it would never cross their minds to break the social *mores* of the society because they are helping their neighbours and themselves.

INTEGRATED PROGRAMMES

It is self-evident that family planning is wider than the truly negative aspect of preventing births. The policy of integrating family planning programmes with other aspects of health or socio-economic development appears so attractive at first sight that the limitation of this approach needs to be emphasised.

There is an artificial polarisation of views concerning the relationship between family planning and development. The examples of Bali, Northern Thailand and to a greater extent that of mainland China demonstrate that fertility can decline in advance of major economic changes. The *per capita* income in Northern Thailand is lower than other parts of the country, transport is difficult and there was nothing to encourage the belief that fertility would plummet down so rapidly. Probably infant mortality rates have dropped during the years of rapid fertility decline, but no more quickly than in any other traditional society where fertility has remained high. Because fertility control causes such a marked reduction in maternal and infant mortality and has a marked impact on economic development, the possibility of shortcuts of this type are exciting and welcome. To state this is not to say that all those who are professionally engaged in family planning and have experience of the developing world do not see and subscribe to the need to promote development in as many ways as possible. Family planning is not a solution to all problems, but it assists in solving a great many.

When complex and expensive programmes linking family planning with other aspects of health or social development have been planned, using high level resources, they have often been disappointing. When several ministries, such as Health, Education, Economic and Social Affairs are involved, then it is difficult for any single one to take the necessary leadership. The more stools that are available, the less likely it is that anyone will notice when a programme falls between them.

Sometimes, as in the case of Kenya which has been quoted, the pressure to integrate family planning with other services seems little more than a crude attempt to deflect any genuine possibility of success.

The Danfa project in Ghana is an example of a rural health project in which family planning was an important part. In an area (population: 60,000) typical of many developing countries with unmade roads, poor water supplies, low literacy and high infant mortality (100 per 1,000 live births) and where three-quarters of the babies were delivered by traditional midwives, a variety of test areas were created. The birth rate of 48 per 1,000 is one of the highest in the world, and the total fertility rate is 7.8.

The acceptance rates for contraceptives was higher than predicted and 20 per cent of women between the ages of twenty and thirty-four in the most intensively-covered areas attended a family planning clinic at least once in the first two and a half years. Male acceptors were more common than female, reflecting a male-dominant society. It is interesting to speculate whether the Pill would have been more widely used had it been distributed freely, rather than tied to medical services. Indeed, the need for women to travel to clinics which were only open at a limited time, which required the embarrassment of a pelvic examination and yet were unable to offer abortions should a contraceptive method fail, are examples of the limitations common to a great many family planning programmes.

One of the purposes of the programme was to see if delivering contraceptives within comprehensive health care increased acceptance. The evidence so far is that this has not been the case, although in the areas where health and family planning were most closely linked the balance of female to male acceptors changed to the former.

It is often asserted that couples in the developing world will not plan their families until infant mortality declines, a view that has been challenged in recent studies by Chowdhury and Taylor (*see* p. 96). The latter concludes that infant mortality is not a necessary condition for fertility decline but that family planning services, which he sees as essential in most countries, "can be more effective, as well as politically more acceptable, if appropriately integrated with maternal and child health and nutritional services".

Integrated services hold much more promise when organised from below, upwards. A village distributor who has handled Pills and condoms for six months or a year can readily be trained to assist in another aspect of development. It is proposed in Thailand to make such distributors the centre of small rural credit schemes. Nutrition supplements may well be distributed along with contraceptives to women with four babies. In Brazil, schoolteachers have been very successful in providing Pills for the mothers of children they teach.

A suitable mixture of realism and compassion in those that plan programmes, combined with the good sense of the poor who live in villages and shanty-towns, will throw up an ever increasing list of possibilities for what Mechai Viravaidya has called "fertility-related development". The grandiose schemes which all too often come out of the air-conditioned offices of ministries and international agencies need to be approached with much more caution. Commonly they flounder on the grounds of expense.

BEYOND FAMILY PLANNING

The uneven performance of many family planning programmes has given rise to a literature of so-called "beyond family planning" measures. Singapore has developed the most complete system of social legislation related to family limitation of any country in the world. In 1968 paid maternity leave was limited to the first three births, in 1973 to the first two; in the latter year income tax relief on fourth and later children was withdrawn and children of small families and of parents who had been sterilised were offered preferential admission to the most sought-after schools.

The total fertility rate in Singapore fell from 4.498 per woman in 1966 to 2.098 in 1975—in other words, Singapore has reached biological replacement level, although there is still population growth which will continue to the year 2030 A.D. as a result of the large number of young women in the population, reflecting high fertility in the recent past.

Is this rapid fertility decline related to the deterrents to large families which Singapore has introduced, or is it due to an improved availability in fertility regulation services?

A voluntary family planning programme had been in existence for many years when the government entered the field in 1966, but both were limited to clinic-based, reversible methods of contraception. The number of acceptors for this conventional and limited approach reached a peak in 1969. In that year the additional option of abortion was added, but only with great caution. Approval by a board was necessary and less than 2,000 operations (3.6 per 1,000 women of the ages fifteen to forty-four) were performed in the first year. Only in 1972, one year before the more punitive of the social legislations was introduced, did abortion become available on request for couples with three children. By 1975 there were 12,000 abortions (23.2 per 1,000 women of the ages fifteen to forty-four). Sterilisation followed a similar path and even in 1972 was only approved for women with three or more children. Therefore, the paradox existed that, while the State was penalising couples who had more than two children, they were refusing sterilisation until a woman had three. Even by 1970 the obstetricians whispered that the maternal mortality had risen slightly following the introduction of charges for fourth and subsequent deliveries in hospitals. The possible long-term effects of depriving children of equal educational opportunities also seem unfortunate.

Singapore is a modernising society which, after Japan, has the highest *per capita* income in Asia. There is a rising age of marriage and by 1975 42 per cent of women were economically active outside the home. These changes and access to the full range of fertility control methods were probably sufficient to bring the population down to replacement level. The political leadership rightly saw the importance of population limitation, but perhaps was not fully aware of the logistics of fertility regulation or that the family planning programme was being held back by the fine print of the regulations and the restraint of the medical profession. As the implementation of services until 1975 was consistently one step behind the social incentives that were introduced, the interpretation of these "beyond family planning" measures seems unproven (*see* Fig. 64).

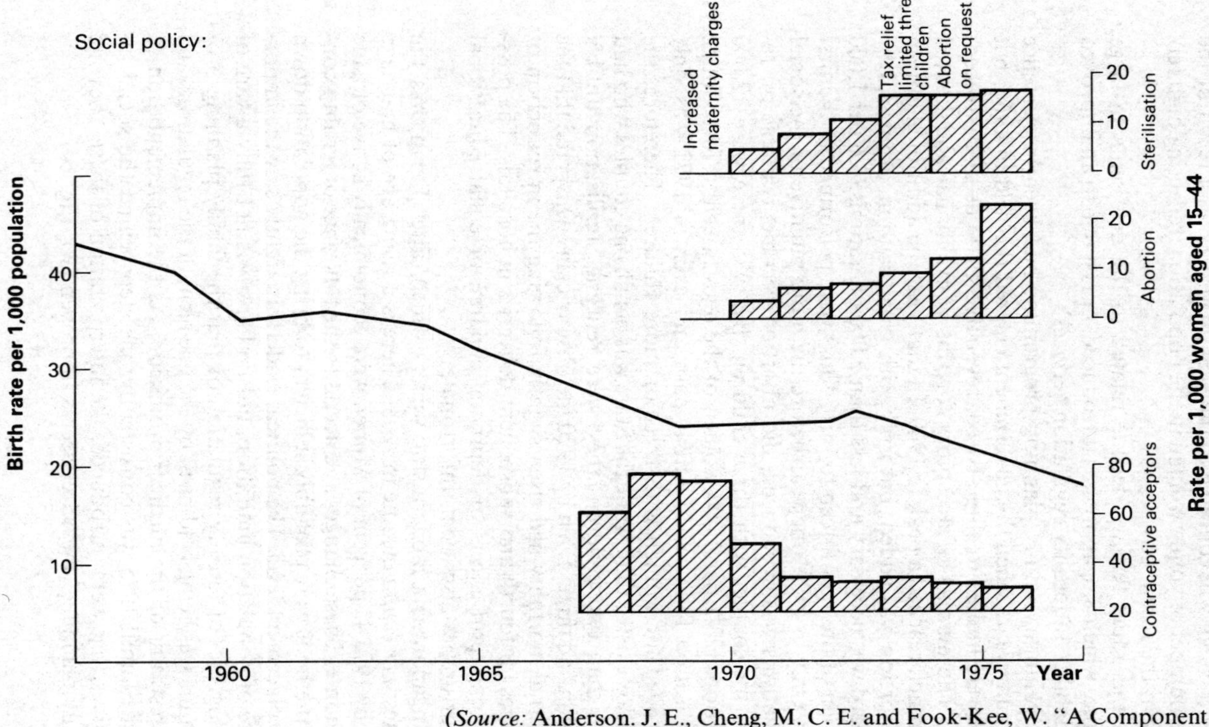

(*Source:* Anderson. J. E., Cheng, M. C. E. and Fook-Kee, W. "A Component Analysis of Recent Fertility Decline in Singapore." *Studies in Family Planning.* 8 (11) 1977)

Fig. 64. *Singapore: disincentives or access to fertility regulation?*

COSTS

The gap between developed and developing countries is especially wide in the case of the resources available for social welfare programmes. Most developing countries spend less than $1.1 per year on all aspects of preventive and curative medicine. In 1972 the average cost of one day's admission to a U.S. hospital was $103—a sum exceeding the total *per capita* income of many developing countries. The Planned Parenthood in the U.S.A. spends more on recruiting and serving a single acceptor in family planning over a year than the *per capita* income of neighbouring Haiti.

The available resources are unequally divided nationally as well as globally. There is a beautiful hospital in a provincial capital in South East Asia, where the electricity bill for running the lighting and air-conditioning is equivalent to 25 per cent of the national malaria eradication budget; one hospital in a certain West African country consumes one-quarter of the total health budget for that country. Family planning programmes can and must be cheap. Each method and each channel of distribution has a price tag attached to it. It may be higher in Brazil than in Bangladesh, but for developing countries as a whole generalisations can be made.

The provision of the reversible methods of contraception through family planning clinics is expensive. Premises and professional personnel cost money and facilities are often in the wrong place or open at the wrong times and poorly used. In addition, services become clogged with check visits. In Latin America in the early 1970s between three-quarters and nine-tenths of all family planning clinic visits were re-visits.

The cost per new acceptor in 1972 varied between $8 in Chile and $29 in Mexico. The medical and clinical services of the Family Planning Association (FEPAC) in Mexico had a budget of $850,000 but only recruited 18,000 new Pill and 12,000 new I.U.D. acceptors in a twelve-month interval.

Family planning services that are integrated with other activities, such as maternal and child health, are even more costly. A simple division of total programme costs ($36 million) by target numbers of acceptors (640,000) in Kenya over a five-year period gives a figure of $56 for each acceptor to be recruited. The cost of averting a birth is estimated at $240. The *per capita* income of Kenya is well under $200 and clearly there is something wrong with a system in which the cost of averting a birth equals what a man can earn in a year. The Danfa project in Ghana is more realistic but still expensive. A crude division of programme costs by number of family planning acceptors recruited gives a value of $28. Each clinic visit costs nearly $10.

But, it could be argued, an "integrated" programme provides many things in addition to family planning, and therefore they will be expensive. However, this sidesteps other issues—if a country spends only $1 a year per head on health, is it reasonable to expect that it should spend $20 *per capita* on an integrated health programme which has a family planning component?

Korea is a country where, a decade ago, the government spent less than one dollar a year *per capita* on health, yet was bold enough to spend one-fifth of this small total on family planning. It required courage to maintain such a level in the face of very pressing demands from other quarters. The problem is that preventive and curative medicine are remarkably cheap and for a tiny input of fifty cents *per capita* Korea has a death rate of 8 per 1,000. In family planning, relatively large initial investments may only bring marginal returns. However, while clinic-based services often prove impossibly expensive, the community-based distribution of contraceptives is within range of most economies and the surgical means of fertility control can be made available on a very wide scale. When purchased in bulk the Pill can be obtained for less than $0.2 a cycle. Community-based distribution costs run at $1–5 per person served per year. In some schemes consumers pay up to $0.25 a month for Pills which will cover half or more of programme costs. In Thailand, where C.B.F.P.S. services have existed for three years, some districts now cover the whole of their distribution costs and are paying back initial start-up costs.

National and international funds for family planning in the developing world already exceed $400 million annually. This would provide a free supply of contraceptives to meet any foreseeable need into the 1980s. Unfortunately, a disproportionate share of present funds goes on administration, clinical salaries and so-called information and education programmes. For example, in 1971 the United Nations Fund for Population Activities (U.N.F.P.A.) spent $30,600,000 in total, of which $800,000 went on equipment and supplies. Almost as much went on meetings and seminars, over $2,200,000 on education and training and $21,900,000 on "comprehensive projects".

Sterilisation is usually performed in the early thirties and gives ten years or more protection against pregnancy. Vasectomy can be performed for as low as $5 per case and is without doubt the most cost effective option in family planning. Female sterilisation requires a greater input of skills and more complicated facilities. Even so, it can be carried into rural areas, as the work of Kamheang (from the Ramathodi Hospital, Bangkok) has demonstrated. Having established an adequate programme in the capital city with a high turnover of patients, this was used to train key personnel from a peripheral level who were encouraged to set up satellite services. 10,000 female sterilisations have been performed in this programme, largely at a village level and at an average cost of $12.5. A service of this kind is probably offering protection against pregnancy at approximately $1 a year.

First trimester abortion is offered in private clinics in India at $10. In parts of Indonesia and the Philippines, although abortion is illegal, some doctors offer menstrual regulation for as little as $6. In Calcutta traditional practitioners who have been trained in menstrual regulation make it available for as low as $1. The drive towards abortion is so strong once a woman is unwillingly pregnant, that there is no reason why nearly all abortion services should not be financially self-sufficient.

POLITICS OF FAMILY PLANNING

NATIONAL

In anything as controversial, yet as rapidly changing, as family planning, it is inevitable that governments should lag behind the need of their peoples. This was true in the West and is bound to be true in the developing world, even though the latter is setting a better record. Tunisia, for example, went from modest availability of the reversible methods of contraception to abortion on request in approximately a decade, travelling a distance that Britain or the U.S.A. took a century to cover. As has been noticed, on the whole, latecomers to family planning move more rapidly than the early starters. Although Indonesia still has to recognise sterilisation and add abortion to her national programme, progress has been relatively quicker than at a comparable stage in India.

The facts of population change are such that even the most stubborn and obtuse must, eventually, recognise the problem as did Peru in 1976. Always conservative, it was quick to claim that family planning was a genocidal, imperialistic, American policy and to applaud the most extreme of Vatican statements. Yet with a birth rate of 42 and a population which has grown from 7 million in 1940, to 16 million in 1976 and may reach 36 million by the end of the century, something must give. 45 per cent of the population is under the age of fifteen and only 3 per cent over the age of sixty-five. One in five now live in squatter communities (*pueblos jovenes*) which double in size every fifteen years. The cities receive two-thirds of the country's investment and the top 10 per cent of the population controls 40 per cent of the national resources, while the bottom 30 per cent only get one-tenth of the national cake. Half the children are poorly nourished, despite the fact that the world's richest fishing grounds are off the coast of Peru. The Peruvian Indian tries to sell beautifully handcrafted articles for a few cents off a plastic sheet on the pavement, while descendants of the conquistadores buy electrical equipment or an outboard motorboat from air-conditioned, plate-glass and chromium shops, not six feet away.

These inexorable demographic and economic facts forced the government to pass a series of Population Guidelines, partially drafted by a far-sighted and courageous Jesuit. In an eloquent flight of political fantasy, the document defends itself from the Church and from the right and left wings of politics, by claiming the new policies are to be qualitative and not quantitative, "demographic effects should be anticipated and quantified but in no way do they constitute an objective in themselves". In itself this is a harmless game with words, but when so complex a mythology must be created to make family planning politically acceptable, it tends eventually to be believed. The Peruvian guidelines exclude the use of abortion and sterilisation for "birth-control purposes". Even the availability of the reversible methods is likely to remain limited.

In Paraguay, the most that the non-governmental family planning association can do to help people control their family size, is to follow the tortuous path of offering cervical screening tests for cancer and then passing a sheet of paper to the woman, suggesting a number of additional services, such as "the prevention of abortion" and "responsible parenthood". The social security only provides family planning for women with five or more children. Not surprisingly, one in four pregnancies in Ascencion, the capital, is thought to end in illegally induced abortion. In everything to do with family planning fear of disturbing the social elite always counts for more than the need to serve the poor.

But crude political opposition to family planning *per se* is now rare and the constraints are of a more subtle kind. Countries which adopted family planning policies generally chose the soft option of associating contraceptive services with doctors and health. As a consequence an increasing army of so-called information and education personnel were required to make a significant number of acceptors leap over the cultural hurdles that this route of distribution itself represented. Experience shows that the majority of women able to attend a family planning clinic usually live within half an hour's transportation time. In the Philippines, 30 per cent of the women attending clinics stopped using the method they were given the following year and 22 per cent became pregnant. Before the end of the war in South East Asia, Laos adopted a family planning policy. It was then a country of 3 million people, nearly all of whom lived in villages. To "help" Laos, an international agency built a single clinic in one village. It happens to express all the physical and social limitations of this type of approach; second only in size to the school and larger than the temple, it was the only building in the village with its own water supply and sewage and without doubt the most expensively constructed building in the area. Heavily built of red hardwood, it stood out aggressively beside the flimsy but charming houses raised on stilts with thatched roofs. Even from the road it was possible to see the culturally-inappropriate posters which lined the veranda and depicted the anatomical details of a midline section of the male and female pelvis. To complete the picture, it was surrounded by a barbed wire fence and only opened for a few hours each week. Technically, nothing was ever required of that clinic which could not have been performed on the immaculately kept bamboo floor of any house in the village.

Instead of working backwards from the need of potential consumers and asking common-sense questions, most family planning programmes are heavily overengineered. The political wrappings cost much more than their technical contents. As a consequence, the cry went up in the 1960s that governments must be involved in family planning services, as only they were perceived to have the necessary resources.

All too often governments fell into the political traps awaiting them. In the late 1960s, family planning bureaucracies burst forth like flowers in a desert after a freak rainstorm. These bureaucracies institutionalised the limited spectrum of methods which politics permitted to be available. In turn, they resisted the emergence of new channels of distribution and the addition of new fertility regulation options. In one country of more than 10 million people, an experienced and creative family planning worker devised a scheme whereby the reversible methods of contraception could be distributed throughout the country, using the existing infrastructure of wholesalers and retailers and employing a staff of ten people—including a girl to answer the telephone. But at the time this practical plan was set forth, the Ministry of Health related family planning programme already had more than 100 full-time personnel and, needless to say, the simpler, culturally more appropriate, more cost-effective scheme never saw the light of day.

Too many national family planning programmes in developing countries have become highly territorial. It sometimes seems as if society should not be allowed to control its fertility except by permission of the relevant ministry. In one part of Asia, a senior official in the Ministry of Health used political influence to prevent the nationalised metropolitan transport system carrying advertisements on contraception—because they were promoting a scheme run by a non-governmental agency. Many innovative and practical projects have been strangled at birth by small-minded and insecure people, concerned with their empires and their status, rather than with the needs of the community, or the opportunities for carrying forward vigorous, effective and cheap family planning services. Inside and outside government programmes, the boldness and flexibility which is required in so important a subject is all too often replaced by over-anticipation of possible "backlash" and extreme degrees of caution.

Governments and non-governmental agencies need to see problems in a wider perspective. No one agency or institution controls all the variables determining human fertility. Most family planning services require an excess of records. These are often inflated by local officials who might otherwise get the sack for poor performance, or who are sidetracking resources for fictitious acceptors into the pockets of minor (and sometimes major) bureaucrats. In one Asian country, it is thought that 70 per cent of family planning reports are falsified. While staff waste their time by filling in the details of women given the Pill, street vendors sell condoms without any system of registration, men practise coitus interruptus without a record of the age or parity of their wives and illegal abortionists rarely keep clinical notes. To compound the unreality of many situations, birth rate statistics are sometimes misleadingly low because of deficient registration. For example, in one country the birth rate appeared to fall at the time of the initiation of a national family planning programme, but those close to the situation knew that there had been a change of leadership in the Institute of Statistics where a competent director had been replaced by a less hardworking one.

Family planning programmes accelerate trends. They are a humane and necessary contribution to the welfare of every nation. In poor nations there is an obligation to make programmes cheap and to devise ones that can be built into the structure of society and are eligible for rapid replication should they succeed, as has happened with C.B.F.P.S. in Thailand.

INTERNATIONAL

Whatever political problems attend family planning programmes at a country level tend to be multiplied internationally. The work of the World Health Organisation (W.H.O.) illustrates this clearly. In 1951, the then Indian Minister of Health, given to ideals of sexual restraint, approached W.H.O. for technical assistance in developing a programme based on the rhythm method. The W.H.O. got the American, Dr. Abraham Stone, to visit India. At the end of his tour, clearly disassociated himself from his W.H.O. mandate, he spoke of alternative methods of contraception. When the W.H.O. assembly met a few months later, this mild excursion into reality had created an international crisis. The Scandinavian countries alone backed India in the need for the provision of family planning services. The Catholic countries, led by Eire, threatened to withdraw from the organisation if any aspect of family planning was pursued. The major countries, such as the U.S.A. and the U.K., much to their discredit, decided the simplest thing to do was to bury the topic altogether. They sided with the fanatics and relegated family planning policies to the scrapheap: it took sixteen years for these initiatives to be revived.

The shadow of the past hangs over the present. Conferences and research all too often prove simpler than the support of direct services. And even these require their 'political packaging'. In the early 1970s, the W.H.O. set up task forces on new contraceptive development. Of the initial budget of $1.6 million, approximately $600,000 was spent on obtaining consultant advice on how to spend the remainder of the money. The administration, conference and volunteer support of the I.P.P.F. absorbs 25 per cent of the Federation's budget before a dollar is spent in any country. The World Bank usually launches a programme in a country with several outside consultants, whose fares and support approximate to $100,000 a year each. Many advisors have come from Western nations, unfamiliar with the problems facing the Third World.

The sociology of international agencies is interesting. They often use a variety of sophisticated techniques to look at the behaviour of family planning acceptors, but rarely turn these techniques upon themselves. However, the knowledge, attitudes and practice of the provider of family planning services is equally as important as that of the recipient. A further inhibition to analysis arises because those most eligible to comment are those usually receiving support, and in the real world of human affairs there is a natural reluctance to criticise one's possible sponsors.

Donor agencies tend to support professional groups of their own kind—doctors and civil service administrators—although the influence of such groups may not extend in a meaningful or acceptable way to the poor of the nation concerned. Where civil service salaries are low, corruption becomes an almost essential element if administrators are to achieve a living wage. Where governments are overburdened with bureaucracy, many officials are more interested in keeping their jobs until the retirement age than in doing them well and bettering their communities. International agencies put staff into this sphere whose salaries may be ten times those of their in-country colleagues. Not only is liaison in a country difficult but, not surprisingly, Third World nationals are easily tempted into the international agencies, which often employ the best leaders in any country, as well as some dead wood which they are rarely able to cut out later.

Korten has drawn attention to the significance of managerial skills in implementing family planning programmes. Lack of management is a major problem at many levels of development. In family planning the problem is particularly acute because goals are often vague and achievements difficult to measure. If family planning concentrated on the provision of services, its success or failure might be easier to manage. International agencies have no wider constituency to which they are responsible. The mass media often ferrets out the worst bungling in national bureaucracies, but in the case of international agencies, beyond the cosy sense that they are attempting to do something for the welfare of mankind, there are few who look critically at their performance. Boards of management, international assemblies and volunteer bodies that fly from corners of the earth for two-day, jet-lagged meetings, are easily misled. The W.H.O. is not primarily a family planning agency but it illustrates some common problems. By 1977 it employed 5,000 professional staff—2,000 at the headquarters, 2,000 in regional offices and only one in five in the field. With tax-free salaries running from $260 to $800 a week, six weeks holiday and first class travel for annual home leave, an offer of employment from the W.H.O. like one from the Mafia, is rarely refused and few are likely to resign on matters of principle.

BUCHAREST—WORLD PLAN OF ACTION

The World Population Conference in 1974 illustrates the difficulties which countries and, above all, international agencies have in handling the topic of fertility. It was the product of a political orgy, not the child of responsible parents and it is malformed—perhaps because some unsuccessful attempts were made to abort it. The deformity is simple: a limb is missing—there is no awareness of global demographic problems. Like many loving parents, those nearest to the World Plan of Action do not even recognise its defects. "Population growth," writes one international commentor, "must not be represented in terms of global crisis which every country must urgently contribute to solving. The role of the international community is to assist all interested countries in formulating and achieving whatever population goals they set."

The responsibility of the United Nations was to the world, not to rationalise the selfish aims of individual nations, whether rich or poor. The original draft plan had numerical targets, including the humane one of attempting to extend family planning services to all those who need them by the years 1980–5. Ultimately, to ignore global statistics, as the Bucharest Conference did, is also to show reduced respect for individuals.

The World Plan of Action did call for more research. It is characteristic of modern agencies to steal armour from the genuine province of scientific investigation, in order to manufacture shields to deflect political criticism. In anything to do with human sexuality, a call for research is more likely to be a hallmark of a poor political decision than the outcome of a rational choice.

The role of the People's Republic of China at Bucharest was deliberately inscrutable. While offering their own population the full range of fertility regulation choices and pursuing strict demographic targets nationally, they contributed to the blunting of family planning programmes internationally by overemphasising the links between socio-economic change and fertility, and encouraging "integrated programmes". They must have realised that these, in most countries other than their own, swallow up resources. This, however, may have been the objective. After all, Latin American communists were delighted by the Papal encyclical *Humanae Vitae*, knowing it would exacerbate the social problems of many countries.

CONCLUSION

Fundamental breakthroughs in contraceptive technology are unlikely. It may be that vaccination against pregnancy will be perfected or that a predictable medical way of inducing a late period will be found, but the future of the world cannot hang on such possibilities. Fortunately, it is possible to control human fertility with the means currently available, even in poor societies. However, this cannot be achieved unless sterilisation and abortion are available beside the reversible methods of contraception.

Family planning is not like agricultural development or educational extension services; it has the unique property of being related to sexual activity. Therefore it is controversial. Usually, a small group of pioneers take a few options from the many that are required to control fertility and perform some miracles of political cosmetic surgery to make services available. But the most useful services are the most difficult to introduce. The evidence of biology, sociology and economic analysis suggests that perhaps the first service a rural community needs is sterilisation, because pregnancies are often adequately spaced by breast feeding. In a rapidly urbanising community, an easily accessible, safe, humanely-run early abortion service is the first need. Contraception can and should be added to these first steps. Unhappily, the poor of the world, crucified by their own overfertility, who cried for water, were given the vinegar of culturally inappropriate, geographically inaccessible, clinic based services, such as I.U.D. insertion and doctor-prescribed Pills.

Paradoxically, although this expensive packaging blunted programmes, it did not deflect political criticism. "It is believed by most of the influential and responsible circles in the developing countries," writes Yusuf Ali Erej, "that the birth-control campaign is organised by powerful pressure groups with headquarters in rich countries who want to prevent the poor from breeding because they fear that the poor might one day thrust them aside with their sheer bulk. Whether this belief is right or wrong, it is my opinion that the people in the developed nations should accept its existence."

Fortunately, the second half of the 1970s is escaping from some of the frustrations of ten years earlier: programmes can work and agencies can change.

China, the largest single collection of human beings on earth, has controlled its fertility with astonishing rapidity and discipline. Other areas in Asia also show that fertility control can precede major socio-economic changes—or to rephrase this generalisation, sufficient control has already taken place in society to trigger new patterns of fertility regulation. The need is to take the known successes and enlarge them. To do this the agencies with the resources also need to change. In 1977 the W.H.O. Assembly transferred $40,000,000 from the Geneva administration to field programmes and promised to cut 300 staff jobs in the foreseeable future. Other agencies need to do the same.

For millions, these adjustments may come too late. In the next twenty years Bangladesh will grow from around 80 million to over 140 million, with an inescapable implication of mass starvation. Indonesia will grow from over 140 million to nearly 240 million, with the implication of massive unemployment and landslide poverty. Nigeria may grow from over 65 million to over 135 million and it is doubtful if the wealth of its oil can carry such an explosive population forward to any degree of dignified life.

From the point of view of family planning and a number of other parameters, the developing world can be divided into the difficult and the desperate. As a broad generalisation, India, Bangladesh, Pakistan and Ethiopia fall into the desperate group, characterised by low *per capita* income, poor literacy rate and rigid family and religious structures. China, Latin America, the rest of Africa and Asia fall into the difficult group, but even here, if economic change and population growth are to be brought into any kind of harmony, realistic services will have to be made available as rapidly as possible, including abortion and sterilisation.

In sociological terms, the difficult countries, such as the Philippines, Thailand and Colombia are sufficiently far down the road of socio-economic development that, given the opportunity, individuals can adapt themselves to the stresses and opportunities of modern urban living in one generation. But in the desperate countries the pattern of life is so remote from that of the twentieth century that such change is impossible for the bulk of the population—even in the improbable circumstances that they have the economic and social opportunities to do so. In the difficult countries, patterns of decision-making are not totally removed from those of the Western world. They can be analysed in conventional sociological terms. Individuals are aware of the possibility of making personal choices in a number of aspects of life, even if poverty and lack of opportunity greatly restrains their choices. In the desperate countries, the bulk of the population has practically no choices presented to it and is bewildered and unable to deal with the situation where choice becomes a reality. A girl of sixteen in Bangladesh was employed as a servant in a house. She was brutally beaten by her "owners". By chance she was rescued by the director of a small nutrition project, who became the first person in her life to treat her with any respect or equality. She was given a tiny income, had some freedom of choice as to what to do with her life, yet within six months she had run away as the sexual partner of an unmarried man, breaking every convention of her culture and embarking on a course which could only lead to her self-destruction.

Another, older woman of twenty-nine, also a household servant, but with more humane employers, had five children and was using oral contraceptives. She and her husband were sure that she did not wish to have any more children and she was offered a tubal ligation. She understood the nature and consequences of the operation, but when asked if she wanted it, turned to her advisor repeatedly and said, "You decide for me."

SELECTED REFERENCES AND BIBLIOGRAPHY

Davis, K. "Population Policy: Will Current Programs Succeed?" *Science*. 158, 730 1967

Piotrow, P. T. *World Population Crisis; The United States Response*. Praeger, New York 1973

Potts, D. M. "The Implementation of Family Planning Programmes." *British Journal of Hospital Medicine*. 10, 288 1973

Proceedings of the Tokyo International Symposium. Japan Science Society, Tokyo 1977

Salas, R. *People: An International Choice*. Pergamon, Oxford 1976

Stycos, J. M. *Ideology, Faith and Family Planning in Latin America*. McGraw Hill, New York 1973

Suitters, B. *Be Brave and Angry*. I.P.P.F., London 1973

Symonds, R. and Carder, M. *The United Nations and the Population Question*. McGraw Hill, New York 1973

Tyrell, D. A. J., Burkitt, D. P. and Henderson, W. *Technologies for Rural Health*. Royal Society, London 1977

Chapter 13

Adapting to Modern Needs

We think that it is reasonable to speculate about our way of life as a species before language and cultural evolution replaced the Darwinian pressures which had moulded biological evolution since the origin of life. We may presume *Homo sapiens* had a low density of population and lived in small, roaming, food-gathering bands in which the males "in their prime" generally had a number of mates, but possibly not more than two or three, with whom they developed individual emotional bonds lasting several years. Adolescent males may have been deprived of mating opportunities for at least some of the time and perhaps homosexual relations occurred between some individuals at this interval. Men may have had a higher mortality than women. Co-operation between family groups almost certainly took place.

Sexual maturity probably did not occur until the late teens and in the female a number of anovulatory menstrual cycles probably took place before the first conception happened. During this interval intercourse probably began and the female may have begun to learn some of the mechanical and emotional aspects of sexual behaviour, prior to assuming the burdens of motherhood. The human female is unique in developing breasts at puberty and not during the first pregnancy, as occurs in other mammals (even apes), suggesting that this was probably a time when sexual attraction for the males commenced and sexual activity would begin. Probably the first pregnancy was more likely to end in a stillbirth or an infant death than later ones.

If the baby survived, breast feeding would have gone on for perhaps two years and for most of this time ovulation would have been suppressed. Lactation was nature's contraceptive. If the baby died ovulation and the possibility of conception were resumed more rapidly. A woman might have had ten or more births if she survived until the menopause, but on average only two or three children would live to replace themselves. The population probably grew slowly but had to face episodes of food shortage due to the circumstance of climate. The simplest societies that survived prehistoric times are more complicated than what has been covered in the above summary, but none were in serious discord with it. At an early stage society had to begin to evolve rules for this first Eden. They probably had the dual benefit of ritualising fighting between males over partners and permitting a further trimming of fertility to meet local conditions.

CONTROL OF FERTILITY

We have argued in the preceding pages that sexual behaviour and reproductive patterns are moulded by many social pressures and that in nearly all societies factors exist which reduce achieved fertility below the biological maximum. Moreover, societies adapt to new needs by evolving new mechanisms, which although not necessarily consciously designed, tend to fit human reproduction to the exploitable resources available. The explosive technical, social and public changes which accompanied nineteenth-century industrilisation in the West and the modernisation of contemporary living on a global scale, have placed very serious strains on the ability of societies to adapt their sexual and reproductive patterns to new needs. At no time in the past—and at probably no time in the future—was the adjustment of reproductive patterns as critically significant for the welfare of contemporary mankind and his descendants, as in the second half of the twentieth century.

Tragically, the years between 1945 and 1965 when the rich world should have taken action to extend access to family planning to individuals in so-called developing countries were wasted. The reasons were partly the inherent conservatism of society in anything related to sexuality, but were also a hangover from the conflicts of the Western world concerning family planning, which totally negated the constructive influence the developed world might have had as former colonisers, advisors and as leaders in international agencies.

Today, fertility is declining and the evidence is that the Third World may pass through the demographic transition more rapidly than did the West. Certainly, the abilities of governments in Asia, and even in Africa and Latin America, to handle fertility regulation services is superior to that of Europe or North America at a similar stage in population history. However, even this optimistic assessment will leave numerical problems of unique and threatening proportions.

We have discussed the costs and benefits to individuals of controlling family size. In broad terms, the factors that influence fertility are well understood and income, education, urbanisation and work opportunities for women are more important than religion and ethnic groupings. In the last analysis, couples will determine their own family size regardless of any public position the state may adopt. On the one hand, the demographic transition in the West was largely completed in the face of opposition from the Church and medical profession; on the other, pro-natalist policies in contemporary Eastern Europe or in France and Canada in the 1950s and 1960s, if they achieved anything, brought about only marginal increases in achieved family size.

The problem of family planning in the developing world is partly one of the unequal diffusion of innovations. A good deal is known about the way in which technical, organisational and even educational innovations diffuse through both modern and traditional societies. Sometimes, an innovation which appears to benefit society is taken up or discontinued for unexpected reasons. In New Mexico, a hybrid strain of corn was introduced and adopted by the Spanish/American community within two years, but then dropped again when wives of farmers objected because the flour it produced did not prove suitable for making *tortillas*, the staple way of eating grain in the area.

Some of the most important means of death-control have been remarkably simple to diffuse. For example, the W.H.O. estimates that in ten years it has spent a total of 83 million dollars to eradicate smallpox. It is worth remembering that some of the larger international family planning agencies spend more than this in one year without achieving a fraction of the impact on birth rates which smallpox control has achieved on death rates.

Not only are the techniques of family planning often tiresome to use and somewhat uncertain in their outcome, but most family planning programmes have made a difficult problem even harder to solve by demanding the simultaneous diffusion of two unrelated innovations. With all the cultural barriers that any new idea has to overcome and the possibilities for failure which face even the best thought out plans, it is not surprising that progress has been irregular. Family planning programmes to date have demanded innovations in technology, such as the use of oral contraceptives or the insertion of I.U.D.s, and have depended for their spread upon medical and organisational innovations, such as so-called field motivators on a government payroll. Or they have involved the use of doctors in clinics, which also represents a considerable innovation for a community cut off by economic and geographical factors from Western medicine. Although a traditional community may seek, and indeed spend, a considerable part of its disposable income on Western forms of medicine, it always finds it difficult to obtain. It is not surprising when the same society is suddenly offered contraception from Western trained doctors in clinics that the potential recipients are confused. At a minimum, they are likely to infer that the methods being offered are very dangerous or the government would not use these high quality resources to distribute them. Often methods are made available in conflict with the traditions of the community, for example, when the Pill was given to Iranian women from very poor socio-economic backgrounds the discontinuation rate was very high, but when the same contraceptive was given to their husbands to pass on to their wives the continuation rate was remarkably successful: in a Muslim Iranian society the man is the decision-maker within the family and he should receive the contraceptives whether they are anatomically related to the opposite sex or not.

So the community-based distribution of contraceptives which has been successful in many countries works well partly because it removes one-half of the problem of diffusing fertility regulation innovations: it uses distribution networks which already exist and limits the process of adopting any new technology to the methods themselves.

Paradoxically, what is probably the easiest part of fertility regulation to improve has been studiously avoided in all programmes. Illegally induced abortion, through a variety of traditional means and traditional practitioners, is universal throughout the developing world. If this technology were to be upgraded, existing practitioners trained and extra ones brought in, there is every likelihood of a rapid acceptance leading to a marked fertility decline. The barrier lies not with potential recipients, but with social elites and decision-makers who have ambivalent, largely Western attitudes and perceptions towards induced abortion. Methods of fertility regulation need to be reviewed not only from the point of view of their clinical side-effects and the administrative costs of their distribution, but in relation to their political advantages and disadvantages (*see* Table 40).

Some superficial remarks have been made about the cultural acceptability of the various methods of family planning. On the whole, there are more similarities than differences in the way in which societies respond to various family planning options. The reversible methods that have done best are those that can be eaten or injected and, no doubt, vaccination would have an appeal and usefulness if it could be perfected. Reversible methods which involve the vagina and uterus have not been widely used with one or two exceptions such as the highly successful use of intra-uterine devices in Bali. However, all women of all cultures are willing to submit to any type of genital invasion once there is a conceptus in the uterus, and the resort to abortion and the usefulness of modern methods of early abortion are universal.

The sheer strain of carrying and attempting to bring up a large number of children makes sterilisation an attractive option for women, wherever it has been made available. The fear of operation and misinformation about possible long-term consequences have not dampened enthusiasm as much as many predicted. Vasectomy very rarely shows the instant appeal of tubal ligation but when it is consistently and patiently made available an increasing number of men come to accept it. Similarly the use of the condom has never climbed as rapidly as that of oral contraceptives but over a number of years it can become a significant method.

The most remarkable fact of the second half of the twentieth century is the homogeneity of the culture that is arising all over the world. From the hills of New Guinea to the wastes of Alaska, from

TABLE 40: CLINICAL, ADMINISTRATIVE AND POLITICAL ATTRIBUTES OF FERTILITY REGULATION OPTIONS FOR POOR COUNTRIES

	Pills	*Condoms*	*I.U.D.s*	*Vasectomy*	*Tubal Ligation*	*Early Abortion*	*Late Abortion*
Use-effectiveness	good	fair	very good	excellent	excellent	very good	fair
User safety and freedom from side-effects	fair	good	fair	good	fair	very good	poor
Cost-effectiveness	fair	fair	good	excellent	good	very good	poor
Simplicity of organising facilities, training and follow-up	good	good	poor	good	poor	good	very bad
Political acceptability	very good	good	very good	fair	good	very bad	disastrous
User acceptability	good	fair	fair	fair	very good	excellent	poor

the traffic-choked streets of Lagos to the traffic-choked streets of Bangkok, and from the villages of Colombia to the villages of Indonesia, Western twentieth century influences are increasing every day. The town, and increasingly the countryside, are changing visibly; jeans and T shirts, wrist watches and transistor radios, Honda scooters, Mercedes lorries, Ford *collectivos*, jeeps and minibuses, plastic sandals, brassières, cigarettes, detergents, ballpoint pens, sunglasses, an ever-increasing number of television sets, refined sugar, plastic stickers, bottle feeding, Western, Indian and Chinese films, pop records, cheap cameras, plastic buckets, billboards, imitation leather briefcases, lipstick, false teeth and aspirins, Coca-Cola and 7 Up, thermos flasks (mainly to keep things cold), rubber stamps, the power of the police, identity cards, and irregular but life-saving access to antibiotics, sanitary towels, primary education, loud hailers from Mosques to Catholic churches and into the market place—all these things and a thousand other tools and influences of Western twentieth century civilisation have invaded and will continue to invade the developing world at an accelerating rate. In family planning the problem is also how rapidly techniques will spread. The paradox is that international organisations offer, and local organisations seek, the least effective methods (such as the clinic distribution of the reversible methods of contraception) before they permit the most effective (which are early abortion and sterilisation). The quest for public respectability rather than private acceptability halts and maims practically every private and public programme, disadvantaging the weakest in all communities and compounding already serious problems of population growth.

The attitude of society towards access to the means of fertility control and the subsidisation and promotion of those means to the poorer sectors of the community makes a great deal of difference to the dignity and happiness and ultimately the efficiency with which people plan their families. Societally approved access to culturally meaningful and economically (and geographically) appropriate family planning services can accelerate the trend which individuals will pursue towards new fertility goals.

POPULATION PROJECTIONS

One of the main tasks of demographic analysis is to estimate future trends in the size and age-structure of a population, by projecting the current size and composition into the future on the basis of assumptions about the course of mortality, fertility and migration. Such techniques involve projection rather than prediction. Any set of projections is based on a particular set of assumptions which are almost certain to prove incorrect to a greater or lesser degree.

Extrapolations often include consideration of the likely influence of social and economic factors and in such cases we often talk of a "population forecast", which may be compared to a meteorologist's prediction of future weather conditions. One reason why demographers have been even less successful than the "weather men" is that the forecasts they make are themselves likely to influence the very events they aim to predict.

Population projections have taken many forms. In the nineteenth century simple linear extrapolations of existing trends in population growth were used. More sophisticated approaches were developed to allow for fluctuations in many basic trends. In the inter-war period it was fashionable to use gross and net reproduction rates in an attempt to overcome errors derived from a neglect of the influence of existing age-structure on crude rates. This led many demographers to proclaim the inevitability of future population decline. The population of England and Wales for the 1970s was assumed on the highest projections to be about 40 million and on lower projections nearer to 30 million. A decline to 10 million by 2000 A.D. was suggested. None of the writers of the time seemed to bear in mind the possibility of a reversal in the pattern of birth rates and, in particular, very few seemed to be aware of the potential increase in fertility that existed as a result of the relatively late age of marriage and high number of women remaining unmarried at that period.

In developed countries today, projections are usually made by what is known as the "component" method, in which the total population is divided up into its separate parts and then reassembled at successive future dates: the number of persons of a given age and sex who will be in the population a year after the starting date is taken as the number a year younger in the original population minus the number of deaths during the year, and plus or minus the number of migrants. To obtain the number of children under the age of one, an estimate is made of the survivors of births assumed to occur in the year. The number of births is obtained by applying fertility rates to the total number of women in the population for each age between fifteen and forty-nine. The process is then repeated for each successive year until the date for which the projection is required has been reached.

Changes in fertility present the greatest problem in making population projections. Failures to anticipate changes in fertility patterns lie behind most of the failures of projections in Britain and the U.S.A. over the last forty years. In the short term, projections of births are usually based on recent trends in fertility, but these become increasingly open to error as assumptions are made about future changes, linked to the spacing and timing of births. For this reason, projections increasingly contain two elements:

(*a*) assumptions about period factors likely to influence the number of annual births in the immediate future, including any change in the age composition of the population;

(*b*) assumptions about the average level of generation fertility rates, which have historically been relatively stable. These can then be broken down by age to give possible timing of births.

Making long-term projections is acknowledged to be difficult, as for any one generation guesses have to be made about total achieved family size in which relatively small changes today can be associated with important fluctuations in the population tomorrow. High and low estimates of future populations are usually made, but are often a long way apart. For example, within the last decade projections for the British population for the year 2000 have varied between 80 and 50 million. While the ability to handle variations in long-term projections may have improved since between the war years, we are now faced with a community which has access to improved family planning and therefore can react even more quickly than previously to changes in the economy and other influences affecting fertility. In the 1970s the birth rate in most Western countries is at a record low, but this is being achieved by a postponement and spacing of births and it is still difficult to guess what the present generation will achieve in family size by the time the woman leaves the fertile years. It would be possible both to restrict fertility further, or for a quite rapid rise in the birth rate to take place. This presents obvious difficulties at the community level when decisions about training teachers or any type of long-term investment have to be made.

In the developing world the very high population growth-rate which has taken place since the Second World War makes projection less difficult in some respects. The large numbers of people already born, not yet at the age of reproduction and not yet at the time when they require employment, represents a problem which has already arrived. In some developing countries, even if biological replacement was achieved very rapidly, there would still be an expanding population as more and more already born children reached the fertile years. The post-war population explosion will lead to major growth in the global population of the world well into the twenty-first century.

Frejka shows that the world's population of 3,600 million in 1970 would have settled at about 5,600 million by the middle of the next century if the then current N.R.R. of 1.9 fell to 1.0 within a few years. Writing at the beginning of 1978, with the population already well past 4,000 million, it is clear that this will not happen and that Frejka's second assumption of replacement fertility by the early 1980s and a population of 6,400 million by 2100 is equally unrealistic. The alternatives of a more gradual decline in fertility to a N.R.R. of unity by the end of the century, the first quarter of the twenty-first century, or as late as 2040, lead to stabilised populations of 8,000, 11,000 and 15,000 million respectively (*see* Fig. 2).

Clearly, the world has to accommodate an unprecedently rapid increase in its numbers and to do so at the very time that modern technology is pressing at the limits of certain of the planetary resources and the ability of the biosphere to tolerate man-made pollution.

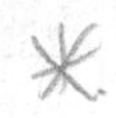

IMPLICATIONS OF POPULATION CHANGE

The ability of the world to offer any sort of acceptable life to its rapidly increasing population is partly dependent on the rate at which fertility declines to match falling death rates: the less the lag period, the greater the chance of society adjusting to the formidable problems before it.

Unfortunately, societies respond somewhat slowly to changes in population, just as they do to changes in individual sexual behaviour which may be at variance with past experience.

The population projections of the 1930s and 1940s led to publications such as *Twilight of Parenthood*, *Parents Revolt* and *France faces Depopulation*, all of which suggested not only the supposed facts of "imminent population decline" but forecast dread social, economic and political implications. Today, the same fears are being expressed about recent falls in fertility. To take the British example, commentators are already speaking of a "geriatric society". Indeed, declining fertility, rather than increasing longevity, leads to an ageing population, but the implications of current low levels of Western fertility need closer examination.

Two outstanding points require stress: the actual number of old people in the foreseeable future is already determined by the fertility of the past half-century or so; secondly, the burden of dependency is not simply a question of the proportion of old people, but also of the number of dependent young in a community. The immediate prospect for industrialised nations with a low birth rate is of a diminishing proportion of dependants in contrast to the potentially productive adult population. This is illustrated for Britain in Table 41 which looks at the implications of four possible patterns of fertility, ranging from very low (assuming an average family size of 1.6) through low (net reproduction rate of 1.00) to high (gross reproduction rate of 1.37, the mean level for the period 1961–5). On all except the very low assumption, the projection is of an actual increase in total population. The proportion of old people is highest with the very low fertility projection, but the over-all burden of dependency, expressed by a dependency ratio is in fact lowest on this assumption.

If the very low fertility model is projected until 2051, when the population of Great Britain would have fallen to 39 million, the proportion of old people would have risen to 27 per cent, unprecedentedly high, but the over-all dependency ratio would be similar to the present.

Since 1971, the birth rate has fallen further, so that the 1976-based principal projection is for a population of 56 million in 2011, less than the Population Panel's low variant. Even so, the pattern of dependency over the next forty years shows no major shift. The proportion of old people rises marginally, but at a very slow pace, while the fall in the proportion of young people, which proceeds rather more rapidly, leads to a steady decrease over the period in the dependency ratio.

If such a course were to be followed, there would be little reason to panic, but the provision of social services might need to pay more attention to the priorities of the aged, especially the oldest amongst these, the total number of whom we know will increase steadily in coming years. Uncertainty about short-term trends in fertility, even if the long-term low variant proves correct, should make us cautious about too hasty decisions concerning future primary school needs or

TABLE 41: PROJECTED AGE-DISTRIBUTION OF BRITISH POPULATION IN 2011

Age-Group	*1971 (actual)*	*Very Low*	*2011 Low*	*Medium*	*High*
	%	%	%	%	%
Under 15	24.1	15.4	20.4	23.1	26.8
60/65+	16.1	19.4	16.7	15.4	13.7
15–60/65	59.9	65.2	62.9	61.6	59.5
Total projected populations (millions)	54.1	52.3	60.7	66.1	74.3
Dependency ratio	.671	.534	.590	.625	.681

(*Source: Report of the Population Panel.* H.M.S.O., London 1973)

maternity services. The wisest course may well be to introduce a larger element of flexibility into the use of both personnel and buildings. The major changes over the next generation are likely to result from different patterns of employment opportunity (and lack of opportunity) rather than shifts in population structure.

Looking further ahead, the possibility of a declining population with a growing proportion of elderly should be approached in a positive way. Improved health care should mean that our view of the aged as "dependent" can be modified and their role in society rethought. This would certainly be in the interests of the elderly. Again, the need is for a more flexible approach to what we mean by old age and what we see as an appropriate time for retirement. We seem prepared to hand over the government of our country to men in their sixties, but to apply rigid rules for retirement elsewhere. At the same time, there remains the anomaly of women retiring five years earlier than men, while having a life expectancy that is five years longer. In Britain miners are still having to battle for an earlier age at retirement, which their European counterparts have long since won. With high levels of unemployment, it seems sad that we cannot permit an earlier move out of work for those whose potential years of retirement are all too often cut short by the ravages of coal dust.

On a wider front, the arguments for and against having a smaller population will no doubt continue. We can personally see no reason to be other than optimistic at the prospect that the population of Britain and most Western countries has at last ceased to grow, as long as the achievement of a stable population or a declining population is not seen as some sort of cure-all.

For developing countries the problems of adjustment to their more massive population changes is going to be even more formidable. Politically, most developing countries now espouse the cause of family planning as well as pressing for socio-economic development. In examining the demographic transition theory and its relevance to developing countries, we suggested any simplistic interpretation of the theory which asserted that in all cases economic development will "take care" of population growth matters is unjustified. There are important differences as well as similarities between what happened to population in the West and what may happen in the Third World.

CONSUMERS AND PROVIDERS

In adapting to new conditions human society can act in a paradoxical fashion. In nineteenth century Europe and North America and in twentieth century Latin America, Africa or South East Asia the social élites (who are always the first to restrict their fertility and use the more modern methods of family planning) can also act in such a way as to restrict the access of others to these same methods. The sociology of those who provide and administer family planning services is important as well as the behaviour of the consumers of those services.

While the reversible methods of contraception involve some do-it-yourself methods, such as coitus interruptus and the over-the-counter sale of contraceptives, the option of elective sterilisation and the choice of abortion on request is determined by others.

The actions which couples take to control their fertility will be fitted into an interlocking whole according to:

(*a*) the policies of those providing services, which in turn may be related to statute law, although they can be independent;

(*b*) the degree of public approval (or condemnation) as expressed through the media and political or religious leadership.

One key to understanding family planning programmes is to see them not so much as rational approaches to the needs of individuals trying to plan their families, but as compromises partly determined by the tolerance of social élites and the perceptions of decision-makers concerning the political consequences of overtly supporting certain services.

When a nation adopts a national family planning policy, it does not necessarily mean that its citizens now have access to meaningful family planning services. A programme may be tailored to meet the perceptions of the nation's religious leadership. For example, in the Philippines there is a tacit agreement between the Catholic hierarchy and the Population Commission that the former will not criticise the current family planning programme too harshly if the latter studiously avoids meeting the need of Filipino women for safe abortion services.

One consequence of pressure of this type is that family planning programmes in Third World countries are often more expensive than they need be if the full range of fertility regulation services could have been made freely available through appropriate channels. The most straightforward and successful family planning services that meet with the greatest approval from consumers include:

(*a*) elective sterilisation;

(*b*) abortion on request;

(*c*) adequate distribution of the reversible methods of contraception.

Experience shows that in poor societies the social marketing of Pills and condoms (as in Bangladesh) is the most cost-effective method of distribution. Where an inappropriate but nevertheless real limitation of oral contraceptive distribution to medical prescription still exists, the community-based distribution of a method using trained distributors from within the community (as in Colombia and Thailand) may succeed. In selected situations saturation programmes are appropriate (as in the Iglesia ni Cristo programme in the Philippines or pilot projects in Tunisia).

Many family planning services in both rich and poor countries have only reached an intermediate stage in the evolution of the full range of necessary services. Sometimes, as in the case of induced abortion, the missing services are not totally absent but are provided by traditional channels. These non-programme channels need to be viewed more sympathetically and current second-rate or dangerous technologies improved.

The medical profession has an uneven record in inspiring and running family planning services. Individual physicians such as the late Alan Guttmacher have made all important contributions, but others have raised barriers to family planning. A medical training makes it seductively easy to see requests for family planning in diagnostic terms. In reality those seeking help make their own diagnosis: they suspect they are fertile (and their guess is usually as good as the physician's), they note they are having regular coitus (something the practitioner is unlikely to verify), and they have decided they do not want another child (a fact the doctor must accept at its face value). Even the doctor's vocabulary must change: the person seeking family planning advice is no longer a "patient", unless one subscribes to the hypothesis that sexual love is an illness. Some doctors understand this role transformation and are happy to serve. Others are confused or reject it. It is this sudden and, for many, unwelcome alteration of roles that is probably at the root of much of the opposition to abortion from within the medical profession. Doctors, after all, generally remember enough embryology to appreciate the difference between the conceptus at six weeks and the foetus at six months and most do not accept the simplistic assertion that abortion is murder. It is acceding to another person's choice that is often the greater challenge.

As society takes a bigger and bigger role in family planning programmes, so not only the attitudes of medical workers but of administrators becomes significant. At the present time, particularly acute and destructive conflicts are arising, especially in developing countries.

When a national family planning programme is implemented at a stage when society only tolerates a partial availability of contraceptive methods, then a bureaucracy develops to propagate the particular range of methods that are politically acceptable at that time. When society moves forward and other methods become acceptable and are promoted by the medical and family planning leadership of the country, then that same bureaucracy becomes threatened, insecure and may eventually resist the spread of methods or alternative programmes of distribution.

ADAPTATION OVER GENERATIONS

Modern living is altering the way of life of young people particularly rapidly. Education is ever prolonged in an increasingly technical world. Migration to cities puts new strains on family life. Novel biological pressures fall on contemporary young people as the age of the menarche falls. Adolescent sexuality is not a problem in a traditional society. Society once defined maturity by a rite of passage; today adolescence extends over many years.

Adolescents are capable of causing or carrying pregnancies at a time when they are not socially able to become parents. In the past twenty years most developed countries have come to accept pre-marital sexual activity, providing it does not lead to pregnancy. But it has been a painful adjustment for parents as well as for the teenagers who first began to adopt the new ways of behaviour. In developing countries the same evolution has still to occur. Most African family planning associations either refuse to help the unmarried or are split with regard to policies, exactly as was the British F.P.A. in the 1950s and 1960s. The transition is going to continue to be a painful one. The young make frequent contraceptive mistakes and their errors are not the "wanted but mistimed" pregnancies of the newly married, they are often socially catastrophic "unwanted" pregnancies. Therefore, services for teenages, even more than to their parents, must include legal abortion.

REPRODUCTIVE MORALITY

Morals attempt to define the social rule book relating the individual to the community. As we have emphasised, sex and reproductive behaviour are moulded by many social forces but the moral commandments regarding sex tend to be cut particularly deep on the tablets of social behaviour.

Pregnancy outside defined relationships has always been condemned. Prior to effective contraception and safe abortion, and especially in societies where women are totally dependent economically on their partners, sexual activity outside those same defined relationships was defined as immoral. Because the woman was the one who became visibly pregnant, moral sanctions have always fallen most harshly upon her. In the contemporary developing world a form of sexual apartheid currently applies to hundreds of millions of women; their choices, the equal opportunities they deserve and even their physical mobility is restricted. With the rise in infant survival rates they must now suffer the additional burden of unwanted pregnancy and sometimes those who defy the unwritten statutes of sexual apartheid die at the hands of the illegal abortionist.

Today, coitus and conception can be separated. In some societies women are beginning to attain social and economic equality with men and the most privileged can, if she wishes, rear a child alone. Changing patterns of contraception, abortion and sterilisation have been alternately labelled as moral and as immoral, according to the viewpoint of the commentator.

Family planning services have been perceived as an engine of social change, although observation suggests that society adapts more slowly than its technology. There is no evidence that patterns of sexual behaviour among young people have altered because they know they can get the Pill or an abortion. Indeed, they most frequently first adopt a new pattern of sexual activity and only later new patterns of fertility regulation.

It may be reasonable to assert that society benefits from rules and guidelines defining acceptable patterns of reproductive behaviour. But it is also apparent that these can take a number of forms and it seems likely that those most appropriate to, for example, a hunter and food gathering community will differ from those suited to a modern industrialised society. Further, in the contemporary world different patterns and ideas of sexual behaviour exist side by side, as is especially marked in the U.S.A.

As sexual activity expressing love between two individuals is private and innocent of any effect on those other than the partners involved, a divergence of moral codes in this field need not necessarily disrupt society in the long term. The general precept that anything is acceptable providing it does not exploit or offend one partner seems reasonable. Conflicting views on what characterises a suitable environment for bringing up a child could be a more devisive social issue. However, the moral consensus which seeks the welfare of the child is almost as unified as it is diverse in relation to codes governing sexual activity.

In practice, the area which gives rise to the deepest conflicts and the one where, to some, public and private interest may seem totally opposed, is abortion. If abortion was not a moral problem then it would be readily available to people throughout the world, because clinically it is one of the most predictable and (when done early) the safest of fertility control procedures. It is manifestly desired by people of all religions and cultural backgrounds.

For most people abortion is a conflict between the future of the mother, whose life is woven into the social web of everyday life and may be drastically altered by pregnancy, and the embryo, which is genetically unique and on the threshold of development. The minority of the public who shout slogans and carry banners see themselves as belonging to one or other extreme, either upholding the total right of the embryo over the mother, even to the extent of risking the life of both, or asserting the total right of the mother over her own body and the embryo within it. However, in practice neither group finds its simplistic interpretation of the problem tenable. The strictest Catholic will still argue for the licitness of operations for ectopic pregnancy, even though it is possible to demonstrate that in astronomically rare cases an ectopic pregnancy can go to term and produce a viable infant. Similarly, the feminist is unlikely to admit the acceptance of a woman's right to dispose of the growing life within her during the last months and weeks of pregnancy.

What should a society do when deep and sincere conflicts exist over access to abortion services? Fortunately, the problem is not unique: it is basically one of religious tolerance. Those who oppose and those who support abortion may place different emphasis on the biological and clinical facts concerning the operation, but they do not differ on the basic body of information that exists. However, they do make different assertions over the interpretation of that information, just as different religions make different assertions about the theological interpretation of temporal life. In a community which separates church and state, and in particular in those with a strong tradition of religious freedom, it is philosophically reasonable for those who wish to claim access to safe abortion services. It should be no more surprising to find an abortion clinic in a society where a proportion of the population condemns abortion, than it is to find a church, a synagogue and a mosque in the same city.

CONCLUSION

In the last analysis, family planning is about choice. Sir Dugald Baird has called family planning the "Fifth Freedom". The one factor on which it has been possible to unite politicians in relation to family planning has been the ideal of the basic human right to control fertility. The freedom to determine family size, like the other great human freedoms, is one used responsibly by individuals. The aggregate of individual decisions concerning the means of fertility regulation can be as good, and sometimes is better, than society's expertise.

In the current world of change rapid adjustment is necessary. The evidence is that the necessary adaptation is beginning. Unfortunately, part of the process of adaptation is sometimes retarded by community attitudes which tend to uphold the *status quo* in sexual behaviour, which may block access to contraception and sterilisation and which can be intolerant of abortion. Such attitudes have already wasted important decades. There is no historical imperative to guarantee that the traditional checks of famine, war and disease will not return to restore the current imbalance between births and deaths. The fight for extending the choice of family planning to all people as rapidly as possible is perhaps the most important battle for freedom in the contemporary world.

SELECTED REFERENCES AND BIBLIOGRAPHY

Baird, D. "A Fifth Freedom." *British Medical Journal.* 12, 1141 1965

Buxton, M. and Craven, E. *The Uncertain Future.* Centre for Studies in Social Policy, London 1976

Charles, E. *The Twilight of Parenthood.* Watts & Co., London 1934

Frejkà, T. *The Future of Population Growth.* Wiley, New York 1973

Petersen, W. *Population.* Collier-Macmillan, London 1975

Spengler, J. *France faces Depopulation.* Duke University Press, North Carolina 1938

Titmuss, R. *Parents Revolt: A Study of the Declining Birth Rate in an Acquisitive Society.* Secker & Warburg, London 1942

Index

12.12.11